Learning from My Daughter

Learning from My Daughter

The Value and Care of Disabled Minds

EVA FEDER KITTAY

OXFORD
UNIVERSITY PRESS

OXFORD
UNIVERSITY PRESS

Oxford University Press is a department of the University of Oxford. It furthers
the University's objective of excellence in research, scholarship, and education
by publishing worldwide. Oxford is a registered trade mark of Oxford University
Press in the UK and certain other countries.

Published in the United States of America by Oxford University Press
198 Madison Avenue, New York, NY 10016, United States of America.

Excerpts from the song "My Funny Valentine" appear in this work's preface.

Library of Congress Cataloging-in-Publication Data
Names: Kittay, Eva Feder, author.
Title: Learning from my daughter : the value and care of disabled minds / Eva Feder Kittay.
Description: New York, NY : Oxford University Press, [2019] |
Includes bibliographical references.
Identifiers: LCCN 2018031470 (print) | LCCN 2018047893 (ebook) |
ISBN 9780190844615 (updf) | ISBN 9780190844622 (epub) |
ISBN 9780190844639 (online content) | ISBN 9780190844608 (cloth : alk. paper)
Subjects: LCSH: Children with disabilities—United States. |
Child rearing—United States. | Values—United States.
Classification: LCC HV894 (ebook) | LCC HV894 .K57 2019 (print) |
DDC 362.4/043092 [B]—dc23
LC record available at https://lccn.loc.gov/2018031470

1 3 5 7 9 8 6 4 2

Printed by Sheridan Books, Inc., United States of America

*To my children, Sesha and Leo, who each in their own way
guided me through parenting with their wisdom and love*

CONTENTS

FOREWORD: SINGING WITH SESHA

"Just sing to her. She loves music."

I was more nervous about meeting Sesha Kittay than I've ever been about meeting anyone, but Sesha's mother, Eva, alleviated my anxiety with these simple words of advice. I had met Eva some months earlier at a philosophy talk, but it was on my first visit to Eva and Jeffrey's home in Rye, New York, that I met Sesha. Although this was thirty years ago, I still have a vivid memory of the occasion.

I knew *of* Sesha—that she had very significant cognitive and physical disabilities; that she lived with Eva, Jeffrey, their son Leo, and a full-time care provider, Peggy; that she required assistance with just about everything; and that she could not talk—but I didn't know what to expect. How would I introduce myself? Should I shake her hand? Would she be able to clasp mine? What would I say—and in what tone of voice? She was nineteen years old at the time, but with no discernible IQ. Should I talk to her the way I'd talk to an adult? Or to a toddler?

After I said some sort of greeting, Eva and I went for a walk, with Sesha in her stroller, and I sang a Scottish lullaby, "Rocking the Cradle," not because I thought of Sesha as a baby, but because it's a fun tune to sing *a cappella* and it usually gets a good reception.

Sesha listened, politely, but I could tell she wasn't really into it. I started to panic, thinking, "Oh, no, this isn't working. She doesn't like my singing. She doesn't like *me*!" Although she's able to be entranced by music she's never heard before, Sesha prefers—especially when encountering a stranger—music that's familiar, something from her vast repertoire of favorites ranging from "Baby Beluga" (at the time I met her) to Mahler's symphonies (these days). Eva suggested we sing something by Elvis Presley, so we knelt down to Sesha's level and started singing "Love me tender, love me sweet, never let me go," and by the time we got to "tender," Sesha was beaming at me. (I think I had her at "love.") What had seemed to me to be an unfocused, uncomprehending stare became a delighted, adoring gaze. And then she reached out and hugged me! (She also grabbed my hair and pulled me into her, but I'd been warned about that and quickly extricated myself.) I'll never know what she was thinking, but I was smitten. From then on, I was never at a loss for things to do with Sesha.

I didn't know a lot of Elvis songs, but it turned out Sesha also loved Rodgers and Hart, so I sang "My Romance," followed by "My Funny Valentine," which soon became one of her favorites. After getting to know Sesha better, I had to modify the lyrics—"Your looks are laughable, unphotographable / Yet you're my favorite work of art"—because Sesha is one of the most photogenic people I know. I also found it increasingly hard to sing "Is your figure less than Greek? / Is your mouth a little weak? / When you open it to speak, are you smart?"— because I was learning so much from Sesha, so I would, with a gesture or an incredulous look, indicate that I thought those questions were ridiculous. But the ending has always rung true: "Don't change a hair for me / Not if you care for me / Stay, little valentine, stay / Each day is Valentine's Day." And it *is* with Sesha. Whenever I see her, it's a lovefest.

My husband, Tom, and I became regular visitors to the Kittay household, and Jeffrey, who is a very talented jazz pianist, would accompany me in a command performance for Sesha every time. She was, and is, the best audience I've ever had and that's because, I came to realize, I'm not performing when I sing with her. Music is something we do together. Whether we're listening to music or playing rhythm instruments or clapping our hands against each other's hands, she's completely engaged. Singing with her is like singing with a jazz combo in that it's a kind of improvisation, and she's totally present in the moment. She's not, as I once heard someone describe most people, "temporarily abled and permanently distracted."

Her ability to focus so intently enables Sesha to appreciate many things with an unusual intensity—the colors, shapes, and smells of flowers; the tastes of her favorite foods; the slippery coolness of water on her skin when she's in the pool. Georgia O'Keeffe wrote that "nobody sees a flower—really—it is so small it takes time—we haven't time—and to see takes time, like to have a friend takes time."[1] I can't know how Sesha sees flowers or hears music, but I can see that she takes more joy in them than many, if not most, people ever take time to do. Likewise, to learn these things about her, to be her friend, has taken time. My main purpose in writing this foreword is to give those who haven't had the opportunity or time to get to know Sesha a sense of who (I think) she is and of what it's like to be her friend.

---

[1] This quote is attributed to Georgia O'Keeffe and dated 1939 in *O'Keeffe: Georgia O'Keeffe Retrospective Exhibition and Catalogue*, edited by Lloyd Goodrich and Doris Bry (New York: Whitney Museum of American Art, 1970), 17.

It's difficult to convey the delight those of us who know Sesha take in her company. She cannot speak, let alone have a conversation or engage in witty banter. But in her presence, one comes to realize that these things are not really necessary for communication, after all. It's said that people will forget what you said, people will forget what you did, but people will never forget how you made them feel.[2] Here, as in so many other matters, what one can learn from interacting with Sesha gives one a deeper understanding of one's interactions with people who *aren't* Sesha—and new insights into one's own self, as well.

At that first meeting, Sesha made me feel like she wanted us to become friends. I'm not saying that's how *she* felt—how could I know?—but the way *I* felt was enough to motivate me to figure out how to relate to her in spite of my awkwardness. Getting to know her has taken time, as getting to know someone always does. I had to learn how to listen to her various silences, how to read her expressions and her movements, how to tell when she's not feeling well, when she's not in the mood for me to sing, and when she'd prefer the company of Eva or Jeffrey or another of her long-time care providers.

It took me many years to realize how much I was learning from Sesha, and it was only after reading *Learning from My Daughter: The Value and Care of Disabled Minds* that I came to appreciate just how much Sesha has taught me about philosophy and about how to live. Much of this knowledge was second-hand, taught to me by Eva, who has been an invaluable teacher and mentor of mine from the time we met. This book not only expands and deepens Eva's previous work on care ethics and what she calls "dependency work," but also raises metaphysical questions about what it is to be a human being; epistemological questions about how we come to know one another; ethical (in the Greek sense) questions about what makes a life a good one, a flourishing one, one worth living; and questions about the role of emotions and other attitudes—joy, gratitude, curiosity—in our lives. What Eva has learned from her daughter and shares with us in this book are transformative lessons for anyone interested in philosophy, feminist theory, contemporary politics, or simply how to live a fully human life.

Philosophers have long pondered what it is to be a human being, a person, a member of "our" moral community. This question—what is it to be human?—has often been conflated with the question: What is it that makes human beings different from everything else in the universe? I don't share this preoccupation with discerning what makes us humans different from everything else in the universe. Consciousness? A soul? language? The ability to use tools? To laugh? To play? To be honest, I never felt the need to say just what makes all human beings

---

[2] It's often said that Maya Angelou said this, but this is apparently a misattribution.

of equal moral worth until the moral worth—the full humanity—of people like Sesha was called into question by some of my fellow philosophers.

Licia Carlson observed, after studying what philosophers have had to say about severe cognitive disability, that "Plato decreed that 'defective babies' should be left to die. Locke and Kant defined those who lack reason as less than human. And most troubling of all," she noted, "when I looked for contemporary discussions about this group, most of the references I found were in discussions of animal rights, asking pointedly whether the 'severely mentally retarded' could be distinguished from non-human animals in any meaningful sense."[3] It's not wrong to ask this question, just as it's not wrong to speculate about whether there's any morally significant difference between human beings generally and nonhuman animals. But it's deeply misguided to assume a priori that there isn't—and couldn't be—any such difference.

Some prominent contemporary philosophers have asserted, without any empirical support, that those who, like Sesha, lack sufficient cognitive abilities, have the moral worth of a pig (which is less than that of nonsimilarly-impaired persons).[4] Jeff McMahan asserted, in a 1996 article, that "the profoundly cognitively impaired are incapable . . . of deep personal and social relations, creativity and achievement, the attainment of the highest forms of knowledge, aesthetic pleasures, and so on."[5] I can confirm Eva's testimony, lest some think it's skewed by a mother's bias, that Sesha is capable of all of these things, except for "the attainment of the highest forms of knowledge"—but, then, I suspect most of us are incapable of this.

If we agree that philosophy begins in wonder, as Plato and Aristotle thought, how can some philosophers lack the curiosity needed to learn even a few basic things about people like Sesha? How can they not take any interest in the lives such people actually live? This lack of curiosity is profoundly unphilosophical, an oddly anti-intellectual attitude for those who value the intellect above all. It isn't just the moral failing of not caring; it's the epistemic failing of not paying attention. Philosophers who assume that Sesha has nothing to say, for no better reason than that they have not taken the time to understand her or to listen to those who have, are like children who assume speakers of a foreign language are talking gibberish. This is willful, culpable ignorance.

[3] Quoted in Eva Feder Kittay and Licia Carlson, eds., *Cognitive Disability and Its Challenge to Moral Philosophy* (Malden, MA: Wiley-Blackwell, 2010), 396.

[4] See, for example, Peter Singer and Jeff McMahan's exchange with Eva Kittay on this issue at the Conference on Cognitive Disability: A Challenge to Moral Philosophy, held at Sony Brook University, Manhattan, in September 2008, quoted in Kittay and Carlson, *Cognitive Disability and Its Challenge to Moral Philosophy*, 407–9.

[5] Jeff McMahan, "Cognitive Disability, Misfortune, and Justice," *Philosophy and Public Affairs* 25 (1996), 8.

"The unexamined life is not worth living," said Socrates before he drank the hemlock. Some may think that this, if true, implies that the examined life *is* worth living, but it does not. For some, the examined life is worth living, but the examination of a life need not be what makes it worth living. When I advise first-year students at the beginning of the academic year, I urge them to think not only about how to fulfill distribution requirements and to plan majors and minors. "Even more important," I say, "is to find out what is going to sustain you in hard times—and then develop and nurture that. You may end up being a teacher or a doctor, but it may be painting—or dance—that you turn to, to get you through difficult times. As important as anything else—and, at times, *the* most important thing in your life—is to know what makes your life worth living."

Not long after I met Sesha, I had to figure out how to carry on after a near-fatal rape and attempted murder. My intellect, my ability to reason, was of no help. At our lowest point, a few months after my assault, I turned to Tom, who was struggling with his own trauma, and said, "Just give me one good reason to carry on," and he couldn't. We talk about taking terrible twists of fate "philosophically," as if stoicism were the only game in town, but I found no consolation in philosophy. Things had stopped making sense, and life was unbearable.

My self-esteem plummeted. I couldn't write, teach, or even walk down the street by myself, and I didn't know if I would ever be able to do these things again. I was dependent on Tom for so much and felt of no use to anyone. Coming to appreciate what Sesha had to offer helped me to carry on when I felt worthless. If I didn't value *her* for her ability to be self-sufficient, productive, and gainfully employed, then why should my own self-worth depend entirely on such things? In addition, Sesha had what I lacked and needed most at the time: the ability to experience joy and to bring joy to others.

I had to relearn how to take pleasure in life. I had to *work* at it. It wasn't philosophy that sustained me then. It was music—and learning, in a deeper way than I'd known before, how to care for, and *be* cared for *by*, other people.

My friendship with Sesha also enabled me to navigate my relationships with loved ones who became cognitively (and otherwise) disabled. In the last several years, as my parents' health failed and my father developed severe dementia, I was immensely grateful to have learned from Sesha how to communicate with them in ways I wouldn't have known before. Of the many things I've learned from Sesha, perhaps the most significant was how to be with my father as his dementia worsened.

There were times when losing my father by degrees to dementia was agonizing. He'd had a keen scientific mind and had, from the time I was young, encouraged me in my intellectual pursuits. At first, his dementia revealed itself as paranoia and anxiety, as well as short-term memory loss. As it became more severe, however, and robbed him of his ability to talk, it brought him a kind of serenity I'd never seen in him. Especially after his dementia had progressed to the point where he didn't realize he had it, my father took great pleasure in things he hadn't taken pleasure in before. I would walk around the grounds of the memory care facility where my parents lived, with my dad in his wheelchair—just as I walked with Sesha in her stroller—and, though he couldn't speak, he would marvel at mundane things: cars going by, airplanes overhead, people walking their dogs. He would pause to look, really look, at a flower, pointing to it and turning to me with an expression that said, "I've never seen anything like this in my entire life! Have you?"

My father's severe cognitive disability brought out in him an intense delight in music. The staff at the facility were aware of the importance of music in the lives of people with dementia and not only had many musicians come to perform, but also arranged for the residents to sing along with the staffers every day. For the last year or so of his life, even though my father couldn't talk, he could sing and, to my astonishment, sang lyrics to songs I didn't realize he'd ever known.

Music, Naomi Scheman once commented in a paper of mine, "expresses the joy of being alive, [and] part of the joy is the shared intelligibility of it." My friendship with Sesha taught me how to experience that joy with my father in his final months and enabled me to see that he was still present and very much himself, even when he could no longer take care of himself or say a single word.

I've enjoyed hearing Sesha's musical tastes change over the years, as tastes do. She developed a love of opera as a child, having been exposed to it by Peggy in her early years. Jeffrey and Eva played classical music for her, as well as lots of kids' music, including Peter, Paul, and Mary and, later, Raffi. Jeffrey tried to get her to like jazz, but Miles Davis just wasn't her thing. In time, she refined her own tastes, growing tired of children's songs and choosing composers she really loved. She was fortunate to have been exposed to many varieties of music, but *she* chose the musical genres and idioms that she wanted played for her again and again.

We have similar musical tastes. We both enjoy musicals—"My Fair Lady" is a current favorite of hers—and she loves Glenn Gould's performance of J. S. Bach's Goldberg Variations, as I have since my youth. She gets a kick out of hearing variations on songs she already knows and laughs when one does something unexpected. She thrills to Beethoven's "Ode to Joy" and, at times, finds the frenetic protracted finale of the movements of his Fifth Symphony hilarious, as do I. When Jeffrey spoke with Oliver Sachs about Sesha's musical tastes and sense of humor, Sachs said, "It is not that she has just musical sensitivity. She has musical intelligence," which she surely does. Her seemingly spontaneous delight in music comes from a highly sophisticated appreciation of it.

None of this implies that the ability to appreciate music is a uniquely human quality. And the fact that my deep and abiding friendship with Sesha is grounded in, though not entirely based on, our mutual love of music doesn't imply that her musicality is what makes her human or is the only thing that makes our friendship possible. To be sure, music helped me come to appreciate Sesha's full humanity, and it continues to give our friendship the unique form that it has. But noting that does not mean that I am substituting one individualistic trait—an ability to appreciate music and musical humor—for another one—rationality or a measurable IQ—as a criterion for full moral personhood. Sesha's musicality is more than an individualistic trait; it is thoroughly relational. She couldn't have developed it on her own, without Jeffrey, Eva, Peggy, and others. It's one of her ways of being in community with other human beings.

In presenting this portrait of Sesha, I'm mindful of the hazards of speaking for others and the special dangers of speaking for the cognitively disabled. I'm not here attempting to speak for Sesha, but, rather, talking about the ways she's informed and enriched my life, because I think that's something that those who would deny her full humanity need to hear. Like the imperative Rilke heard upon seeing an ancient Greek sculpture—"You must change your life"[6]—the lesson I learned from Sesha was, "You must change how you think about your life."

With this book, Eva has given a gift to the philosophical community and beyond—a sense of wonderment at the extraordinary person who is her daughter, Sesha. I urge you, who are holding this book, to take the time to read it and to take what's said in it seriously, even if you end up disagreeing with some of it, because it has invaluable lessons for you, whoever you are and whatever you're thinking about. Even—especially—if you're inclined to disagree with it, it's imperative for you to read it, because you *can't* reasonably disagree with a position if you don't know what it is and what the evidence for it is.

Now, when I see Sesha, I'm not nervous, just excited to see a dear friend I don't get to see her nearly often enough. Even before I greet her, when Eva announces I've arrived, she grins in anticipation. I hug her and kiss her cheek and tell her how happy I am to see her, and she pulls me close (without grabbing my hair, something she's thankfully learned not to do), and I sing, softly, so only she can hear, "Don't change a hair for me / Not if you care for me . . . ." Then she throws her head back and laughs as only she can laugh—a swiftly inhaled breath that sounds like pure joy—and I think, oh Sesha: "You're my favorite work of art."

Susan J. Brison
September 8, 2018

---

[6] Rainer Maria Rilke, "The Archaic Torso of Apollo," in *The Selected Poetry of Rainer Maria Rilke*, ed. and trans. by Stephen Mitchell (New York: Vintage Books, 1984), 61.

PREFACE AND ACKNOWLEDGMENTS

Sesha is my daughter. Her significant cognitive and physical disabilities have challenged my understanding of philosophy even as I first became a professional philosopher. The life I have led with my daughter has provided me with a set of lessons that I have shared with readers for well over two decades. These are lessons that I believe are worthy of, and require, philosophical meditation and reflection. They touch on some of the most profound and fundamental questions philosophers have raised. In putting them forth, not only do I interject myself into the discourse of disability, but I also make room for Sesha in philosophical discourse.

This work can be viewed as a follow-through of many of the themes I articulated in *Love's Labor: Essays on Women, Equality, and Dependency*. There I put the narrative of Sesha in the last two chapters. Only when the philosophical points had been argued in the earlier chapters did I want to put forward the motivating concerns, thoughts, preoccupations, and life experiences that informed my arguments. In the present work, however, Sesha moves front and center, along with my personal voice, the voice that brought up the rear in the previous volume.

The ideas in *Love's Labor* were bookended with the concepts of equality and dependency. By working through a dialectic between equality and dependency, I urged that if women were ever to share the world with men in true equality, we needed an equitable distribution of labor and a different, nonstigmatized relationship to inevitable human dependence. The persons caring for people with significant dependency needs were the focus (though not the exclusive focus) of that volume. In the current project, which spans two books (of which the current volume is the first), the emphasis is reversed: the place of those who are inevitably dependent because of lifelong significant disabilities is primary, although the roles of care and caregiving are not eclipsed. In this project, love and dignity are at the fore in the quest for a philosophy concerned with what matters.

Love and the specific relations we bear to others displace rationality and other elements of cognition as essential to a life lived with dignity.

Individualistic and rationalistic conceptions of the person are put to (and fail) the test of theoretical adequacy when they try to include those with serious cognitive disabilities. In *Love's Labor*, I proposed that the only universal and morally significant property that all humans possess is that we are all some mother's child. That is, we are born of two human parents, and to survive and thrive we require a nurturing person (or persons) to adopt our welfare as their own, at least minimally, through infancy and early childhood. A child with disabilities, who lacks intrinsic properties that philosophers have defined as essential to equal moral standing, is no less a mother's child and no less entitled to become a member of our moral community than any other child. When we hold moral equality to reside in the relation that each human being has or has had to a mothering person that enabled the child's survival, we recognize that care must be at the center of our morality and politics. It is through the care of a disabled child that I have had to turn around my own understanding of a good life and a just society.

I couch these new understandings as what I have learned from my daughter Sesha. These are offered up as arguments and as stories. Through them, I mean to convey the transformations of thought and self-understanding that have come out of encounters with my daughter, with her needs, her body, her mode of communication, and her relationship to me and the world.

What I have learned from my daughter has taken place in the context of my family, my students and colleagues, friends, caregivers, and institutions that have allowed me to pursue this work. My first and deepest thanks are then to my husband Jeffrey, my daughter Sesha, my son Leo, and my daughter-in-law Kim. Leo and Kim have allowed me to see parenting afresh; and Micah, Asa, and Ezra have enlarged Sesha's world as she has enriched theirs. Seeing their relationship has allowed me to see, all over again, how many riches Sesha provides to our family. A close second are those caregivers who, with Sesha, have served as my teachers in the practice of care. The longest and deepest relation is with Margaret Grennan (Peggy), who came to help us when Sesha was five and stayed until Sesha left to live in the Center for Discovery at the age of thirty-two—twenty-seven years of a remarkable friendship and project in co-mothering. I am fully aware that few are as privileged as I have been to find and be able to retain such a devoted, skillful, and persevering caregiver.

The good fortune in finding and keeping Peggy by Sesha's side has been followed by another gift, the Center for Discovery in Harris, New York. In the Center for Discovery, we have found the essence of a caring community— a community, as the Center likes to say, inspired by the lives of people with disabilities, where people with even the most significant disabilities can live lives of fulfillment and dignity. Their work has deeply informed my own. The Center, led by the genius of Patrick Dollard and sustained by the exceptional work of Dr. Theresa Hamlin, Richard Humleker, and so many others too numerous to name, has been Sesha's home since 2001. We hope she will be able to live out her life there. At the Center, we have also found parents who share our own passion for their disabled children and with whom I have had the opportunity to share some of my work as well as the joy and hard moments, especially Denise and Art Thomson, Patty and Danny Abelson, and Karen and Eric London.

I must thank Suzie Nair, Dr. Philip Wilken, and Dr. George Todd from the Center, who helped us through some dark days of Sesha's recent illnesses, as well as Dr. Orrin Devinsky, who finally (and we hope forever) conquered her seizures. I would be remiss not to mention some particular individuals who have assisted Sesha individually for over fifteen years: Maria Sorto and Julia Brosius. Learning from such talented and devoted caregivers never ceases.

But this book is nonetheless foremost a work of philosophy. Philosophy has been my intellectual home since I was in college, and as many times as I have run away from home, I have returned. Like a prodigal child, I had to reconcile myself to that home. Fortunately, I have had mentors and supports. I am deeply indebted to Edward Casey, as well as others in the Department of Philosophy at Stony Brook who supported my unorthodox work, especially Mary Rawlinson, Allegra de Laurentiis, Jeff Edwards, Gary Mar, Bob Crease, and Lee Miller. Stephen Post at the Center for Compassionate Care and Bioethics was always willing to take me in if I ever were to decide to finally reject philosophy—which I never did. Much of my willingness to remain in the field had to do with the amazing students I met and had the privilege to teach and mentor at Stony Brook. Many of them took an active part in my research by reading my manuscripts, assisting me with research, and engaging in dialogue on the topics discussed. Many have gone on to successful academic careers exploring their own passions in philosophy. So, many thanks to Barbara Andrews, Ellen Feder, Sarah Clark Miller, Serene Khader, Jean Keller, Bonnie Mann, Chris Kaposy, Danae McLeod, Michael Ross, Cara O'Connor, Katie Wolfe, Nathifa Greene, and, more recently, Phillip Nelson, Andrew Dobbyn, and others in my last seminar at Stony Brook where we combed through the book manuscript. A very special acknowledgment goes to Lori Gallegos de Castillo and Oli Stephano for their invaluable assistance doing research for and editing the manuscript itself, and to Alyssa Adamson who took on the daunting work of preparing the index.

Among those outside the department who have been influential in my pursuit of this project have been remarkable philosophers and disability scholars. Anita Silvers was an especially important interlocutor, and while we don't always agree, we always learn from one another. Sarah Ruddick was a central inspiration for my work on care, and Bill Ruddick was an important discussant for issues of care and parenting. Two chapters, "The New Normal and a Good Life" and

"The Ethics of Prenatal Testing and Selection," were occasioned by workshops at the Hastings Center for Bioethics, which both were spearheaded by Erik Parens. Adrienne Asch, who sadly is no longer with us, was a formidable interlocutor for discussions on prenatal testing. The extended workshop on prenatal testing was formative, as were the many discussions I had there and in the meeting on surgically shaping children with Bruce Jennings, Jamie Nelson, Hilde Lindemann Nelson, Bonnie Steinbock, and the rest of the participants at the Hastings Center. Benjamin Wilfond and Sara Goering invited me to a meeting concerning Ashley X and growth attenuation, thus spurring me on to writing what is now chapter 9. At various points in my thinking and writing I have also had help and inspiration from Martha Nussbaum, Michael Bérubé, Virginia Held, Michael Slote, Licia Carlson, Simo Vehmas, Owen Flanagan, Sophia Wong, Nicolas Delon, and John Vorhaus. I had the opportunity to discuss my ideas with Elizabeth Lloyd and Christia Mercer while we work-vacationed in White Lake, and with Nancy Vermes, wherever we were. Several read and commented on one or more chapters in earlier versions. Additionally, Adam Cureton, Lawrence Becker, and Tom Shakespeare read and commented on the entire manuscript. Richard Rubin read several chapters with care and offered helpful suggestions; Stephen Campbell provided massive and invaluable editorial commentary for chapter 5, and Dana Howard provided insights on an early version of the chapter; Gina Campella commented on an abbreviated version of chapter 8, and Vrinda Dalmiya carefully read and commented on a later version. Throughout, Susan Brison encouraged me when the writing faltered, offering the kind of support possible only from someone with whom one feels a deep intellectual and personal affinity.

Invitations to visit and participate in lecturing and teaching at other universities have variously informed many of the chapters. Among these, a thanks goes out to the faculty and students at the University of Newcastle (special thanks to Janice McLaughlin and Jackie Scully); University of Miami (thank you, Michael Slote); Stellenbosch University (thank you, Leslie Swartz); University of Waterloo (thank you, Carla Fehr); the University of Hawaii (special thanks to Vrinda Dalmiya); Emory University (gratitude to Rosemarie Garland-Thomson and Joel Reynolds); and the University of Malta (thank you especially to Anne-Marie Callus, Maria Victoria Gauci, and the Fulbright Foundation). There were students and faculty at numerous institutions and meetings over a ten-year period at which I read parts or versions of chapters whose comments figured in the final transformation of these portions of the book.

Lucy Randall, my editor at Oxford, has offered important guidance and encouragement. My sincere thanks for this much-needed assistance.

Finally, I want to express my deep gratitude to the National Endowment for the Humanities and the Guggenheim Foundation for their generous fellowships. These allowed me to spend undiluted time focusing on the manuscript. The rewards of these fellowships are still only half-realized in the current volume. The rest remain as a promissory note for the volume to follow, *Who's Truly Human? Justice, Personhood, and Mental Disability*.

Learning from My Daughter

PART I

LEARNING TO BECOME
A HUMBLER PHILOSOPHER

We seldom hear at academies the comfortable and oft times reasonable "I do not know."

It is wisdom that has the merit of selecting from among innumerable problems that present themselves, those whose solution is important to humankind.

—Kant, "Dreams of a Spirit-Seer" (1902, 2:368)

Overview: The Journey and Its Ends

On a *Washington Post* editorial page, one parent of a child with severe disabilities wrote that having a child with a severe disability made of every parent a philosopher (Cohen 1982). What if you are already a philosopher and are raising a child with multiple and severe disabilities, including severe cognitive disabilities? You become a *humbler* philosopher. Having a child with a severe disability makes of every parent a philosopher because it makes one search anew for what makes life worth living.

In part I of this book, I introduce the reader to the journey I have taken as a philosopher and mother of a daughter who, while lacking the characteristics so valued by philosophers—the ability to reason and fashion arguments—has taught me many unique lessons about what matters in life. Chapter 1 recounts how I came to recognize the significance of what I was learning raising a daughter with very significant cognitive disabilities, how I came to understand that what this experience was teaching me was knowledge that I needed to share with my philosophical community, and how caring for my daughter altered my understanding of philosophy. At the end of the chapter I outline the argument that runs through the chapters of this book, and I adumbrate the arguments in a subsequent volume that is a continuation of the same project.

Chapter 2 jumps into the argument of this project at the beginning—that is, at the outset of the discovery that one's child is not "normal." It attacks the question that arises for every parent raising a child who, in Andrew Solomon's words, "falls far from the tree": Can my child have a good life if she is not what we call "normal"? It pursues the question by asking what it is that we desire when we desire normalcy for one's child. In coming to answer this question, we see that the attempt to answer the age-old philosophical question "What is a good life?" requires that we step back from prideful answers and look more humbly at the lives of those who do not measure up to vaunted philosophical ideals. We can gain a new insight into the ends that we seek in a well-lived life.

1

On What Matters/Not

Philosopher Susan Brison (2010) has remarked that while she is not sure if an unexamined life is not worth living, she is sure that an unlived life is not worth examining. That is, it is the reality of lived lives that bears examination, not idealized lives. The reality of a disabled life and of a life with a disabled person is the life I hope to examine.

To do so, I must take the reader on an expedition into a scarcely traveled philosophical terrain. What I offer is both a story and an argument. The story begins with a fundamental life contradiction that comes in the form of a beloved baby. The argument is directed against the devaluation of human life lived with intellectual disability. The argument, together with the story, is about a fierce parental love for a vulnerable, dependent, and stigmatized child; a love that has moved this philosopher/mother to want to impart lessons I have learned to an uncomprehending world. Sarah Ruddick speaks of one of the demands of motherhood as the need to socialize one's child so that the child can grow into an adult that is accepted by her community (1989). But when one has a child like my daughter, the demand is to socialize the community to accept her as an individual worthy of moral parity with all human beings. In these pages I track a journey: as a mother, a caregiver, and a philosopher.

1.1 The Story—The Beginning

A work of philosophy normally begins with the birth of an idea, but we begin instead with the birth of a child. It was two days before the Christmas of 1969 when this child—my child—was born. She emerged with a startled expression, a head full of black hair and a perfect little body. Her cry—a slow transition from the shock of birth to a full-throated protest—assured us that all was well. I was, as the title of the "natural birth" primer said, "awake and aware." No drugs muffled the pain or the joy of childbirth. Without sedatives, we had a fully alert infant. She had a perfect Apgar score of ten. The elation was dampened only as my baby was wheeled away and my husband was escorted out. I lay there surprisingly not tired, wanting only these two beloved persons by my side. I waited to be told I could visit my child in the nursery. And I waited for them to bring her back to my room as they were supposed to after a brief time. But I waited, waited, and waited. At long last she was brought to me, along with the news that she had experienced a cyanotic episode and the assurance that nonetheless all was well. I was to go home with her after three days.

We named her Sesha (properly spelled Cesia, the diminutive of the Polish name, "Czesława") to honor a cousin of mine who, while only a young child, perished in the ovens of Treblinka. Our Sesha was our first child—and the first grandchild of two Holocaust survivors. Her birth marked the bright future even as it carried the heavy load of the past. When we learned of her disability, I was painfully aware that under the Nazi regime, disability was a death sentence for the child, and often for the mother as well—especially if they already belonged to a despised minority. It was not until I began writing about disability that I discovered the intimate connection between the fate of Jews in general and the fate of those with mental disabilities (Kittay 2016). But on that December day, looking out at a snow-covered New York City with my baby sweetly nursing, I knew nothing of what awaited us. We were lulled into thinking that her perfect form, bright gaze, and sweetness meant all was fine.

Sesha was serene but alert, and she melted in my arms. I didn't know then that this lovely sensation was caused by her hypotonia, her lack of muscle tone. She slept for long periods of time, and as a new mother I didn't know whether to feel lucky or worried. She was not a vigorous eater, but she was gaining weight. She did surprisingly few tricks—we waited for her to roll over, to pick up her head, and to meet the other milestones of early infancy. Today I realize that these should have been warning signs, but at the time I had only baby books, and I preferred to think that Sesha had her own timetable. When I queried my pediatrician about Sesha's struggle to lift her head and turn it from side to side, he feigned ignorance, urging that the reason Sesha had not yet been able to lift her head was probably because she had a large head—a feature most likely inherited from my husband. Foolishly we accepted the explanation, even measuring my husband's head to assure ourselves that this was the reason for Sesha's inability at nearly four months of age to do what my son was later to manage in the first few days of his life. The pediatrician failed in his duty to be truthful; my husband and I allowed ourselves to be soothed by the deception. How desperately we new parents wanted our child to be normal.

Our bliss was disturbed when a college friend visited with her five-month-old baby. The baby was so much more active and capable than our beautiful, placid Sesha. On the advice of a friend who had quietly watched our daughter's lack of progress with trepidation, we made our first visit to a pediatric neurologist.

He made us understand, as gently as possible, that there was cause for concern. However, he indicated that the most troubling possibility was a progressive deterioration, one that could only be detected by observing her for a period of time. This was hard enough to digest. On his suggestion, we consulted another pediatric neurologist in San Francisco while on holiday there. It was no holiday. A doctor with Hollywood looks greeted us, did a very brief exam, told us that our daughter was "severely to profoundly retarded," then excused himself to see his next patient. It was brutal. Returning to our hotel room, nausea overtook me, but there was no way to expel this unwelcome news. From then on, we lived with the reality of her severe cognitive impairment. In *Love's Labor*, where I first chronicled my life with Sesha and raised the first of the many questions this experience posed to my chosen métier, I wrote:

> Sesha would never live a normal life. . . . the worst anticipation was that her handicap involved her intellectual faculties. We, her parents, were intellectuals. I was committed to a life of the mind. . . . This was the air I breathed. How was I to raise a daughter that would have no part of this? If my life took its meaning from thought, what kind of meaning would her life have? Yet throughout this time, it never even occurred to me to give Sesha up, to institutionalize her, to think of her in any other terms than my own beloved child. She was my daughter. I was her mother. That was fundamental. Her impairment in no way mitigated my love for her. If it had any impact on that love it was only to intensify it. . . . We didn't yet realize how much she would teach us, but we already knew that we had learned something. That which we believed we valued, what we—I—thought was at the center of humanity—the capacity for thought, for reason, was not it, not it at all. (1999)[1]

Two features of this brief recounting of the first few months of our life are worth remarking upon. The first was how desperately we clung to the idea that there was nothing the matter with our child. The second was my eventual realization that the child I loved, and whose life meant more to me than my own, could never share in the life of the mind. Though this realization was painful, the love of my child won loyalty over my love of the mind. Still, a philosopher (or rather a graduate student in philosophy) I remained. Philosophy served me well as an escape. The dissonances between what I knew from philosophy and what I experienced with Sesha were present from the start, but I was yet to confront these

---

[1] Much of the rest of the tale is recounted in my essay "Not *My* Way, Sesha, *Your* Way, Slowly." The narrative comprises the last two essays of *Love's Labor*. I will recount bits and pieces of my life with Sesha as they pertain to the concerns of chapters that follow.

and acquire a new understanding of philosophy in light of my passionate love for my daughter. The amazing and wonderful outcome is that what I learned from my disabled daughter is what I had been searching for in philosophy: an understanding of things that matter.

1.1.1 Sesha

To do justice to Sesha, I first need to introduce her. But I have already done her an injustice. I have introduced her as my disabled daughter. She, however, like everyone else, is first someone with her own distinctive characteristics, an individual, a presence in this world that should be expressed in positive terms. I prefer to tell you about Sesha in terms that any mother wants to speak of her child—that is, with pride in the special and singular qualities that we cherish. Had I begun to speak of her as I would have preferred— telling you of her ability to light up a room with her smile, the warmth of her kisses, the fastness of her embrace, her boundless enjoyment of the sensuous feel of water, and perhaps most of all her abiding and profound appreciation of music—one might reasonably have asked: So why is Sesha not speaking for herself?

Sesha's inability to speak (and so to speak for herself) is but a synecdoche for all that she is unable to do: feed herself, dress herself, toilet herself, walk, talk, read, write, draw, say Mama or Papa. When asked about my daughter, I want to tell people that she is a beautiful, loving, joyful woman. But then people ask me, "And what does she do? Does she have any children?" So, I soon have to tell them what she cannot be, given her profound cognitive limitations, her cerebral palsy, and her seizure disorders. When people ask how old my daughter is, I always hesitate, wondering whether to give her chronological age and speak of her as a lovely and intense forty-eight-year-old woman, or to speak of the indeterminate age that reflects her level of functioning and her total dependency. The positive set of responses is truer to who she is. Knowing her capabilities, one gets a glimpse into the richness of her life and the remarkable quality of her very being. Nonetheless, the limitations shape her life and the life of her family, so we all must address them if we are to realize her possibility of flourishing. At the same time, it is only by considering Sesha in the fullness of her joys and capacities that we can view her impairments in light of her life, her interests, her happiness— and not as projections of her "able" parents or of a society biased by what some have dubbed "ableism."[2]

---

[2] For the idea of "ableism" see Campbell (2009).

1.1.2 An Apologia: Speaking for Another

As I try to articulate through philosophy the understandings I gleaned of the things that matter from my relationship with a person with an intellectual disability, I will be speaking not only for myself, but also for my daughter. What I wish to impart are not my lessons, but hers. She cannot speak for herself. Yet speaking for another rather than allowing people to speak for themselves is problematic: to what extent do we truly understand what the other is telling us? To what extent are we being ventriloquists, using another's visage to voice our own concerns? To what extent are we suppressing the other's voice as we raise our own (Khader 2011a)? Speaking for people with disabilities is especially problematic since the agency of people with disabilities has long been suppressed. Disabled people have insisted on no longer being silenced, on having their voices heard. The mantra is simple: "Nothing about us without us."

For most all people with significant mental disability, such a demand for voice appears futile. Although advocates of disability rights have argued that their impairments are disabling only in an environment that is hostile to their differences and that has been constructed to exclude them, some impairments (particularly those that affect our cognitive capacities) are not easily addressed by environmental changes and even social changes. Of all disabled people, those labeled "severely intellectually disabled"[3] have least benefited from the inclusion fought for by a disability community that is dominated by people who are able to speak for themselves (Ferguson 1994).

Many with significant mental disability cannot ever hope to be independent or capable of participating in rational deliberation. Those who speak do so in a language not recognized—and even demeaned—by those who speak in the language of the public sphere. Without a claim to cognitive parity, even those who can speak are not recognized as authors or agents in their own right; that is, their voice is given no authority. Those who cannot speak must depend on others to speak for them. Perhaps there is no more disabling disablement.

To be heard, to be recognized, to have her needs and wants reckoned along with those of others, the mentally disabled individual requires an advocate—a role that has voice at its center. As the mother of a daughter, now an adult, who is disabled in this fashion, I speak as an advocate. Otherwise, my daughter and those who share her disability will be doubly disabled and silenced. So, I am left in the awkward position of speaking of an individual with a disability—needing to speak not only *about* her but, contra the disability dictum, *for* her, and to speak for and about her in a way that captures who she is and does her justice.

---

[3] When Sesha first was diagnosed the term was "severe mental retardation." The "R" word is now not acceptable.

1.2 The Story Meets the Argument: The Lived Life Matters

I was attracted to the field of philosophy because, having been born in the shadow of the Holocaust, I wanted to know if one could be a good person in an evil world. It was not the question I ever pursued, however, as a professional philosopher. But the ethical impulse never left me even as I avoided the field of ethics. And I returned to it in large measure because of my experience as a woman and as a mother.

But when I decided, after Sesha's birth, to enter graduate school, it was not to resolve the ethical dilemmas I anticipated as the mother of a disabled child. Instead I entered graduate school to pursue a discipline rigorous enough to offer me a diversion from mothering. Adrienne Rich spoke about her poetry as a place where she was nobody's mother (1995). I too needed to be someplace where I was no one's mother, where hard intellectual work would distract me from the pain of my growing understanding of all that Sesha's life could not be. I cordoned off these unwelcome thoughts by pursuing philosophy of language, philosophy of science, and the most demanding philosophical work at hand. Yet as I pursued the study of the philosophy of language, explored the puzzles that metaphors posed to semantic theory, and worked to help develop a nascent feminist ethics and political philosophy, the experience of parenting my daughter hovered about me like Socrates's gadfly.

How can one repeatedly read and teach texts that give Reason pride of place in the pantheon of human capabilities, when each day I interacted with a wonderful human being who displayed no indisputable evidence of rational capacity? How can one view language as the very mark of humanity, when this same daughter can speak not a word? How can one read about justice as the consequence of reciprocal contractual agreements, when one's own child is unable and will apparently never be able to participate in reciprocal contractual agreements? My daughter gave the lie to most of my professed philosophical beliefs. Were they merely dogmas I accepted? Could they be made compatible with the lived reality of existence with a beloved person such as my daughter? These questions lay fallow in my mind; I placed them on a back shelf there labeled "FUTURE PHILOSOPHICAL PROJECT: SESHA." The dissonance might change my relationship to philosophy. It could not, however, change my relationship to my daughter. That was my fixed point of reference.

Mothers, with few exceptions, do want an open future for their child; they want their children to have good health and to thrive. Under the long shadow of "mental retardation"—to use the term that was long used to describe her situation—this appeared to be an impossibility.

Time healed the initial pain and shock. Our love and appreciation of Sesha *as she was* grew and became more expansive. Sesha has taught me that a profound love of another can change one's values and priorities.

At a certain point, philosophy could no longer be a distraction from life with a person with severe disabilities, and instead, what Sesha had taught me had to become my philosophical project. This has meant using philosophy against itself to engage in a deep critique. Thanks to the sort of work done in feminist philosophy, critical race theory, and the scholarly work on disability (only just starting in philosophy, but well developed in other disciplines), there was a small opening to examine this unexamined feature of life.

Philosophy is a stolid, hoary discipline. Its greatness derives from its embrace of a long-lived and venerable canon of thinkers, writings, and problems. Its weakness, its fading centrality to both our daily and even our intellectual lives, can be traced to the same source as its greatness—a reliance on canonical thinkers whose lives are so distant from our own and whose questions are so abstract, so far removed from all that is quotidian. Disability and especially intellectual disability has never been featured in the problem set of philosophy's canonical works.

The idealized worlds of philosophers have little room for disability, and virtually none for cognitive, as opposed to physical, disability. Philosophers have given the subject even less attention than some of the differences among persons that today take central stage in the academy: sexual/gender and racial/ethnic differences. The disabled individual, if she was mentioned at all in the philosophical literature, was invoked as the exception, as the infant that was to be abandoned, the changeling who was scarcely human, and most recently as the marginal human who moves us to ask about the moral status of nonhuman animals—in short, as the exception that proves whatever rule the philosopher hopes to instantiate.

Despite its conservatism, a critical edge has also always been important to philosophy. Socrates began it with the critical questioning that brought him a philosophical following—and a death sentence. Aristotle took Plato's philosophy as a starting point—but often to criticize it. Since then many of the great marking points in Western philosophy have been based on a repudiation of what previously counted as philosophy: Descartes rejecting all previous philosophical inquiries and claiming to begin anew with the *cogito* as his point of certainty; Kant awakening from his dogmatic slumber and repudiating the use of pure reason to operate beyond the limits of possible experience; Wittgenstein arguing that the perennial problems of philosophy were all a consequence of the misuse of language.

In each paradigmatic philosophical advance, the critical move has been to question the starting point or the perspective from which philosophical inquiry proceeded. Seen in this light, the challenge of philosophy's claim to universality by feminists and race theorists is in the great tradition of philosophical critique.

Yet when I contemplate the challenge that my silent daughter poses to steadfastly held convictions of philosophy, I must wonder if hers is not the most profound critique of all. How does one include cognitive disability into the disciple of philosophy? Philosophy is the love of wisdom. Wisdom is primarily, if not exclusively, an intellectual achievement. If Western philosophy has rested on any certain foundation, it has been on the importance of the capacity of reason for all that is human. I do not know if my daughter can reason, but I do know that many causal sequences appear to elude her. As she cannot speak, can do little with her hands, and must be wheeled about in her wheelchair, her agentic skills are attenuated. Her ability to follow directions is limited, and discovering what she understands can be inferential at best. While I cannot say that she lacks the power to reason altogether, I cannot assume this ability. Reason is the philosopher's major instrument and highest good. By its light, we delve into the mysteries of the universe. Improving our ability to act in accordance with reason is often posited as the quintessential telos of human beings. Our ability to reason grounds our moral and political obligations to one another. Does it then even make sense to examine philosophical questions by contemplating the life of someone who might not merely reason poorly, but who might not reason at all?

And yet philosophers can fall too much in love with things intellectual and with humans' cognitive abilities. The philosopher who looks at the nature of the mind, Kant told us, is like a surgeon doing surgery on himself, and Kant warned of its difficulties and constraints. But that enterprise has more than the obvious limitations. When we train the mind's eye to concentrate on what is too close at hand, everything else outside that focal point is a blur. The brain surgeon, after all, sees only the brain. But the brain exists in a body, which exists in a larger physical and social context. A surgical, myopic vision misleads us into thinking that what we can know in this fashion is all we need to know—that what we see is all that we need to see. Coming to know an individual such as Sesha can serve as an invaluable intervention to a narrow focus on the intellect. Such an intervention is made possible by an openness to encountering more than meets the eye, and it is facilitated by love, attachment, and acceptance.

The opportunity to start this thinking came with an invitation by Sara Ruddick to contribute to an interdisciplinary book of essays by scholars whose experiences of mothering were atypical.[4] I conceived of my contribution as a narrative, not a work of philosophy. The essay, "Not *My* Way, Sesha, *Your* Way, Slowly," was simultaneously the easiest and the most difficult writing I have ever

---

[4] That book became Hanigsberg and Ruddick (1999).

attempted. The ease was in the writing itself, yet the material remained difficult to confront. At the same time, I was invited to participate in a project on prenatal testing and selective abortion for disability at the bioethics institute, the Hastings Center. The Hastings Project resulted in an essay that was in the form of a series of email letters I exchanged with my son on the topic (Kittay and Kittay 2000).

Both the Hastings essay and the chapter for the mothering volume required revisiting those early days when my partner and I had to come to terms with the fact of our daughter's serious impairments. Each project had to be approached with unsparing honesty. Otherwise they would be served up with too much sugar or too much tragedy. Once I began to write on the topic, my philosophical and my personal life were joined. I had broken the prohibition of subjective inquiry, and my life with Sesha could not be put back into the genie's bottle.

1.2.1 Writing Philosophy in a Personal Voice

From Socrates onward, the personal or autobiographical have been essential tools for pushing beyond fixed views to insights not otherwise accessible. However, in philosophy generally the personal voice tends to be viewed with suspicion. It is the impersonal voice that has the mark of objectivity, of truth that transcends the subjective and particular.

Scientific theories are presumably tested (or testable) through empirical methods, ones that are meant to establish their truth and objectivity. Philosophy is not an empirically based inquiry. It models itself instead on mathematics which, starting with self-evident truths, uses valid inferences to establish objective truths. Using the model of the mathematical proof, philosophers depend on intuitions that are presumably widely, if not universally, shared. But intuitions in moral matters can be unreliable, leading some philosophers to distrust them entirely and others to accept them only provisionally. What philosophers rarely do is acknowledge the autobiographical origins of all intuition that they appeal to, as well as the autobiographical source of their predilection for one theory over another.

The autobiographical is not merely an individual's idiosyncratic narrative. With every life experience, with every choice we make, with each set of circumstances that we find ourselves in, we take up an interpretive work that becomes our autobiography. From this interpretive matrix arise intuitions, motivations for inquiry as well as action, and biases that incline us to one theory or another. Here the personal and the autobiographical can facilitate and be a resource for the enlargement of knowledge. The insights derived from the autobiographical and personal may or may not be unique to us. Stanley Cavell urges that the personal voice needs "neither to claim uniqueness for oneself nor to deny it to others" (Cavell 1994, 12). That is, on the one hand, the knowledge we claim from our individual perspective need not be uniquely available from our own perspective alone; on the other hand, another's perspective may reveal a different truth that, in fact, is unique from the other's perspective.

Cavell's recognition is underscored by the feminists and race theorists who have led the way. Their works have been a powerful and often explicit manifestation of how the personal is at once political and philosophical. Feminists, race theorists, LGBTQ philosophers, and Latinx and Native American philosophers have used their autobiographical positions explicitly both to enlarge the scope of philosophy and to broaden our understanding of how to do philosophy. Reading Patricia Williams's *The Alchemy of Rights and Race* was transformative. Although a legal theorist and not a philosopher, the modes of argumentation are closely aligned. Williams broke open the constraints of argumentation in this work. The personal was interwoven into the legal arguments she put forward. For example, in speaking of property, she invoked her own ancestors who were legally property, allowing her to have a different perspective when examining property law. Her subsequent works have been similarly peppered with personal anecdotes that directly demonstrate the necessity of looking at the law through the lens of race. Iris Young was another important and early practitioner of this method of philosophical discussion. She regularly introduces a personal experience as impetus for philosophizing about issues that sometimes have been considered only tangentially philosophical. Here are but a few examples: the meaning of gender in how we throw a ball, identity as embodied in the pregnant body, the home as a political space.[5] María Lugones's work also gave us the courage to open the scope and voice of philosophy. In an early influential work, Lugones (1987) makes the relationship to her mother the axis around which revolve issues such as identity, intersectionality, and difference. Equally influential was her conversation with Elizabeth Spelman (1983). Not only does it matter who speaks, but it also matters who the interlocutor is. Of course, dialogue has a noble tradition in philosophy, but in Lugones and Spelman's essay, the ability to converse across their differences is the very subject of the piece. The influence of this work should be apparent in chapter 4 of this volume. Another important and relatively early example of how the personal can transform the philosophical is Uma Narayan's work (1997), where she philosophizes from her dual position as an Indian woman with a training in both feminism and Western philosophy.

---

[5] These essays are "Throwing Like a Girl: A Phenomenology of Feminine Body Comportment, Motility, and Spatiality," "Pregnant Embodiment: Subjectivity and Alienation," and "House and Home: Feminist Variations on a Theme," respectively. These essays and others that are equally illustrative of the idea that the personal is philosophical are collected in Young (2005).

Her own experiences of life as an Indian woman of a certain class and education are fundamental in allowing us to grasp the philosophical conundrums in a
postcolonial world.

Among the contemporary philosophical works, Susan Brison's essays and her
book *Aftermath: Violence and the Remaking of a Self* (2002) have been pivotal.[6]
Here the personal voice takes center stage and becomes a powerful and *essential*
part of treatment of classical as well as newer philosophical issues. Among the
concepts that are revisited in *Aftermath* are the relation between the mind and
the body, the nature of personal identity, oppression, masculinity, and sexual
violence, the role of narrative in the construction of the self, and a deep reflection
on the relational nature of the self. Unlike my discussion of my daughter in *Love's
Labor*, Brison does not confine her story to the last pages of her book. She forth-
rightly and courageously places her searing experience as a survivor of sexual assault
in the front of the book. Every page is informed by the experience of violence and
the effort to retrieve a self out of victimhood. The spirit of that work especially—but
also along with other feminist, race, and gender philosophers—infuses the entirety
of my own effort in this project.

When I speak of what I have learned as the parent of a child such as Sesha,
I do not mean that this knowledge can be gleaned only in this way. But it is to
say that this perspective is of value in gaining insight that can then be shared. At
the same time, I can acknowledge that I will have only limited epistemic access
to knowledge gleaned from other vantage points. In locating the autobiographical in our approach to more abstract questions, we can better understand our
different views, accept the limitations of our own understanding, and recognize
new sources of insights and arguments.

In philosophical literature it is in times of paradigm shifts, as Thomas Kuhn
defines these, that the autobiographical mode surfaces. Kuhn maintains that
the shift from an Aristotelian world to a Newtonian one, and from Newtonian
physics to Einstein's relativity theory, involved a shift in paradigms that "are the
source of the methods, problem-field, and standards of solution accepted by any
mature scientific community at any given time" (2012, 103).

While philosophy is generally less likely to discard the old in favor of the new,
philosophy too has its paradigm shifts. When our world is expanded, when our
times demand new substantive and methodological frameworks, we find that
the philosophical figures who try to comprehend these moments interject their
lives into their philosophical arguments. As the "I" comes face to face with the
limitations of past knowledge, the interjection of the "I" signals a search for a

---

[6] She began publishing essays demonstrating and speaking directly to the question of the personal as philosophical many years before the book's publication (1993; 1995; 1999; 2002).

new epistemological authority. Socrates's life and circumstances are essential to his philosophical displacement of the Sophists. Augustinian thought, a paradigm shift in theology and religious philosophy, is not comprehensible without the Confessions. At times, self-revelation can serve as the justification for changing the subject. Descartes inserts the "I" most vividly in the *Meditations*, as he motivates his new quest for knowledge, established not on authority or tradition but on the individual mind. At a similar historical moment, Spinoza begins his *Essay on the Improvement of the Understanding* with a self-revelation that leads us directly to his rejection of teleological thinking:

> After experience had taught me that all the usual surroundings of social life are vain and futile . . .; that none of the objects of my fears contained in themselves anything either good or bad, except in so far as the mind is affected by them . . . I finally resolved to inquire whether there might be some real good . . . of which the discovery and attainment would enable me to enjoy continuous, supreme, and unending happiness. (Spinoza 1996b)

By means of that personal voice, Spinoza sought to motivate the philosophical impulse anew at a time when Scholasticism had failed to address tumultuous times and new strivings for individual understanding and happiness. Rousseau's *Confessions*, indulgent as they are at times, mark another of many such moments of revolutionary philosophical fervor. Even Kant, the very model of the impersonal voice, begins his critical philosophy by telling us of how he awoke from his "dogmatic slumber."

The personal voice in philosophy often tells the journey of a singular soul. But sometimes a relationship marks a turning point. John Stuart Mill credits his departure from the utilitarianism of his father and Jeremy Bentham to his companion and wife Harriet Taylor. Taylor, a substantial thinker in her own right, directed him to the importance of liberty and women's rights. She was the intellectual interlocutor who, in opening his eyes to women's situation also altered his narrow understanding of human life.

My own turn to the personal and autobiographical, while not as momentous as any of the figures I have cited, shares with other feminists, race theorists, LGBTQ philosophers, and disability scholars a turn away from the hegemony of the largely white, largely male voice in philosophy.[7] That turn is also an

---

[7] The personal voice as such is not always necessary in the way it is in Brison's work. The mere fact that the philosopher lives a certain sort of life, has experiences and expectations that differ from philosophers who have come before her, can have a profound effect on the philosophy that is done. I can scarcely begin to enumerate the powerful influences in my own work, from the analytic analyses of Alison Jaggar (1983), Marilyn Frye (1983), Claudia Card (1991; 1994; 1995), Virginia Held

abandonment of the sole individual thinker sitting in front of the fireplace. Like the feminist-inspired work of Mill and many of the feminists of the last part of the twentieth century, my turn also involved more than a solitary "I." My daughter is more than an inspiration, and yet, while she is not an interlocutor in a philosophical dialogue, she, and my life with her, define this philosophical inquiry. The world that she has opened for me forced my own paradigm shift. The questions my experience with my daughter have raised are animated by a philosophical impulse, but the matters provoking these questions are outside the bounds of any extant philosophical framework. The concepts in which to find answers adequate to my experience are absent in the philosophical literature, or they are there only in nascent form, and need still to evolve.

My argument in this book and its sequel is that we cannot give complete answers to questions about our moral obligations and our social and political commitments unless and until we find a way to include people like my daughter. We cannot answer questions about the meaning of equality or even see clearly what gives life its meaning. When we take into account her life, the full salience of its (nontypical) embodiment comes into focus; we find different ways to think about what a good life is; we see how more neglected questions are critical, such as the place of care and dependency in our moral and political lives. All these are without doubt philosophical concerns, but, in attempting to address them, we run up against the inadequacy of our current tools.

Therefore to redress this exclusion presents a philosophical challenge. There are two obstacles. First, there are no evident concepts available that can be used to this end. Second, one must introduce empirical information, which is rarely viewed as relevant to conceptual problems. Without knowing something of the lives of people with significant intellectual disabilities (indeed, without knowing some*one* with such disabilities), there is no way to formulate concepts adequate to demonstrate the moral value of these lives. Having such an acquaintance helps to clear a space for the mind to question certain philosophical dogmas. The hope is that within that space we can begin to broaden our understanding of what it means to be human, what moral action requires, and what human perfection may look like. My ambition is only to point the way, to help redirect our moral gaze. This modest project involves both critique and constructive work,

(1987; 1993) and Diana T. Meyers (1989; 1994), to the phenomenological (Bartky 1990), historical (Mercer and O'Neill 2005), and political writings (Benhabib 1987; Fraser 1989) and the writings of philosophers of science and epistemology (Harding and Hintikka 1983; Alcoff and Potter 1993): the debt is enormous and my own work would not have been possible without this groundwork. This shifting of the paradigms and parameters in philosophy goes on unabated today. I hope to capture some of this richness in the works I discuss and cite in the pages that follow. Even so, the works truly are too numerous to cite adequately.

taking seriously the limitations of our current assumptions about what matters in life.

I am not alone in this effort. As early as 1982, Loretta Kopelman and John Moskop organized the conference "Ethics and Mental Retardation," and subsequently published the proceedings (Kopelman and Moskop 1984). While not strictly speaking a work of philosophy, Michael Bérubé's *Life as We Know It* (1998) is an extremely thoughtful and philosophical reflection on many of the same questions from the perspective of a father of a son with Down syndrome (DS). Simo Vehmas (1999), a Finnish philosopher, has been writing about philosophical issues concerning intellectual disability since 1999, taking a relational approach to moral status not dissimilar to my own. Anita Silvers (1994) was an early pioneer in introducing philosophers to questions in disability, and, along with Leslie Francis, has developed views on justice and intellectual disability (Silvers and Francis 2000; 2005; 2010). Martha Nussbaum (2006) has since done significant work on many of the questions I have raised. Licia Carlson (2009; 2010) and Sophia Wong (2008) have brought their feminist and personal concerns to bear on questions of cognitive disability. These are but a few who have joined the discussion. Philosophical theologians have contributed important work early on as well, including figures such as Jean Vanier (1982), Robert Veatch (1986), and Hans Reinders (2000; 2008). So, as I wind my own way through the set of ideas on offer here, I want to acknowledge the joint effort to make visible a set of philosophical preoccupations too long neglected.

Much of what I have to say is based on the fact that we know as yet so little of the possibilities that disabled lives present. We can imagine our knowledge as represented by a fire surrounded by darkness, a darkness that represents our ignorance. As the fire grows and extends, the larger the circle of darkness becomes. The more we know, the more we are aware of how little we know. The more people in all their variety are included in our philosophical deliberations, the wider is the circle of knowledge, and with it the greater our appreciation of how much in the dark we still are. Once we move beyond the charmed circle of those whose intuitions and experiences have until now shaped philosophical discourse, we grow humbler and humbler about the certainty of our deliberations. We cannot grow wiser until we assume a humbler posture in philosophizing about matters of disability. We will never even know the many ways our ignorance is hindering the life prospects of people with disabilities unless we shed prejudices and our adherence to fixed beliefs, particularly those about the human organism and how personal, social, and political relationships shape its prospects.

1.3 The Argument

The argument that defines this project spans two books, the current volume and one that is soon to follow. The current book, *Learning from My Daughter: The Value and Care of Disabled Minds*, constitutes the first half of the project. The concepts developed here will lay the groundwork for claims of justice for people with significant disabilities, and for conceptions of dignity and moral personhood that will not exclude people with these sorts of disabilities. These ideas will be the subject of the second volume, tentatively titled *Who is Truly Human? Justice, Personhood, and Mental Disability*.

Some will object that using outliers like my daughter as reason to question traditional philosophical views is misconceived. They will insist that people with such significant disabilities are 'hard cases,' and just as hard cases make bad laws, so too do hard cases make bad philosophy. My retort is that hard cases make better philosophy. Hard cases challenge philosophical dogmas. They are a subset of tools that are philosophers' stock in trade: the counterexample. The counterexample unmoors us from presuppositions that are otherwise left unexamined and challenges us to find better formulations—and hard cases do just that. But the hard case can do still more. It can provide us with more adequate models for our theorizing. The hard cases considered here broaden the scope of our understanding of the human—for the limitations that Sesha lives with can come to be the limitations of any human being. I hope the skeptical reader will allow me to demonstrate the importance of learning from these hard cases.

Part I of this book, "Learning to Become a Humbler Philosopher," speaks to the transformational effect of living with and learning about my daughter's disability. Chapter 1, "On What Matters/Not," begins by recounting the challenges life with my daughter posed to my beliefs of what constituted a life worth living. It has begun with the story of Sesha's birth and how I came to see that I must bring my experiences with Sesha into my philosophizing. But doing so has required a sort of philosophizing different from what my training prepared me for. It calls for a more personal approach and a humbler sort of philosophizing. It is the start of the story of how I have needed to reconfigure thoughts about what matters most.

Chapter 2, "The New Normal and a Good Life," begins with the shock felt by most parents in learning that their child has a significant disability. I had taken the ability to reason as central in a good life. That was a baseline assumption, that is what I took to be normal. But Sesha, I was told, was not normal, and her ability to reason was not a given. Often the first thing felt by an able parent who is confronted with the information that her child has a disability is the terror that her child will not live a "normal" life. It is a fear insofar as we take normalcy to be a prerequisite for a good life. What is this desire for the normal, and is normalcy needed for a good life? I argue that we desire the normal because we desire to be loved for the unique individual that we are, and that normalcy provides a standard against which our singularity can be perceived and appreciated. The difficulty many able people have with imagining a good life with a significant disability (a belief contradicted by studies of disability and well-being) arises from conceiving of normalcy as having a fixed set of norms. Rather than having one specification for *the* good life, I call for more capacious norms that give us room to have *a* good life and be ourselves, in all our multivariate forms.

The desire for normalcy weighs heavily in choices made possible through advances in reproductive technologies. Learning from my daughter, my discussions with my non-disabled son, and the writings of disabled people, I consider the philosophical and bioethical issues that swirl about these new technologies. In part II, "Choosing Children and the Limits of Planning," which consists of three chapters, I insist that reproductive choices around disability need to remain, like all reproductive choices, in the hands of the woman who carries the child. But *how* we argue for any position that tolerates selecting against disability matters. I begin, in chapter 3, "The Limits of Choice," by posing the question of choice itself and pointing out that our ability to freely choose is limited not only by our circumstances, but also by inherent paradoxes of choice in the face of uncertainty. Rather than trumpeting a triumphal celebration of reproductive technology, I urge that we more humbly understand that the unpredictability of fortune is ever with us.

In chapter 4, "The Ethics of Prenatal Testing and Selection," I dispute a central argument put forward by many in the disability community: that those who sanction and encourage reproductive choice to select against disability send a message—that is, *express* the belief—that life with a disability is not worth living, or alternatively that disabled people are not welcome in this world. The various formulations of the view, all of which are thought to be discriminatory and harmful to existing disabled people, are known as the *expressivist* objection to selective reproductive decisions. Although I argue against the expressivist objection in chapter 4, in chapter 5 "How Not to Argue for Selective Reproductive Procedures," I also contend that certain arguments about reproductive selection, especially those that maintain that we are *morally obligated* not to give birth to a disabled child (whenever we can help it), are also problematic. The arguments in these two chapters are sometimes very detailed and exhaustive. A reader who wants only the gist of the positions can safely skip some of the more elaborate argumentation.

The position which I favor is that we do not put a moral onus on a woman's choice based on whether she chooses for or against disability. It is imperative that we encourage a woman to make her decision in a thoughtful manner, considering the available evidence about the likely impact of the disability on the child, the woman herself, and the other members of the family—all considered in the context of the society in which she lives. It is the woman herself who will be responsible for raising that child herself or assigning that obligation to another, and her choices might depend in good part on the social supports available to her. It must be her decision whether or not to bring a child into the world. If there are any morally significant messages sent by decisions to prevent the birth of a disabled child, these are that our society fails people with disabilities and their families by providing such scant resources to make their lives go as well as they can.

To say that those charged with the care of the child should be the ones who make the morally significant decision to have the child is to underscore the importance of the relationship of *dependency* of the child to the carer. Not until feminist philosophers articulated an ethics of care have questions of dependency and care received much attention from philosophers. As my daughter has remained dependent through her adult years and is in need of care all the time, I have long occupied a distinctive perch from which to view the centrality of care to a life well lived. I have concluded that a philosophy that fails to consider dependency and care cannot be a fully adequate one.

In part III, "Care in Philosophy, Disability, and Ethics," I adumbrate an ethics of care. My intention is not to lay out a complete ethic, which would be at once too ambitious and may not address the intersection of disability and philosophy that I target in this volume. Instead I want to consider aspects of the concepts of dependency and care that will both make salient their importance for philosophy and address the distaste for both dependency and care that have been voiced by disability activists and scholars. The dependency of disabled people, these activists and scholars want to insist, is a construction of an ableist society that is used to stigmatize and exclude them (Barnes 1990). I propose instead that it is not dependency but independence that is a social construct.

Part III takes up these lessons of the inevitability of dependency and the centrality of care in human life in four chapters. In chapter 6, "Dependency and Disability," I suggest that rather than striving to join the "independent" citizen, disability offers up the occasion to question the presumption of independence as the requisite for equal dignity and worth. In chapter 7, "An Ethics of Care," I discuss the distinctive features of an ethics of care and address some of the concerns that disability scholars have had with such an ethics. An ethics of care, I argue, is especially fruitful in thinking about how one can flourish *regardless* of ability or level of dependency. A complaint that disabled people often launch against an ethic of care is that care is paternalistic and thus disrespectful to adult people with disabilities, denying them the full dignity of persons. In chapter 8, "The Completion of Care—The Normativity of Care," I counter this objection to care by discussing an underappreciated aspect of care: what Nel Noddings called "the completion of care" (1984). I argue that when we take this aspect of care seriously, we can get a fully normative ethic of care that is not only compatible with, but requires respecting the individuality and the dignity of the other.

In chapter 9, "Forever Small: The Strange Case of Ashley X," I discuss the case of Ashley X, who was a young girl of six when she was subjected to large doses of estrogen to attenuate her growth, given an hysterectomy, and had her breast buds removed. The idea was to keep her forever small, and presumably forever a size that could allow her to remain cared for by her family. I use my experiences as a mother of a daughter with disabilities similar to Ashley as part of a philosophical argument against the "Ashley treatment." Central to my argument is that an ethic of care such as I articulated in the previous chapters shows the treatment not to be justifiable. That is, there are good reasons to think that, contrary to the claims made by Ashley's parents and physicians, the care that enabled the Ashley treatment fell short of care in the fully normative sense, and the parent who believes that this is the best care for a child has been misled.

We can know little of what Ashley and others with her disabilities know, what they sense, and what they feel. We must always be alert to the fact that the lack of expressive language does not preclude the possibility of receptive language and understanding. And we must respect the right of bodily integrity. Recognizing another's bodily integrity is not only a matter of rights, it is also an essential part of caring. Only by recognizing the need to care for and respect Ashley's bodily integrity can we allow for the possibility that she is more aware than we can know. The case of Ashley X allows us to see an ethics of care in action. It brings together questions about care and disability in a way that illuminates why an ethic of care is the ethical theory that complements the demand of rights for people with disabilities. We see again that care and rights are not oppositional, that both relationality and the integrity of the individual need to be operative, and that a love that flows from the horizon of ability must be in dialogue with the many corners of the disability community. This first book of a two-book project concludes with A Final Reflection, "My Daughter's Body: A Meditation on Soul."

The second book, *Who is Truly Human?*, continues the project of rethinking philosophical concepts through the lens of cognitive disability. There I argue for the moral personhood of people with significant cognitive disabilities and for their equal claim to dignity and justice.

Portions of the public, and a number of philosophers, have argued that there are not justifiable reasons to devote resources to the care of people with significant *cognitive* disabilities.[8] Using current theories of justice and theories of

---

[8] See exemplars in the works of McMahan (1996; 2003; 2005; 2006; 2008; 2009), Rachels (1990; 1998), Singer (1979; 1994; 2007; 2008; 2009) and Singer and Kuhse (1985).

personhood, they argue that people with these disabilities do not partake in the cooperative venture that is society, and so they are not properly recipients of its benefits. Others argue on utilitarian grounds that the concerns of those with significant cognitive abilities have less priority. And some arguments maintain that the special needs of these individuals constitute a bottomless pit, diverting resources from the rest of society's needs. Jeff McMahan (1996) has even made the argument that whatever theory of justice one espouses, people with significant cognitive disabilities do not deserve the same entitlements and protections we grant to other members of society.

Theories of society as a system of social cooperation underlie the distribution of resources in a liberal society. I argue that if one starts only with the assumption that justice presumes a society in which everyone is a rational, independent, fully functioning person who can be a social cooperator, one cannot get to a conception of justice in which people with significant disabilities are included. We cannot get from "here" to "there" with our present theories of justice. Rather than conclude that the protections and resources demanded by justice are not due these individuals, I maintain that the inability to justify devoting resources to people with significant cognitive disabilities is a failing to be remedied in *any* theory of justice. If we accept that justice is a virtue of social structures, then we need a theory of justice that can do better.

In *Learning From My Daughter* I make the case that an ethic of care is best suited to handle relationships of dependency and to promote the idea that living with a disability is compatible with living a good life. In my next book I will reject the idea that care and justice are necessarily opposing perspectives, and suggest principles for a conception of justice that requires our basic institutions to conform to values and principles of care. Rather than consider, as John Rawls would have us do, that justice provides the fair terms of social cooperation, we recognize that much of this cooperative labor serves to nurture and care for the very young, the ill and significantly disabled, and the frail elderly, as well as to maintain us in our cooperative ventures. While some cannot join in these, others can do so, given additional supports and care. Some may not be 'cooperators' as that term is used in political theory, no matter the supports. Yet all people need to be part of any vibrant and just society. A theory of justice that is fully inclusive would determine not just the fair terms of social cooperation among those who can be cooperators. It would consider the facts of *inevitable* human dependency and *inextricable* interdependency in determining fair terms for *all* to live together in a just society. If we take an ethic of care as the one we want to promote in our daily interactions, then we need to build a theory of justice where social structures embody this ethic even as they remain suitable to other requirements of a just society.

Essential to all arguments that people with significant cognitive disabilities are not due justice is the view that only *persons* are subjects entitled to justice, and people such as Ashley and Sesha are not *persons with equal moral status*. In countering these views, which have a deep history in Western philosophy, the overarching argument begun in the pages of *Learning from My Daughter* reaches its climax: What is a person? In *Who's Truly Human?*, I will attempt to provide different grounds for both personhood and dignity based on the care-ethical conception of the self as relational.[9] I mean to displace the centrality of intrinsic properties such as reason as definitive of personhood and dignity. I will draw on conceptions developed in *Love's Labor* and *Learning From My Daughter*, especially the idea that we are all "some mother's child." This, not our rational capacities, is the source of our moral dignity and moral parity, as well as our entitlement to the resources and protections of the state. Appealing to our relational property as 'some mother's child' does, however, not mean that the entitlement of people with significant mental disabilities to justice and dignity is for the sake of those with whom they are in relations. Instead we recognize that the morally significant relationality is possible only because the people in question are the sorts of beings who can have the dignity and moral standing of persons. A teacup cannot be a "mother's child." Nor can a member of another species be the child of a human mother. Our species membership, I argue, *is* morally significant— but not because it gives us license to misuse or abuse members of other species. It is morally important because of the sorts of morally weighty relationships only human beings can have to one another. We can agree that we have moral relationships to nonhumans without denying that that our relationships to other humans carry special moral weight that must apply to all humans, regardless of an individual human being's intrinsic attributes. I argue for *human* dignity, not for the claim that only humans have dignity.

Human dignity has been regarded by many as the very basis of human rights. I make a case for a dialectics of dignity and care, by reflecting on an incident in which the director of the agency that runs the residence where my daughter now lives objected to the fact that Sesha was wheeled into the hallway of her residence after her bath wrapped only in a towel. The director strongly felt that this was an affront to her dignity. The virulence of her response, she explained to me later, was due to her experiences at a state institution that housed people with mental disabilities. There she saw naked men marched into the washrooms where they

---

[9] For a different use of care as necessary for a definition of personhood, see Jaworska (2007), and Jaworska and Tannenbaum (2014).

were washed down with water hoses. Such treatment heightened her awareness to the indignities that can befall people with mental disabilities. The consideration of disability, and the dependency which accompanies most forms of bodily disablement, leads inexorably to the need for an ethic that recognizes both the dignity of care and the place of care in a life of dignity. Such an ethic is one based on the fully normative conception of care for which I argue in *Learning From My Daughter*. In such an ethic, dignity is grounded in relationships of care.

When we care for another in the fully normative sense, we understand that this individual's ability to flourish is an end in itself, one that is worth promoting for the sake of that person. To promote the equal dignity of all human beings, as I will argue, is nothing other than the recognition and affirmation of the inherent, equal, nonfungible, and noninstrumental value of another as an embodied, relational, and enculturated human being. It is that conception of the person which must guide the caregiver, and, in a dialectic of dignity and care, care at once confers upon and recognizes the dignity of another.[10] An ethical theory based on a fully normative sense of care has as its goal the recognition and maintenance of the equal dignity of all.

To conclude the argument in *Who's Truly Human? Justice, Personhood and Mental Disability,* I will look at the historical treatment of people with mental disabilities during a period when their personhood was systemically obliterated: Nazi Germany. The noncontingent relationship between the Nazi eugenics movement and racism is exemplified in the figure of a single man, Irmfried Eberl. He was first the physician-in-chief of Brandenburg and Bernburg Hospitals, where the murder of the mentally disabled were carried out in a program known as T4, and subsequently the Commandant at Treblinka, the Nazi death camp where the racially based killing of Jews was undertaken with unsurpassed efficiency. The members of my own family who perished in the Nazi Holocaust were all killed by the same man whose hands were first bloodied by the murder of German as well as Jewish children and adults like my daughter, Sesha.

I use this exemplar as a grim reminder of the ultimate consequences of the refusal to acknowledge the full dignity and equality of *every* human being. The Nazis themselves believed that there was little to differentiate between their "medical" and racially based exterminations. The eugenics program of the Nazis is often characterized as negative eugenics—the evil sort—in opposition to the positive eugenics employed in improving human beings. Such positive eugenics, it is averred, can harness technology to augment and enhance human capacities. It is at one with the triumphalism that we encountered in the debates around

[10] In *Who's Truly Human? Justice, Personhood and Mental Disability*, I will follow the helpful distinction between equal dignity and group dignity offered by Deryck Beyleveld and Roger Brownsword (2001). Equal dignity demands the recognition of that equal value of each individual.

selective reproductive procedures. The people who deride the idea of human equality as speciesist and question the dignity of people like my daughter often are the same who hold the belief in positive eugenics. The pairing of these two views should give us pause. Who decides which characteristics are worthy of value and should be enhanced? Who decides which characteristics land some humans outside the moral boundary reserved for the possessors of valued traits? I argue for extreme caution in proceeding to develop enhancements, and I propose that the best way to "enhance" human beings is to draw on their capacity for shared caregiving. Caring, not culling, is the way to a better future—one that will include people with widely varying abilities and disabilities. When we accept cognitive disabilities as within the spectrum of that diversity, we learn new things about what matters. The lessons my daughter has taught me can be summed up in the appreciation for our ability to give, receive, and share care and love, and in our acceptance of the rich diversity of human capacities for joy.

2

The New Normal and a Good Life

Wednesday morning. The morning after. I awoke feeling sore internally, somewhat nauseated, somewhat as if I were recovering from a physical torture. I had spent Tuesday at the Hastings Center in a workshop on prenatal testing and selective abortion for disability. It was my first efforts to engage professionally with the question of Sesha's disability. On Tuesday evening, a dam burst and the floodgates came undone. I sobbed deep, deep sobs from the interior of my soul. I cried, I cried for Sesha. I felt the hurt for her impairments, for the profound limits of the life she could experience, for the multiple aspects of life she could never know or even know that she couldn't know. I wept for Sesha— not for me, not for Jeffrey [my husband], not for Leo [my son], but for her, her sweetness, her limitation, and the pain of knowing what a small aspect of human life she could inhabit. It is a hurt that doesn't dare to be felt, almost all the time, and it is a hurt that cannot be felt in her sunny presence. But it is there and at moments like the post-Hastings meeting, it floods in.

Now what is this mysterious pain? Mysterious because ... who is hurt? I don't know that Sesha is aware of her limitation. I have to think more about this.

—from my Diary: October 23, 1996

2.1 Desiring the Normal

"Normal" is such a benign word when things are normal. It is a cutting one when things are not. When the norm of normal is met, the term is deceptively descriptive. When it fails to be met, the normative and judgmental meaning is apparent, sometimes brutally so. When used against an individual who fails to meet that norm, the word can feel like a bludgeon, an excuse to accuse, condemn, exclude, or denigrate. As autistic writer Clare Sainsbury observes, " 'normal' people take it as a basic human right to be accepted as they are, while the rest of us are viewed only in terms of what will make us more acceptable to them" (Sainsbury 2000). What is it about normalcy that can so denigrate those judged not normal? Why is normalcy desirable, desired, and presumed so often to be essential for one's life to go well? Is a good life compatible with a life that is "not normal"?

The object of investigation in this chapter is the *desire* for the normal. I will attempt to untangle the knot of a desire that throws into question one's ability to construct a good life against a constricting norm.

From a child's as well as a parent's perspective, I feel that I have a particular claim on the question, "Why do we desire normalcy?" For as a child of two Holocaust survivors, I wanted above all to be normal. Born into a time when the world was recovering from a second worldwide war, stability and normalcy was the order of the day. In the aftermath of the chaos and disruption of war, there is a profound desire to achieve predictability with rigid norms. The United States of the 1950s was such a time. Conformity to a singular norm was reinforced by television, movies, and theater, policed by scrutinizing neighbors, and maintained by stigmatizing and excluding those who did not fit (Feder 2007). It was a stifling atmosphere in which immigrants, Holocaust survivors and their children, people with disabilities, homosexuals, the political left, and so many others could scarcely breathe the air of the freedom for which the war was fought.

The fifties gave way to the sixties, and the vistas opened. In this historical moment, it seemed as if all those excluded took center stage. Their cares became the subject of popular songs and popular culture. Their movements captured the headlines. The "normal" met defiance; in meeting the resistance, the normal changed. More problems promised to be addressed than were in fact resolved. Nonetheless, some like me suddenly felt as if we belonged to the great American narrative.

When I became the parent of a child who, as it happened, turned out to have very significant cognitive disabilities, the desire for normalcy once again held me in its thrall. The desire for normalcy was at the heart of the pain and despair that so tore our hearts in those early days. Few individuals and still fewer parents escape a similar anguish when confronted with the news that they or their child has some impairment, some anomaly, that threatens to make a "normal" life impossible.

Donna Thomson writes of her experience learning about her son's disability:

> Tears glistened on the doctor's cheeks as she told me my baby was severely disabled. "Never be normal" are the words I remember. . . .
> I looked down and something red caught my eye. Blood was oozing from the edge of my thumbnail where I had bitten it. (Thomson 2010)

Thomson compares her response to that of a grandfather of a young family that perished in a terrible road accident. The dazed grandfather said, "I don't understand—we brought them up so carefully so nothing like this would ever happen." Like him, she had "the experience of falling victim to random tragedy and a serious derailment of one's life plans," which "caused such profound shock and questioning of all I believed was solid and true" (Thomson 2010).

Another mother, Jane Bernstein, recounts taking her unusual child to a behavioral psychologist who informed her that her daughter was "extremely disfluent":

> When I told him in a moment of frustration that the thought of her like this in the future was devastating, he said, "It's going to be devastating." I wept when I left the office as if the world was coming to an end. (Bernstein 2010)

Why does the news that your child is not normal involve such a profound shock, such an upheaval of everything?[1] The worst fear is often that the impairment will be to the child's cognitive abilities. The shock, the unravelling of all that you had based your expectations on, the "terrible news" of the abnormality, is immediately comprehensible to most. But why, when the source of the anguish is not death, but abnormality?

Perhaps only someone who is habituated to asking "why" would ever challenge the seemingly indisputable loss that significant disability brings. We want health, opportunities, and general well-being for our child. How will this child grow into an adult that others can love and cherish? Will she be viewed as a valuable and valued member of society, included as a full citizen, not merely a pitiful charity case? All are questions that are especially poignant in the case of significant intellectual disability.

We humans may simply be creatures who have deep psychological, as well as practical, needs to be normal. The pragmatic desire is not puzzling—it is simply easier to move through life without being viewed as "abnormal." But there is a depth to the desire that goes beyond the evident advantages. I will suggest that even the purely psychological desire can be de-psychologized, that the desirability of the normal lies in the concept of normalcy itself. That is, we may not be able to escape a desire for the normal because, at least on some interpretations of the concept, the normal is precisely that which is desirable and to be desired.

---

[1] Andrew Solomon (2012) studies families in which a child is different from the "normal" parents. He attributes his own fascination with the cases he studies to his own deviation from the norm of heterosexuality. In a fascinating discussion, he reflects on his own parents' reaction to his coming out, and his own thoughts and concerns as he becomes a parent. Solomon couches them in terms of a difference between the vertical identities that mark the parental relationship and the horizontal identities that characterize those children who are apples falling far from the tree. The norm here is identified with the parent; the deviation from the norm (and from the parental identity) on the part of their offspring is the core of the parental shock of "abnormality."

Not to desire the normal would be not to desire what is desirable. The simplicity of this formulation, however, belies a complex notion and our own ambiguous relationship to it.

With rare exceptions, there is little philosophical acknowledgment of the wide variety of human possibilities, and the "normal" human subject is presumed when human beings are discussed.[2] Normalcy is derided only when its antithesis is excellence, not when "normal" is opposed to a difference that is interpreted as a deficit. The child who is not "intact" may justify infanticide at worst, exclusion at best. The adult who falls outside a normal range of capacities is considered a poor wretch, a burden, and at times implicitly (and sometimes explicitly) excluded from the protections, demands, and privileges of justice.[3] As much as philosophers extol the examined life, the desire for normalcy goes unexamined. When one's life is touched by disability, however, then living an examined life demands interrogating the concept and desire for normalcy. As a parent, that inquiry begins by questioning the desire that your child be normal.

2.2   Examining the Desire for a "Normal Child"

Sara Ruddick, who has developed one of the finest philosophical discussions of the practice of raising a child (a practice she calls simply "mothering"), spoke of the three fundamental demands children make on parents: preservative love, fostering growth, and socialization for acceptance (1989). A parent's understanding of her role and her expectations of her children take shape in relation to the three demands. Ruddick later confessed (Ruddick n.d.) that in formulating her theory, she had assumed "an intact" child, and she came to acknowledge the importance of considering a child's disability for the expectations and responsibilities of parental practice (Hanigsberg and Ruddick 1999). As Joseph Stramondo and Stephen Campbell (2015) put it, disability is a "high impact trait." The nature of the disability too will make a difference, and cognitive differences have a profound effect.

The child's claim on the mother's preservative love perhaps requires the greatest vigilance from all parents, regardless of the child's abilities. A young child has little understanding or awareness of danger that can lead to a life-threatening situation. One mother I know referred to mothering in these early

---

[2] Nietzsche is a prominent exception, as is Michel Foucault. Some of the attractiveness of their philosophies has been their ability to see "normalcy" as a repressive ideal.

[3] The question of who is entitled to the protections of justice is treated in *Who's Truly Human?*

years as being on "suicide alert." A child with significant cognitive impairments, however, often has accompanying neurological or other physiological disorders which are ever-present imminent threats to the child's immediate survival and ability to thrive. For instance, between 40 and 50 percent of children with Down syndrome will have heart impairments that will shorten life if not end it (Bull 2011). Babies born with severe developmental disabilities will often have difficulty swallowing and require surgical interventions so that they can take in nutrients (NIH 2014).

While a parent's preservative love for children without disabilities is also intense at the start of life, it grows less demanding as the child herself acquires more skills of self-preservation. In the case of a child with cognitive disabilities, the suicide alert doesn't end in early childhood, nor does the constant proactive care cease. In Sesha's case, her utter helpless dependency meant (and continues to mean) that without constant care and protection, she would simply die. While she has no life-threatening conditions, her feeding was not as robust as it should have been, and, had her condition not been noticed, she might well have failed to thrive. We must always be hyper-attentive since she has no way of letting us know where she has pain, or that she feels unwell. The vigilance must be constant. In the blink of an eye she can get into a dangerous situation. Without someone's preservative love (and the resources to meet its demands), a person with very significant cognitive disabilities simply cannot survive.

The first demand, Ruddick notes, is in constant tension with the forces of nature, which must be resisted or they will destroy the dependent infant or young child (with or without disabilities). The diseases that kill, the pull of bright and poisonous berries, the seduction of water—all must be managed or guarded against. The second demand, fostering growth or development, in contrast, has a more harmonious relationship to nature: a species-typical child will grow whether or not the nourishment is optimal, will learn without constant tutelage, and in general will develop as long as she is not hindered. But the struggle for such development to proceed in the case of severe disability and especially cognitive disability is ceaseless. Parenting a child with such disabilities doesn't feel like giving nature a nudge. It feels instead like moving mountains. Educational processes need to be intensive, specialized, and purposive. They will need to extend well past childhood. And success often is measured in very small increments: "My child smiled today." For the mother of a child with autism, this can be a major accomplishment. When Sesha learned to hug (at age five), the accomplishment was equivalent to another child her age playing a sonata with fluency.

The third demand, training a child so that she can be a socialized member of her community, is never easy even for the most "normal" of children, but the difficulties are daunting when the child has disabilities. Here the social model of disability is especially illuminating.[4] Only so much training of the cognitively disabled child will be possible. If there is a misfit between the disabled child and the society, the difficulty is less a matter of the child's failure to adapt to what is socially acceptable behavior than a failure of society to acknowledge and accept this individual. The parenting of a disabled child therefore requires the socializing of the community to accept the child even more than it requires socializing the child.

The fact that cognitive disability poses such daunting challenges to the demands of parenting may be explanation enough for the heartache parents experience when told that their child will "not be normal" and will be cognitively disabled. A fear of many parents, one that they experience as "selfish," is that their own lives will be consumed with the care of the disabled child. Michael Bérubé, in a memorable passage where he recounts his wife Janet Lyons saying "we can handle this," writes:

> But could we believe our own hope? Could we meet even the simplest of challenges this child might pose? Would we ever have normal lives again? . . . A mere three weeks earlier, the university hired Janet . . . and we thought we were finally going to be "comfortable." But now were we going to spend the rest of our days caring for a severely disabled child? Would we have even an hour to ourselves? . . . These were selfish thoughts, and the understanding that selfish thoughts might be "natural" at such a time didn't make them any less bitter or insistent. (Bérubé 1998, 6)

These concerns are voiced at the very start of a book that celebrates the life of little Jaime Bérubé. Such "selfish thoughts" are quickly supplanted by worries not that it will be more demanding to raise this child ("Would we ever have normal lives again?"), but that the child will not have a normal life. Included in the desire for a "normal" life for one's child is the ability of the child to experience friendship, meaningful dignified work, membership in a community, love, and family.

---

[4] Disability scholars and activists have proposed that it is a mistake to regard disability through a medical lens that defines disability as lodging solely in the individual. They distinguish between an impairment (or an atypicality), which is a characteristic of the individual, and a disability which is a social construction. Proponents of the social model, of which there are many competing versions, direct us to notice that wheelchair users are mobility disabled only in environments that accommodate solely walkers. A sighted person will be more disabled than a blind person when placed in a totally dark environment. And so forth. Although the social model has been hotly disputed, even in the field of disability studies (see, for example, Shakespeare and Watson 2001), the essential point that disability involves a misfit between the body and the environment remains an indisputable insight. See also footnote 9.

The worst ache comes from the concern that the child will not experience these intrinsically valuable and valued experiences, and from the additional worry that the child herself will want goods that no accommodation makes possible, and thus experience frustration and sadness—rejection and exclusion.

2.2.1 The Desire that Refuses to Go Away

When my daughter was diagnosed as having profound impairments, we were urged by well-meaning people to "give her up, place her elsewhere, and live a 'normal life.'" Like so many parents who are faced with their infant's significant anomaly, both my partner and I were already madly in love with our child. In this regard, we felt very much like a normal mother and a normal father. And giving up a child was not part of that norm. That our child did not meet the usual expectations of what a child would be was of far less importance than the fact that this was our child.

Sharing a belief with others who have not directly faced disability, we presumed that a life lived with disabilities was necessarily a diminished life.[5] We desired that our daughter should know the joys of childhood, that she should experience the challenges that give our lives zest, that she be safe and loved. In a word, we wanted our child to flourish. Having a good and flourishing life seemed inextricably linked to having a normal body, a normal mind, and a normal life.

For her to flourish, we as parents would have to be able to respond to the demands Ruddick identified, and we worried about all the complications posed by Sesha's disabled body and mind. Some of our worries were well warranted. She still must be protected at all times. She never learned to put her hands out to protect her face when she falls, and her front teeth were smashed when a teacher's aide in her classroom didn't realize she should be strapped into her chair. She now has a permanent bridge for front teeth. When we asked the dentist what would happen if she fell again, he replied, "She can't fall. Period."

Even when she is secured in a chair she is in danger. Once while strapped into her wheelchair, she pulled a pot of freshly made hot coffee off a kitchen counter and scalded her thighs. She had second-degree burns on both thighs and will always have significant scarring. She had another permanent injury while in the safest place one can imagine. She was in her own bed, complete with railings on both sides, bumpers and a couch that pulls up against the bed's side (so if she ever fell out, the couch would cushion her). One night, she must have had a massive seizure during which her collarbone broke. We came into her bedroom that morning and noticed that her arm was hanging oddly. That was the only way we

---

[5] For a familiar rehearsal of such views see Glover (2006a).

could know that something was wrong. She greeted us with her beautiful smile as she did every morning.

These are only some of the ways she must be protected from hurting herself. More portentous still is the frightening possibility that someone will intentionally harm her—and she is powerless to protect herself in any way or even tell us of what has happened. Yes, the fear for her safety was real then and is real now. Species-typical capacities can be self-protective and are among the tools with which we guard against the fragility of life. This is not to say that we always succeed. We don't. But Sesha hasn't a chance unless others substitute for her missing capacities.

The pain at the thought that she will never have a partner or family of her own is equally real. Whether disabled or not, there are those of us who choose not to settle on a life partner, prefer celibacy, decline having and raising children. For Sesha these will not be choices to forego. I have seen clear signs of her being smitten by some young man, and while she might get a smile and sweet word in return, these are poor substitutes for an intimate love. I have seen Sesha look longingly at a baby. I will never know if she desires a child of her own, but I know that no matter how ardent a desire it may be, it cannot be realized.

The sorrow that she won't know the pleasures of intellectual achievement sometimes flickers across my mind, but for the most part this is no longer a concern. The many heartaches of what she must forego have by now been muted as we direct our attentions to those things that give her joy and make her life rich nonetheless. And no one is more capable of joy and love than my daughter. She may not be able to partake in the wide array of possibilities open to most, but she lives those that *are* available to her fully and with intensity.

In our own development as parents, we have learned to distinguish the common understanding of a good life from "a normal life"—two concepts that seemed inseparable in the early years. In this we were aided, even in those first years, by the wave of rebellion that blew in just at the time of Sesha's birth. Sesha was born in 1969 and we were children of the 1960s. The stifling 1950s were ushered out, along with rigid ideas of comformity and normalcy; looking "freaky" or "funky" was *in*; people took psychedelics precisely to see the world in a way that defied normalcy.

Still, we did not cease to rely on some sense of normalcy. The desire with respect to one's child (I have suggested) is in part a desire that the parent be able to enjoy the various goods associated with a good life, and the desire that the child too be able to experience these. Even as we pry apart the good life from the normal life, there are ways in which the two refuse to come unglued. The desire for the normal persists even as we reject fixed norms to which we are expected to conform. What is the desire that refuses to go away?

Within our own milieu, we fashioned our new normal and enjoyed Sesha for what she had to offer, which was a bounty and a feast. Even after our son was born, and we saw what a baby of typical capabilities was like, the life we all shared with Sesha seemed to be as much normalcy as we cared to have—most of the time. As she passed infancy, her anomaly was evident to everyone, even as we had naturalized—normalized—her situation to ourselves. We came face to face with her difference when we took her to the doctors' office, shopping, or to the park.

The world has a way of intruding on the sense of normalcy one seeks to establish, as Helen Featherstone describes so well. Her son had become so normal to her that she didn't even think to mention her child's disability to the delightful young man she was interviewing to babysit him. When she introduced her seven-year-old, she suddenly found herself seeing her child through the teenager's eyes:

> I saw not the cheerful, handsome seven-year-old whom I care for every day, but a seriously deviant little boy who drools and makes strange, uninterpretable noises. The forgotten terrors of Jody's babyhood surfaced. I saw my son as I might have seen another seriously handicapped child seven years before. (Featherstone 1960, 41)

The dissonance between the norms one establishes in relationship to one's child and those chanced when an uncomprehending stranger encounters one's child can motivate a desire for the "normal" even among the most ardent nonconformist. The confrontation alienates one from one's own child, from the society that we had claimed as our own, and from ourselves in our role as parent. We are, if only for a split second, torn in our loyalties, and we revolt at the very thought that we might be pulled apart so. We are first depressed, then infuriated—and then we feel fear. It is the fear that our child will not be accepted, and so will find neither companionship nor protection by the wider community.

We have now at least a partial answer to why we desire the normal. The desire that refuses to go away is then first a desire to have one's own worth and that of one's children confirmed. Our sense of self-worth depends in large measure on the willingness of others to recognize our worth and that which we value. We require the affirmation of a community that what we are and what we value are, in fact, valuable. Without that recognition, we are in constant jeopardy—both in a psychological and in a physical sense. We are in danger of self-contempt and in being held in contempt by the community. And that which is not recognized as worthy is also not granted the protection of the community.

For social creatures such as humans, the desire for acceptance into a community is hard to abandon. Without acceptance from the community, our projects are threatened with failure. Our projects are not only facilitated by community support, but our flourishing requires the companionship and love only possible together with others. Being denied membership in a community not only can harm us, but being denied affiliation is itself a form of harm. To a large measure, the desire for normalcy is simply the desire to be accepted as one of the community, as "one of us."

2.3 The Paradox of Normalcy

These proffered answers to the question of why we desire the normal, while helpful, are insufficient. For normalcy, desired as it may be, is nonetheless a paradox. As much as each of us desires normalcy, most will, with some cheerful self-deprecation and sometimes with satisfaction, say that ours is not a normal life. There is a certain pride we take in not being normal. We see it in the character of Joy, the protagonist in Flannery O'Connor's "Good Country People." Joy had just one leg and her deviance from the norm was evident. Rather than hide her disability and her lack of normalcy, she, as a point of pride, renamed herself "Hulga" because it was "the ugliest name in any language" (O'Connor 1996, 310).

Like Joy, I too, even as a child, had tasted the ambivalence of normalcy—the desire as well as the disdain for what is common, what is routine, what is normal. I lived with a knowledge that young children in the "golden land" of post-WWII America were not supposed to have: a knowledge of great evil.[6] As I moved in larger and larger circles, I gleaned the multiple ways one experiences oneself as different. The more I learned about those around me, the less I could find anyone who was "normal." (And this I came to realize was normal.)

Claiming normalcy is also admitting to a banality, a lack of distinctiveness and, consequently, distinction. The ambivalence comes from yet another desire—the desire to be recognized and valued for who we are *in our singularity*—not in how we are *like* everyone else, but in how we are *different* from everyone else. If all we can say about ourselves is that we are normal, we have to wonder about the *I* speaking; we have to wonder about the individuality that distinguishes that *I* from all others. At the heart of the ambivalence sits the familiar dialectic of sameness and difference. As much as we want acceptance, so too we know that we cannot always—or may not always want to—meet the norm of sameness that acceptance appears to dictate. Interruptions and disruptions, failings and sufferings may be common enough, but they can motivate us both to reject being judged by an accepted norm and to establish ourselves in opposition to it.

---

[6] I grew up hearing about the United States as "di Goldene Medini"—Yiddish for "the golden land."

2.3.1 The Statistical Norm and the Aspirational Norm

The ambivalent relationship we have to the normal is a reflection of an ambiguity in the concept. The normal provides the basis for what is common, but also for what is an aspiration and perfection. The desirable, Lennard Davis (1995) claims, shifted from the "ideal" to "the normal" in the nineteenth century with the ascendance of statistical analysis, giving the normal a prescriptive force even as it is putatively only descriptive and objective. The center of the Gaussian bell curve (see Figure 2.1) provides this descriptive norm.[7] The normal curve or bell curve is a common way to represent the distribution of frequencies. The norm is represented by a statistical frequency which is a midpoint between extremes, as is illustrated by the IQ normal curve in Figure 2.1.

How frequency becomes the basis for a new sort of ideal can be seen in the transformation of the bell curve into an ogive curve (which represents cumulative frequency).

In an ogive curve, the left side of the bell curve is represented as the bottom half, while the right side is represented as the top half (Figure 2.2). Fifty percent of the population has IQs below 100, while 84 percent have IQs below 115. Whatever is below the midpoint is considered "abnormal," and whatever is above is normal. The closer the IQ is to the top of the curve, the closer it comes to the ideal. The distribution curve thus morphs from an objective representation of statistical frequencies to a value-laden representation of an ideal. To employ the

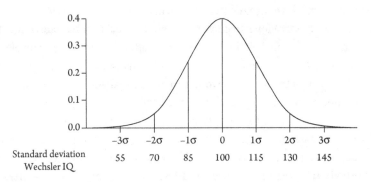

Figure 2.1 The Normal Curve.

---

[7] In a classic article, Edmond Murphy (1972) elucidates seven meanings of the word "normal." These are 1) the Gaussian normal distribution curve; 2) most representative of its class, that is, the average or median; 3) commonly encountered in its class, or the typical; 4) most suited to survival and reproduction, or optimal or fittest; 5) carrying no penalty, or innocuous or harmless; 6) most commonly aspired to or conventional; and 7) most perfect of its class or an ideal. I group the first three under the category of descriptive or statistical norms, and the last four under the heading prescriptive norms.

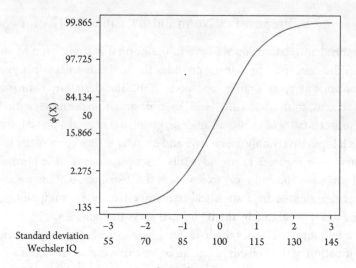

Figure 2.2 The Cumulative Frequency (Ogive) Curve.

terms of the French historian of science George Canguilhem, "normal appears to be an objective 'judgment of reality,' yet it becomes a subjective 'judgment of value'" (1991).

The ancient conception of a transcendent ideal, argues Davis, was less coercive than the modern conception in which the ideal is understood as the normal. No doubt mortal women desire the ideal beauty that is only attainable by a goddess. But to the extent that a lover desires actual women, a woman who falls short is not shut out of the possibility of love. In contrast, when the ideal is not a transcendent one, but presumably is attainable, then our failure to attain it is lodged in ourselves. We are less worthy. The modern ideal of feminine beauty is a superb example. Women come to believe that the images of women in films, magazines, and television are the attainable norm, and they too can look like that if only they buy the right products, do the right exercises, eat the right foods, and so on. True, the models pictured in media representations are not the statistical norm, but they are at the top of the ogive curve; they are the "supernormal." If, even after making an effort, we fall short, the shortfall can come to be viewed as a form of pathology. The nose that is too long, the lips that are too thin, the thighs that are too thick, and the irreversible signs of aging are experienced as forms of disfigurement, not as normal variations. The image purports (even as we know the wonders of Photoshop) to be an image of a real woman not a goddess, and women perpetually feel themselves to be imperfect, flawed—as less worthy of love.

When the judgment of reality becomes a judgment of value, we take the way things are (or suppose that they are) to be an approximate realization of the way things ought to be.[8] We have said, effectively, that what is normal *is* what is desirable, even morally so. The claim that we desire normalcy comes close to being a tautology: "We desire what is desirable." Those who inhabit the space of the non-normal thus do not merely occupy value-neutral positions that deviate from a norm. They occupy positions that take on the stigma of that which lacks value. In this construction of the normal, the desire for normalcy requires no further explanation.

However, when the concept is used *only* to demarcate a statistical norm, that is, when it is simply a judgment of reality, the desirable and the normal cannot so easily slip into a tautological relationship. When the right side of the normal curve indicates only infrequent occurrence and not what is most desirable, it remains puzzling why we should desire what is *merely* common. Medicine provides numerous examples where the statistically frequent condition is less desirable than rarer instances. Older adults who have a blood pressure level that is common for a younger person but rarer in older people are often better off for the deviance from the statistical norm. Still, there are several ways in which even judgments of reality such as those carry surreptitious value judgments.

2.3.2 Pathologies, Anomalies, Variations

One way this happens is when we choose to call an atypicality a pathology rather than a mere anomaly or variation. Canguilhem suggests that the distinction rested on the question of whether functionality was adversely implicated in the deviation from the norm. He writes, "As long as the anomaly has no [negative] functional repercussions experienced consciously by the individual . . . the anomaly is either ignored . . . or constitutes an indifferent variety, a variation on a specific theme" (1991, 135). But whether or not there are functional repercussions can itself be a construct reflecting certain values. Many discussions of disability, especially those based on the social model of disability, argue that at stake is the role of society in turning what can be an indifferent variant into a pathological condition.[9]

---

[8] The "ought" can carry a strong moral valence. In the riveting Ursula Hegi novel, *Stones From the River*, the protagonist is Trudi Montag, born a dwarf in Germany during the First World War. Montag's mother is certain (and is driven insane by the thought) that her daughter's abnormality is actually her punishment for a marital indiscretion committed when her husband was off to war (Hegi 1994). Such a conception of disability is referred to as "the moral model of disability."

[9] The strict version of the social model of disability views virtually all forms of disadvantage as a consequence of social discrimination and obstacles presented by the physical (built) environment. More recent models of disability dispute the the singular focus on the social and call for a more complex and embodied model of disability. See, for example, Shakespeare and Watson (2001), Siebers (2008), WHO (2002).

Some human variations, such as a photographic memory, perfect pitch, or synesthesia, are hardly functional limitations and may even be seen as positive. Moreover, enhancement technologies enhance valued "normal" traits to produce anomalies that are presumed to be still more valued. Few regard such variations as something to rue or something that keeps people from living a desirable, even normal, life.

Other anomalies, such as polydactyly (having more than ten fingers), facial hair on a woman, being of exceptional height, or being a homosexual, are no less mere variations. These involve few if any functional limitations except those resulting from discrimination. To these we can add examples that are called disabilities, but are viewed by many who have them as mere variations: deafness, intersex, autism, and some genetic syndromes such as Turner's syndrome or even Down syndrome. Despite the extensiveness of the anomaly, people with these sorts of conditions can indeed get on very well in the world as long as some accommodation is provided. All these variations, however, do nonetheless carry stigma in some places and in some eras. Once again, the stigma itself often will result in more significant functional limitation than the physiological condition alone. Even though the individual herself may experience the anomaly as a mere variation, not a pathology, the attendant stigma *itself* renders the condition undesirable.

We have seen that to characterize a condition as a pathology is already a value-laden judgment. But to this we can now add that merely *to mark certain characteristics as anomalous* is also not without a value judgment. Why should a minor variant such as female facial hair be stigmatized? Why mark or remark on it at all? That it is remarked on already presupposes that it is a stigmata (a mark). Again, the tautological formula "to desire normalcy is to desire what is desirable" inserts itself and explains why one might want to be rid of the marked trait and simply be normal.

2.3.3 The Norm as That Which Is and Is To Be Desired

One answer to why a variation comes to be stigmatized and, as a consequence, becomes a limitation on functioning is that the statistical norm becomes the basis of social norms and institutions. Because heterosexual men and women are statistically prevalent, social institutions have been ordered to fit them. Attempting to accommodate oneself to institutions not well suited to one's body, mind, and way of life clearly is disadvantageous and affects one's functionality even if, in a different environment, one could function perfectly well. Because the functional limitations of a person of very short stature lies in a built environment that is suited to people who are taller, and in a social environment which is not welcoming, Lisa Hedley, the mother of a daughter with achondroplasia, ponders limb lengthening surgery for her child. She writes:

> There [is] . . . a certain amount of safety in being normal. So as her guardian and protector I am vulnerable to the enticing possibilities of a surgical fix that might bring her closer to that safety zone of normalcy. (Hedley 2006, 43)

The desire for normalcy is at least in part a desire to reside in the safety zone marked out by the normal.

There is still another way in which the seemingly pure descriptive sense of normalcy expresses values that make the normal that which is desirable. Canguilhem argues that "the norm is not deduced from, but rather expressed in the average." The normal lifespan in the United States today is seventy-eight years of age. But were we to receive the sort of care and treatment (improved nutrition, good day-to-day care, appropriate medical care, and good safety measures) that allow us to withstand the forces that kill us today, the normal lifespan would be closer to a hundred years of age. In other words, the standard of care is itself a product of social values, and it determines the statistical norm. Again, Canguilhem: "A human trait would not be normal because frequent but frequent because normal, that is, normative in one given kind of life" (1991, 160).[10]

Nora Groce provides us with a historically documented example. From the late eighteenth century and lasting into the mid-twentieth century, Chilmark, a section of Martha's Vineyard Island in Massachusetts, was home to a large population of deaf persons (Groce 1985). The reason was twofold. The first was biological: a particularly prominent genetic feature traced back to one original settler and subsequent inbreeding. But the second was social: rather than being marginalized or shunned, deaf individuals were allowed to live normal lives. They married and bore children, thereby contributed to the future population of the island. Being deaf was *not* a marked feature of people's lives, and nondeaf persons learned and used sign language as well as spoken English. When asked whether a particular inhabitant was deaf or hearing, villagers had to stop and think and not infrequently couldn't say. Had the norms on Martha's Vineyard

[10] It might appear that the example I use regarding longevity is a poor one for the purpose at hand, for is it not clearly more desirable to live beyond the statistically normal age? In one sense we value longevity, but as we move past the statistical norm, we envision a life that is significantly diminished, where health fails us, and many of our friends and cohorts are no longer alive. Although the desire not to die is powerful, the urge to live much beyond the statistical norm progressively weakens after a certain point.

conformed to prevailing norms of the wider culture, deafness would have been less normal and so less frequent.

The relationship between that which is desirable and that which is most frequent throws a new light on the intolerance of difference. Nothing is desirable if no one desires it. One who expresses no interest in what is prized effectively challenges its inherent desirability. When disabled people make the claim that their disability does not render them tragic, it is shocking; it disrupts the seemingly self-evident desirability of the typical body. Those who refuse a cure—or worse still, contemplate selecting for a child with a disability, as the deaf lesbian couple Sharon Duchesneau and Candy McCullough wished to do—are nothing short of a scandal (Scully 2011). What are we to do with these refuseniks? We cajole, we try persuasion, and if mere inducements are not successful, we threaten, shame, and when all fails, coerce. While we can force people to comply with the norm, we cannot coerce them to desire it—which is, of course, precisely the demand. The larger society does all it can to make these norms self-reinforcing and self-perpetuating.

Doubtless it is more efficient to cater to a narrow set of norms. By presuming a "normal height," we build tables and chairs to a standard height. By presuming mobility using two legs, we build steps. By assuming a standard for intelligence, we pitch tasks, instructions, communications, and so forth to a common measure. And so on. If there are costs to people who try to accommodate themselves to unfriendly norms, there are costs to society at large in accommodating to different bodies, different minds, different structures of behavior. But the demands of efficiency are insufficient if we demand a society that offers its citizens equal rights and equal opportunity to lead flourishing lives.

A more psychological—and less generous—view of the need to conform to a fixed set of norms was offered by Nietzsche, who identified in humans "the herd instinct": a need to obey, to follow commands, to acquiesce to authority.[11] As unattractive as the herd instinct looks in humans, we also need to recognize that, seen through the perspective of evolution, herding is a feature of creatures who are preyed upon. Those who stand out from the herd become the sacrificial beings who allow the herd to survive. While humans are predators, they are also prey. Conforming may be less a desire to kowtow to authority and more a manifestation of the self-protective instinct of a vulnerable prey. Nonetheless, Nietzsche reminds us of what is undesirable about normalcy. Conformity reduces life to

[11] He wrote: "At all times, as long as there have been human beings, there have been human herds ... and very many who obeyed compared with very few who were in command; [obedience] was the trait best and longest exercised and cultivated among men ... It has become an innate need" (Nietzsche 1997, 64).

a blandness, to an oppressive sameness. If conformity—normalcy—is at times undesirable, then the proposition "we desire the normal" is contingent and is not analytically true, as is the tautology "we desire the desirable."

If normalcy comes apart from desirability, why do we remain in its thrall? Perhaps it is simply true that we do, after all, need norms. Norms give rise both to normalcy and to normativity. We need normative standards of behavior to avoid those that can be massively destructive. Without norms of health or proper nutrition, we lack means of assessing conditions that can and should be ameliorated. We risk, in short, unleashing all the dangerous forms of full-fledged subjectivism, relativism, and nihilism.

2.4 Toward More Capacious Norms

At the same time, although we do need norms, we need to be able to challenge *stifling* norms, ones that inhibit the flourishing of individuals and individuality. The way out of the dilemma is to put forward new values that can become the basis of a new normal. We can establish norms that are more capacious—that embrace more varieties of flourishing and that generate their own source of desirability.

2.4.1 Normalcy and Intelligibility

There is still another way in which "the normal" plays a critical role in our social lives. The normal serves as a baseline for intelligibility. In making our norms more capacious we make more forms of living intelligible in ways that enable their flourishing. The struggle of the LGBTQ community to have their unions recognized as full-fledged marriages is part of the struggle to normalize the choice of a same-sex partner. A desire to do so is not only the desire to be included in a set of functionally relevant and valued social norms and institutions, but to do so in a way that does not dissolve one's identity into the statistical norm of heterosexuality. Marriage is *the* framework through which we understand consensual relationships between two adults who choose to make a life together. Its elements include most, if not all, of the following: a sexual affinity, love, the creation of a home, the provision of a home for raising children, the expectation of caring for one another in times of need, and the support of social, legal, economic, and sometimes religious institutions. Private relationships between consenting adults that have some of these elements but lack legal restrictions, protections, and supports are not considered marriages. More importantly still, such affinitive relations may be socially and legally unintelligible: What obligations and responsibilities have the couple assumed toward each other and toward others? What obligations should social and legal institutions assume to-ward them? Are these relationships merely contractual, like business relations, or are they like friendship, kinship, or marriage? Normalizing the relationship via marriage not only addresses the stigma of the same-sex relationship, but it also resolves many of the quandaries that arise because the relationship is outside the frameworks by which we make ourselves intelligible to one another.[12]

If the problems with a life of cognitive disability begin with the frustrated desire for a "normal child," perhaps the prospects for a good life requires us to normalize the hand we have been dealt. Roy Richard Grinker, an anthropologist and father of an autistic girl speaks of "the paradox . . . that a child who doesn't fit in has to be seen as somehow impaired in order to justify an effort to normalise him" (2009, 318). Grinker's point is that he had to acquiesce to labelling the child *deviant* in order to receive services that would help his child (*normalize* her). And so, the paradox arises: We constrict the norm to exclude all sorts of individuals, then we provide means by which we can now normalize what we have placed outside the normal. We could escape the paradox if we simply pro-vide each child with the help they need regardless of how we define them with respect to the standard of normalcy.

The idea of "normalization," first introduced in Scandinavia and made widely known by the Canadian educator Wolfensberger (1972), did try to both hold the content of the norm fixed and find ways to extend its scope. People with cogni-tive disabilities were *not* to be viewed as different or "special," and so segregated and treated like lifelong children. The program called for age-appropriate activities for the cognitively disabled and normal settings supplemented by supports neces-sary for the person to function within such settings. The normalization movement called for de-institutionalization and was behind the idea of inclusion, which has now taken hold as an ideal, if not a full reality. Several of these efforts have immensely improved the lives of many.

Wolfensberger's normalization forced those who serve cognitively disabled people to think more creatively about how to include people who had been excluded by *existing* norms. However, we need more if we are really to include

---

[12] Normalizing and including same-sex affinitive relations by expanding the institution of marriage beyond heterosexual coupling may however strengthen other exclusions, for example sexual affinitive relations between multiple gender-ambivalent or -ambiguous adults. Each attempt to make the institution more inclusive will need to be considered in conjunction with other social norms the society rightfully wishes to preserve. For example, if there is good reason to believe that allowing more than two adults to marry will result in sexist gender relations, we may have sufficient reason to disallow it. (Something similar can be said about insisting that marrying parties must be adults.) If marriage among multiple people who are gender ambiguous does not impede other im-portant and just social norms and will not open the door to regressive forms of polygamy, there is no good reason to disallow it. I owe these reflections to discussions with Oli Stephano.

and allow for the full flourishing of those excluded: we need ways to challenge existing norms that are *stifling*, that repress the individuality and inhibit the flourishing of excluded individuals. We need new values that can become the basis of a new normal, with its own source of desirability. We need to establish norms that are more capacious.

In an essay about the short life of her daughter Isabel who was diagnosed with Tay-Sachs disease when she was one year old, Sabine Vanacker writes: "Knowing Isabel, our perception of that abstract concept 'quality of life' has changed and become more fluid. In our conversations with nurses and doctors they frequently pointed out that we, the nurses and carers who knew her well, were the specialists in Isabel's case and that we knew what normality was for her" (Vanacker 2013).

Establishing norms that are more capacious means recognizing the idea that normality may not have fixed parameters. A child with as disabling a condition as Tay-Sachs still can have a normalcy particular to her. The question then is how we expand social norms and allow for more fluidity in thinking about the normal and quality of life without losing what is valuable in having norms. The task is not without difficulties. Values, like languages, are not merely private. Like languages, they need to be shared and recognized to become intelligible to others. Just as there is no "private language," so there is no value that is not shared (even if by a small community) and is not embedded in some larger practice. Wittgenstein reminds us that "if the mere act of naming is to make sense," there is a great deal that is presupposed. There is a "stagesetting" by a community of speakers who share practices and purposes (Wittgenstein 1973).[13] Similarly, we set values within a "grammar" of cultural valuations that are products of what French sociologist Pierre Bourdieu calls *habitus* (Bourdieu 1990). The *habitus* is the set of dispositions, constraints, implicit rules, practices, and structures from which we derive our understanding of what is normal. Altering norms of normalcy is thus a daunting prospect.

And yet, many of us do it all the time. We do it because we must. For the atypical, the outliers, the ability to lead satisfactory, even flourishing lives depends on setting norms that guide behavior by establishing expectations and providing points of stability. During my childhood, my family created their own sense of normalcy by confining their social circle to those who had shared their own traumatic past as survivors of the Holocaust. In this environment, the members of their circle were not outliers, but normal. They normalized their own experience, however, not only as victims, but as survivors who had insights that others lacked. The consolidation also involved some good-humored self-mockery

---

[13] This point is part of his argument against a "private language" (§258 and onward). The same problems of confirmation exist for values, as do the questions about the intelligibility of the private denotations of meaning.

characteristic of marginal groups. They would poke fun at themselves and each other in Yiddish as "*Greene*": that is, "just off the boat" immigrants. They also felt very much at ease—normal—in their own circle. Their self-esteem resided not only in the strides they had made in pulling their lives back together, but also in knowledge, painfully acquired through their struggles. They knew of the endurance that allowed them to survive, and they knew of the evil of which fellow humans are capable. All this made them feel invincible, and while they envied the ease of Americans—their normalcy—they took pride in the new normal they established for themselves.

Having a child with a disability is not on par with surviving the Nazi concentration camps. But having a child with a disability renders you no less abnormal in the eyes of the wider society. It means you must find your bearings in a new normal, for your own sake and for the sake of your child. Once my spouse and I had digested the difficult understanding that our daughter was never to have a "normal" life, we closed ranks. We associated primarily with those who shared our valuing of our daughter, even if they themselves lacked the first-hand experience. As children of the 1960s flaunting the older generations' sense of the normal, our acceptance of our daughter fell in line with a desire to develop a more creative sense of normalcy.

While we rejected conformity to a convention that presupposed a settled image of a family, we neither rejected the idea of family wholesale nor sought to reconstruct it from scratch. We accepted most expectations of parenting as not just inescapable, but desirable. We never questioned that a parent sacrifices for a child and tries to do the best for the child's well-being. We, no less than anyone, wanted our status as a family affirmed. We wanted others to recognize our wonderful baby and to see us as attentive, loving, and competent parents. We anticipated the grandparents doting, the aunts and uncles speculating on the future career of our child, and the strangers in the street cooing and admiring our new wondrous being. In short, we wanted the whole package.

Grandparents who reject a grandchild because they don't approve of their own child's spouse or who turn away from the baby because she has an impairment, friends who cannot accept the baby and flee from its sight, neighbors who don't know what to say in the face of disability—all these rend the precious fabric woven of familial love, ties of friendship, and neighborly goodwill. When the recognition that one is a family is not forthcoming, one feels undermined as a parent. The acknowledgment is not only necessary for subjective reasons. No one parents in a vacuum. There are critical objective consequences that come with the recognition that a particular collection of individuals forms a family. Absent the affirmation of the worthiness of your child and your parental relationship, the critical supports every parent requires are likely to be withheld.

Even parents with means are vulnerable to the ill effects of the rejection parents of disabled children meet. I have been told by one parent, whose family of origin has substantial means, that unless she and her spouse place their disabled child in an institution and forego parenting this child, they will be disowned and receive not a penny of the family fortune. This is emotionally searing, and it resulted in a terrible struggle for the family as they were cut off from the means that would have eased some of the hardships imposed by disability. Without friends and family to offer respite from the care of a new child, and often from the intensive care a child with disabilities requires, some parents give up and find it impossible to raise their child. The desire for normalcy, for recognition, is then both subjectively and objectively integral to parenting. When the wider world fails in giving the recognition, the only recourse is to create a narrower world that will not let you down. Within that world, the *habitus* is different from but still continuous with that of the larger community.

The analogy of values with language is instructive. A smaller community marked off from a larger homogeneous linguistic community develops a variant or a dialect which is entirely intelligible to the smaller group and may be less intelligible to the larger one. The accommodations become an entirely familiar and comfortable dialect. As dialects can enrich and help develop the more widely accepted linguistic resources, so can the alternate communities of value enrich and expand the norms of the larger society. What is normal for only a few can open a space for political change, a platform from which to contest "the normal."

2.4.2 A Bridge to a New Normal

All the families I had known shaped my own expectation of what it is like to have a child and build a family. Although we had a "non-normal" family, I had gone through pregnancy and childbirth just as most mothers had and now held an infant who needed nurture and love, as all infants do. Starting from some fixed and common points, those who are anomalous in certain regards work to redefine and reclaim the normal, to create their own sense of normalcy, and to locate those from whom they can find validation and support.

That is how my spouse and I did create our *own* perfectly normal family. We found those friends who accepted our family as a family. We worked through the larger familial discomfort with our child and our situation. Along with help from others, we tried to locate our daughter's baseline and her trajectory. We learned to appreciate the small steps in development she did make. We refused the pity of those who could not understand, and we refused the attempts of others to sanctify us, to call us "remarkable" or "saintly," insisting instead that we were doing only what we assumed a parent normally would do: care for, love, protect, and foster the growth of one's child. We tried to extend the sense of normalcy to our other child, and he likewise found his way to normalizing his family by his choice of friends, his understanding of his role in the family, and his understanding of what a sister can be. That normalization has now extended to his wife and my grandchildren. Sesha is their aunt, their dad's sister, and a valued member of our family.

In the backdrop was a growing disability movement that insisted that disability is not merely the result of an impairment or an atypicality, but a consequence of its reception by the larger society. There were inroads being made by a wider understanding that a disabled life was not a tragedy but needed the recognition and support of others to flourish. Nonetheless, a sense of normalcy developed in opposition to that of the wider world is precarious. Recall Helen Featherstone's response when her potential babysitter fled at the sight of her son. Hers is an experience widely shared by parents of disabled children. Her sense of normalcy fell apart—if only for a moment—when she viewed her child through the stranger's gaze. And it needed to be recovered.

It is worth noting what exactly falls apart at these times. What falls apart is the vision of your child as the individual he or she is and not as just someone with the impairment he or she has. What falls apart is seeing yourself first as a parent and not first as a parent of a disabled child. What is imperiled is the connection you have with this singular person, and you must steel yourself not to allow these intrusions to stand between you and the love you have for your child.

When we think of what it is to recover *that* sense of normalcy, I believe we see most deeply what the desire for normalcy is about. True, we want normalcy for the acceptance and safety it promises, for the stability it entails, for the functionality and support it provides. But still more profoundly, the desire for normalcy touches on the self-regard that arises from being recognized as who we wish to be recognized as, and as the distinct individuals we know ourselves to be. That self-regard relies on sharing one's life with others who value us, either the community into which we have been thrown by birth or circumstance or the community that we have chosen to embrace. And lastly, but perhaps most urgently, it is in love that we are most fully recognized as valued.

2.4.3 Normalcy, Self-Esteem, and Love

It is in love that our ambivalence toward normalcy becomes a full-blown paradox. It is fair to say that no one wants to receive the Valentine pictured in Figure 2.3. We want the one represented in Figure 2.4.

At the same time, when we fall outside of the normal, then the unique individual that we are threatens to be obscured by a difference that obliterates our individuality. That is what is so pernicious about a stranger's uncomprehending gaze at our child.

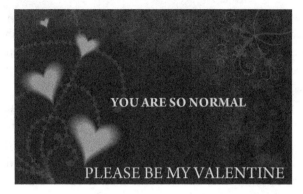

Figure 2.3 The Valentine from Hell.

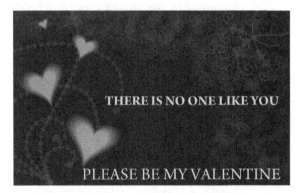

Figure 2.4 The Valentine We Desire.

In "Good Country People," the Flannery O'Connor story to which I referred earlier, the heroine Joy wanted to be loved not *in spite* of her difference, but *because* of it. She refused to be a failed pretty woman. In open defiance of the norms, she not only chose to call herself by a name that she thought signaled an ugly person, but she also refused to comply with standards of feminine beauty. Thus she hoped to transcend the desire for the normal. Yet even as she rejected the normal, she was prey to the most normal desire to be loved, and to be loved for her singularity. By virtue of this desire, however, she was all too easily vanquished. She fell for a man who conned her into believing that he loved her for her uniqueness and that he appreciated, even loved the fact that she had just one leg. But the con artist ran off with her prosthetic leg, mocking her as a freak and exposing the vulnerability of her difference.

Those polar opposites—conformity and individualism—became bedfellows in the historical moment marking the transition of the desirable from the ideal to the normal. That moment is modernity, which brings with it both the modern European's herd instinct that Nietzsche excoriated and the valorization of individualism. Perhaps no nation better exemplifies both the conformity that Nietzsche so scorned and individualism than the United States. Preening American teenagers, who long to look like the TV's Everyteen, want ardently to be loved for who they are as individuals—just as ardently as did Flannery O'Connor's Hulga. And in this desire to be desirable and to have their own desire reciprocated, they too are as vulnerable as Hulga if they fail to negotiate the seeming contradiction of individuality and normalcy.

In setting the *parameters* of the desirable, we also set those of what is the acceptable and intelligible. These become the backdrop against which we see the individual as distinctive, as an irreplaceble being, as the unique person whom we wish to be recognized as and loved for. In contrast, differences that set individuals outside these parameters mark one as deviant and, insofar as normalcy already designates what is desirable, as undesirable. Identified only by these differences, we, as individuals, are erased. There is no longer a unique person to be loved and desired. We see this entanglement of the desire for normalcy and love in Ursula Hegi's novel *Stones from the River*. The heroine, Trudi Montag, is a dwarf, who ardently desired to grow as tall as others. Her father would insist that she was perfect as she was. She thought he lied. She had yet to understand that he did not see her against the backdrop of people with typical height, but against a norm that emerged through his interaction as a parent with her. Viewed against that background, against her role as her father's child, she was perfect. Her differences were merely part of who she was, not a deviation from the norm of a desirable child. Her particularity emerged only against this backdrop of normalcy.

Yet as Trudi reached adulthood, the parental norm was insufficient to buffer her. Only when she encountered another dwarf, and the norms set by dwarfs themselves, could she build on the foundation of her father's love and secure the self-regard she would need to navigate the bigoted and dangerous world of Nazi Germany. When she joined in resisting the Nazi imposition of *their* rigid standard of normalcy, she fully gained the self-regard that sustained her for the remainder of her life, and she could both give and receive love.

The desire for the normal, then, is as much about desire itself as it is about the desirability of normalcy. It is nothing less than the desire to be loved for who one is. As parents of an atypical child, we need to create a new normal for this child to be loved, both by us and by others. If the normal is fixed and unalterable, we are in trouble. But if we as parents who love our children can revise our norms, why should we suppose that others cannot? The community we forge with our child can be enlarged, and love need not be out of her reach. With the love we give to those of our children who deviate from standard norms, we exhibit that they are, in fact, valuable, valued, and desirable. In that challenge lies the start of political and social struggles to alter pernicious norms, norms that exclude the children we love.

The normal becomes tyrannical when it is immutable, rigid, impervious to the fact of its own construction, and blind to the subjectivity with which it is infused. The love of another and the acceptance given by a community makes us comprehensible *both* as unique and as normal. It is the source of the self-regard needed to struggle against a habitus in which we are seen as merely pathologies and anomalies, and it allows us to fashion and enter into a capacious habitus we can fully inhabit. Through love, the paradox of the normal resolves into a dialectic of the normal and the particular.

2.5 Normalcy and the Good Life

We began the chapter with accounts by parents of hearing news that their child was not normal and their devastated responses. And we saw that these families needed to normalize their situation and expand the norms that constitute normalcy to make a life livable. A normal(ized) life is critical for having a good life, but those norms need not be identical to those of "normals." Normals take it as their right to be accepted as they are. Yet we all have a right to be accepted as we are. With such acceptance, a good life is within reach for people with even very significant disabilities. Without wishing to diminish the struggle of the disabled person or her family, I want to end this chapter by conveying how much quality can be had from a life without what so many take to be a normal life. But more than this: we see that when we relinquish norms that exclude the possibility of having a good life when a person's capacities are impaired—capacities thought indispensable for a life that goes well—we see anew what sits at the heart of *any* good life.

Philosophers throughout Western philosophy have of course had much to say about the good life. Today there is burgeoning literature on well-being and what makes one's life go well. There is essentially a tripartite debate. Some, the hedonic theorists, argue that a life goes well when there is more pleasure and less pain. Others, the desire theorists, claim that our lives go well when we are able to satisfy our well-informed and autonomously chosen desires. Still others find both of these theories excessively subjective and argue that a life goes well when it accords with an objective list of goods, goods that define a flourishing life. In addition to this trio, there are also perfectionists, who argue that a life is good when it cultivates some excellence (Crisp 2013).

While we will not survey the many accounts, we can begin with Aristotle's perfectionist view. He spoke of a good life as a flourishing (or happy) life, but this was always a life of a cognitively able individual:

> The activity of the divinity which surpasses all others in bliss must be a contemplative activity, and the human activity which is most closely akin to it is, therefore, most conducive to happiness. . . . Happiness is coextensive with study, and the greater the opportunity for studying, the greater the happiness, not as an incidental effect but as inherent in study; for study is in itself worthy of honor. Consequently, happiness is some kind of study or contemplation. (Aristotle 1908, 1178b21–31)

A more open Aristotelian view is that of Martha Nussbaum, whose views are generally regarded as representative of the objective list theorists. Her list of capabilities includes the opportunity for play, closeness to the animal world, and affinitive relationships, as well as more traditional capabilities philosophers discuss (Nussbaum 2000; 2002). Nussbaum expands the list of capabilities needed for a "truly human life" and includes among these the exercise of practical reason. These capabilities, Nussbaum claims, were drawn from a normative conception of a fully human life, that is, a conception of what people should be able to do in order to have a truly human life—a human life as it *should* be. In other words, to have a good human life. Nussbaum claims that her list of capabilities comes from a widely agreed-upon normative understanding of what a good human life requires, regardless of culture, race, and social or economic status. Lacking the opportunity to exercise any of the capabilities consigns one to a less than fully human life. If Sesha and other folks like her lack something essential like "practical reason," that would mean that they are not living a "truly human life." And that would indeed be tragic.

Happily, Nussbaum has modified that view, and now, while she still insists that a just state must make each of these capabilities available to all its citizens, she no longer insists that a person unable to exercise a capability—not because she is denied the opportunity by her government, but because she lacks the underlying capacity—is to be written off as someone who cannot live "a truly human life," and hence a good life (Nussbaum 2008). This makes Nussbaum's view at least compatible with the first lesson I learned when I had my daughter—namely that, whether or not she could live a life of reason, it was our job to give her a flourishing life—even if what that meant for her still needed to be (re)defined. Although Nussbaum now holds a view compatible with the possibility that someone like Sesha can have a truly human life, others who hold the objective list view of well-being might still insist, contrary to Nussbaum's later view, that the use of reason is a necessary aspect of any good life.

One can argue, as some have, that as life itself is of inestimable value, being alive, no matter how impaired, is better than no life at all. But when we have a child with a disability that takes her so out of the flow of normal life, we seek more than "life is better than no life." We want her not merely to live, but to "have a life," that is to say, a life worth living. Clearly if only the exercise of our rational capabilities makes a human life worth living, then humans with severe cognitive disabilities are excluded by definition. Hedonic theorists might be thought to come to the rescue with the reply that as long as there is more pleasure than pain in that life, that life is worth living. But this is a life worth living in only its barest sense: that is, "a minimally acceptable life," which (as impoverished or as unhappy as it is) is still preferable to death. I am not speaking of "a minimally acceptable life" because, in the view I wish to defend, a good life for people with significant disabilities, especially cognitive disabilities, can and should be much more than minimally acceptable.

The informed desire view could similarly be thought to require an unimpaired capacity to reason in order to assure that our desires be informed. Such positions foreclose the question of whether a person with cognitive disabilities can have a good life. For that reason, I find them wanting, since I do believe that Sesha's is a good life.

Still, there are many ways in which severe cognitive disabilities might be thought to impede the quality of life for the individual herself and for her family. First, there are severe behavioral problems which surely diminish the hedonic worth of that life. We find such difficulties with forms of autism where behavioral problems can be formidable, even when the degree of intellectual disability is not severe. Research into the lives of parents with disabled children has indicated that severe behavioral difficulties, especially hard-to-control aggressive and violent behavior, is highly correlated with familial stress (see for example Olsson and Hwang 2001; Saloviita, Itälinna, and Leinonen 2003; Hassall, Rose, and McDonald 2005). The case of Trudy Steuernagel and her autistic son, Sky Walker who killed her in a fit of rage shows that such aggression and violence impedes the flourishing of the child, as well as the parent—it can even prove fatal.[14] The behavioral disabilities characteristic of some children with autism may be due to perceptual sensitivities that make many ordinary sensory experiences intolerable, or they may be caused by frustration in being able neither to communicate nor to have important desires satisfied. Such suffering should lead us to see that we need to explore the sources of the very difficult behavior and search for ways to help the child and the family manage this aggression—not easy, but

---

[14] Trudy Steuernagel had anticipated that this might come to pass and wrote of the failure of all in providing him the appropriate care (Connors, Joanna. 2009). This case is also discussed in Simplican (2015).

nonetheless an essential task if we are to make a good life possible for all who have disabilities.

Second, high levels of pain may well make life harder to endure and seems certain to reduce the quality of life—and surely diminishes its hedonic measures. Some syndromes—such as Tay-Sachs—are paired with degenerative conditions in which the children experience a great deal of pain and a very short life, though as we have learned, it is possible for even these children to have their own "normal." No one can gloss over these forms of suffering and the consequent diminishment of the quality of life of child and family alike.

Third, some children, including many on the autism spectrum (which we might identify as cognitive disabilities, even when there are not intellectual deficits), have difficulties with physical affection, surely an item on most lists of goods that make life worth living. However, many who are not cognitively impaired live rich lives yet do not appear to want or tolerate much physical affection. Notice that in each of these cases, it is not the cognitive impairments as such that are the source of the diminished quality of life.

So, what of that good life for people with my daughter's disabilities? In what can it consist? Setting philosophical theories aside and looking at what life with Sesha has taught our family, we can say that from her centeredness, her composure, and her strengths we have learned some of the components of a good life. Sesha has interests, desires, and pleasures, some of which have remained throughout her life, and some of which have developed. She is still a gourmet, very appreciative of excellent food. Her tastes in music have matured with her; she no longer relishes Raffi and Barney but Bach, Beethoven, Schubert, Louis Armstrong, and yes, Bob Dylan, Elvis Presley, and Michael Jackson. (Elvis and Jackson she discovered on her own—the rest she picked up from us.) One needs nothing more than to watch this woman—who has no language, who is still incontinent, who cannot feed, dress, or in any way care for herself—listen to a Bach partita, a Beethoven symphony, one of her beloved Broadway musicals, or best of all watch her thrill to the last movement of Beethoven's Ninth, to discern the riches of her life. She listens to music as I do—at my best, that is—in a concert hall. Sesha is one of the privileged in a world full of misery, violence, and privation for millions—lives that are robbed of dignity and quality. To staunch the oozing of pity for this abnormal, severely-to-profoundly cognitively disabled woman, one has only to witness Sesha and me in a round of kisses and embraces and to see the joy that emanates from her. And this is our household's normality.

Parents who read or hear from other parents of children with significant cognitive disabilities feel like we are part of a special club. We recognize each other's sorrows and pain. But what we also hear in each other's voices is a special sort of poignant love for our children.[15] Even in the midst of harrowing stories of pain and the agony and anger of enduring incompetence, indifference, and punishing attitudes on the part of others, there is the terror that we will lose this child. Even while acknowledging the hardships, lack of support, and family breakups, parents speak—almost always—of the joy the child can experience and the joy that the child brings to their lives.[16] In our own development as parents, the concepts of "a good life" and "a normal life," which seemed inseparable in our early years, have become distinct. Many of our original concerns have, for the most part, faded. For example, rather than desire employment for Sesha, we now aim to give her the satisfaction of mastering a skill, or of having some degree of self-efficacy when she succeeds in directing us to satisfy a need or desire. In place of our own concern for the intellectual life, we see her able to have other joys: the enjoyment of water, of food, of music, of love, and of going to see a fun movie.

Spinoza, the supreme rationalist, nonetheless gave joy a pride of place. Distinguishing pleasure and joy, Spinoza said that while pleasure pertains to the body as it is conceived as body: "Joy is a man's passage from a lesser to a greater perfection" (Spinoza 1996a, Bk III, Definition II). Even an examined life, if it holds no joy, may not be a life worth living. With joy, life has a point, a reason to be, a perfection of what it is to be.

We parents of children with cognitive disabilities also tend to have a different relationship to expectations that the child *do* something. Although we and the therapists, teachers, and other professionals involved in their lives are continually trying to teach our children skills, many of us have come to appreciate a life without preconceived expectations. The evidence of a skill or capacity is a surprise and a delight. But so is the ability just to be, to take life in. One of the deepest sources of joy that I see in my very disabled child is her capacity to be. Dave Hingsburger (1998), an educator and writer on cognitive disability, wrote of the moment when he was facing death. He said he realized that his to-do list was quite short, but his to-be list was very long. Being able to be: quiet, good, happy, kind. To be, to derive joy just from being alive and in the world, is a rare gift. I came to see this as I watched my aging mother. My mother was a doer: sewing clothes, knitting, cooking, cleaning, caring for another, and proud of all she could do. As she began to lose her physical and mental capacities, she became increasingly embittered and longed for death. She needed care and refused it as it was she who was supposed to be the carer, the doer. In the last few months of her life, we managed to get her some excellent caregivers and she

---

[15] See also Rapp (2011).

[16] In Solomon (2012), the interviews notably speak of the joy children with cognitive disabilities brought to the parents and those who came to know them. In fact, the term "joy" appears more than twenty times either in direct or indirect quotes from parents.

began to acquiesce and take pleasure from their caring and their company. She would go outside, sit on the seat of her walker, and look around herself, enjoying seeing the plants and trees, the children playing, the occasional breeze. For the first time in my life, I saw my mother just enjoy being. As she adapted to this last stage in her life, the resentment and bitterness left her. She faced her death with equanimity. Sesha has the wisdom my mother acquired only in the last few months of a long, full life: love, joy, and the gift of just being able to be. Perhaps these cut through experiences of cognitive disabilities.

But they also give us a fresh way to understand what a good life consists of. Roy Grinker (2009) writes that he thinks we should judge the value of a life not just by what it can accomplish, but by what it brings into the life of others. When I extol the virtues of being, I do not mean to foreclose the importance of skills—but, as Dave Hingsburger stresses, the skills are to be in service of something the individual can *be*. Borrowing again from Spinoza, what a person learns to *do* should allow her to move to a greater degree of perfection, to more fully *be*, that is, to increase her joy. To love, to derive joy from life, to learn the wonder of being: these are, I offer, the apotheosis of a good life, one that everyone can achieve—and one that, perhaps, even a philosopher can appreciate.

A Meditation on Normalcy Inspired by Camus's *The Rebel*

Camus writes:

> Art, at least, teaches us that man cannot be explained by history alone and that he also finds a reason for his existence in the order of nature. For him, the great god Pan is not dead. His most instinctive act of rebellion, while it affirms the value and the dignity common to all men, obstinately claims, so as to satisfy its hunger for unity, an integral part of the reality whose name is beauty. (Camus 1956)

Human "imperfection," human difference in the form of disability, has the power, like art, of finding a reason for its existence in the order of nature. This is how I am, says the proud disabled person—I exist in the order of nature. I disrupt constructions of history, of a fixed norm of what is human. I exist as the creativity of nature. My existence is itself a vital rebellion, a rebellion "that affirms the value and the dignity common to all men [*sic*]" and "obstinately claims an integral part of the reality whose name is beauty." Camus goes on to say:

> In upholding beauty, we prepare the way for the day of regeneration when civilization will give first place—far ahead of the formal principles and degraded values of history—to this living virtue on which is founded the common dignity of man and the world he lives in, and which we must now define in the face of a world that insults it. (Camus 1956)

PART II

CHOOSING CHILDREN AND THE LIMITS OF PLANNING

> Reflecting now on one participant's memory of when her pediatrician
> told her that he didn't know if her underweight baby would be all right,
> and her recalling this as the most terrible moment in her life, I thought
> what would I have answered had someone asked me, "Was the mo-
> ment you learned that Sesha was retarded the most terrible moment
> in your life?" I would have answered, "No." The most terrible moment
> in my life was when I thought Sesha would die. The next most terrible
> moment was when my mother insisted (or tried to insist) that Sesha
> be institutionalized and that I give her up.
> —from my diary: October 22, 1999

Overview: Choice and Selection

In part I, we asked why we desire normalcy, not only for ourselves but also for
our child. The fear that a good life cannot be possible for those who fail to fit
within the bounds of the normal drives many to consider selective reproductive
procedures to ensure the birth of a "normal" child. In part II we address this
concern and the ethical dimensions of selection for "a child of choice." Issues
raised by medical technologies have recently been added to the problem set of
philosophical inquiry. Attempting to evaluate the desirability of reproductive
technologies and the uses to which they are put raises questions not only about
the ethics of selection in reproduction, but also about the desirability of choice
and intervention in matters of procreation, about the comparative goodness
or badness of a life with a disability, and about how to make arguments concerning these issues in a fashion that is respectful of the lives of disabled people.
In the previous chapter we have argued that those who have even very impactful
disabilities, including significant cognitive disabilities, can have a good life. But
is this a sufficient answer to those who argue that we have a responsibility to our
future children that leaves them with "an open future?" While disability might

allow for a good life, is that a sufficient reason to choose to give birth to *this* child instead of another child who might have the possibility of leading a better life?

The desirability of preventing serious disabilities appears, prima facie, to be an incontrovertible good. We demand that landlords remove lead paint to prevent children from ingesting material that can cause cognitive deficits. Others expect us, and we expect ourselves, to make every reasonable effort to prevent our children from losing sight, hearing, limbs, and mental functioning. We expect prospective mothers today to take folic acid to prevent the fetus they are carrying from developing spina bifida and other neural tube conditions, to avoid unpasteurized milk products that may contain listeria because these can cause congenital diseases leading to blindness, and to stay away from foods and kitty litter that may cause toxoplasmosis, which has serious implications for a baby's health and mental development. Most reasonable people would concur that at least some of these measures to ensure the birth, growth, and development of children without unnecessary disabling impairments are a good thing, and that failing to take these precautions is at best unwise, at worst negligence bordering on abuse.

Can we then take seriously the claim that a disability such as blindness is a "neutral trait," as writer Deborah Kent (who is blind due to a genetic trait) maintains? Kent describes her husband's and parents' relief and joy at discovering that their newborn infant, Janna, can see—and Kent's consternation and sense of betrayal at their reaction. "How do I myself feel about the fact that Janna can see?" asks Kent, and she replies:

> I am glad that her world is enriched by color as well as texture and sound . . . As her mother I want her to have every advantage, and I know that some aspects of her life are easier because she has sight . . . Beyond that, I am glad Janna will never be dismissed as incompetent and unworthy simply because she is blind. I am grateful that she will not face the discrimination that threads its way through my life and the lives of most people with disabilities. But I know that her vision will not spare her from heartbreak . . . disappointment, rejection and self-doubt.

Kent continues:

> I will always believe that blindness is a neutral trait, neither to be prized nor shunned. Very few people, including those dearest to me, share that conviction . . . I feel that I have failed when I run into jarring reminders that I have not changed their perspective. In those crushing moments I fear that I am not truly accepted after all. (Kent 2000, 62)

Kent's words are echoed in the writings of people with a wide variety of disabilities, even those believed to be "severe." A young man with Down syndrome (DS), upon learning from family friends that they just had a child with DS, reacted with great and genuine joy. He made a point of congratulating the family on the birth of a child with DS. Clearly, he didn't think that being born with DS was a cause for distress or consternation; he instead thought it to be an added blessing. And not only are such sentiments expressed by those who have congenital disabilities; they are heard in the statements of those with acquired disabilities as well. If disability is, as John Harris defines it, "a condition that someone has a strong rational preference not to be in,"[1] then neither the young man with Down syndrome nor Deborah Kent regards their condition as a disability in this sense. Can we reconcile these attitudes—even the attitudes of a blind mother about the prospects of her own child being born blind—with the general attitude toward disability expressed in our medical, public health, and prenatal practices? Given these responses from disabled people, can we—ought we—still say that prenatal diagnosis, followed by procedures to select for the unimpaired embryo or fetus, is an ethically justifiable practice and that it is not disrespectful of the lives of disabled people? These are the questions that motivate part II.

I have found myself oddly positioned with respect to these questions in large measure because of my relationship to my daughter. As a feminist who unequivocally believes that women must be able to control their reproductive lives, I firmly oppose any attempts to limit that right by legislating or shaming. Although I resolutely affirm the value of each life, no matter the degree or kind of disability, I also do not believe that women should be made to carry to term a pregnancy they wish to terminate.[2] As a daughter of the Enlightenment and one who treasures the liberal values of equality and freedom—and who believes that having increased control over our circumstances is a good thing on the whole—I nonetheless recognize how little control we have, especially when it comes to the sort of child we bear and rear. Moreover, I have come to appreciate that what we fear in the abstract we might come to cherish when it is embodied in a beloved child. That is, I have determined that an attitude of epistemic humility is appropriate when it comes to making choices about procreative matters. It is difficult to build a set of consistent commitments in this area, since theoretical

---

[1] Cited in Glover (2006b, Kindle locations 141–42).

[2] In places where not only abortion but also contraception is prohibited, in order to avoid the possible birth of a child with a disability, women are faced with the decision of whether to engage in sex at all. This, for example, is the decision women in Brazil and other Latin American nations face in light of an epidemic of the Zika virus, which is believed to cause microcephaly. Since contraception and abortion are in fact available to middle-class and wealthy women, who are also more likely to be able to avoid exposure to the mosquitos who carry the virus, it is a dilemma that mostly poor women face.

commitments fail to foresee the realities and responses toward lived experience. Perhaps this is mere equivocation; or perhaps the truth is as puzzling as quantum theory that tells us that light is both a particle and a wave. In most circumstances, we should champion choice and control; at the same time, we know that choice can be illusory and that we can delude ourselves in thinking we have control.

Part II consists of three chapters. The first of these, chapter 3, is entitled "The Limits of Choice." Before we can discern the ethics of prenatal testing, I believe we need to think about the idea of choice—both why we so value it and how it can lead us astray when we are unaware of its power over us. We value it for the control it gives us to fashion our lives as we see fit. However, choice can be deceptive. Philosophy alone cannot provide us with the tools we need to reveal the illusions and delusions we fall into when we are under the spell of choice. Psychologists, happily, have provided empirical proof that choice is not all it is held up to be.

As we begin to explore the role of choice in reproductive decision-making, we come to understand the complexity of the debates, fed by the multiple perspectives by which we can consider questions of selection. In the next two chapters, "The Ethics of Prenatal Testing and Selection" and "How Not to Argue for Selective Reproductive Procedures," I look at arguments that maintain or dispute the moral permissibility of selecting for or against specific traits of a child, and more particularly for disabling traits. In chapter 4, we are concerned with the position often expressed by the disability community, namely, that we ought not to use reproductive technologies to select against embryos or fetuses that could be impaired and would result in a disabled child. To get a handle on this, I use a conversation I had with my philosophically trained son about the most important argument, the expressivist argument, used by members of the disability community to oppose prenatal selection. The expressivist argument aims to demonstrate that by selecting against disability, we express the view that a disabled life is a lesser life or that disabled people are not welcome in this world. My son and I took opposing sides on the question, shaped in part by our different positions: a mother and prospective care-giver on the one hand, and a sibling on the other.

In chapter 5, I alter the perspective and look at the nature of the arguments that are frequently employed in support of the moral permissibility, and even moral obligation, to select against disability. Although I argue against the expressivist objection in chapter 4, in chapter 5, I argue against a number of philosophers and bioethicists, many of whom admit that disabled people can have good lives, who nonetheless espouse the view that we have a moral obligation to avoid giving birth to a disabled child when we can have an able child in its stead. This, I argue is the

wrong way to argue for permissibility of prenatal diagnosis and reproductive selection against disability. The way in which these arguments are made reinforces
the stigma that disabled people bear and in fact does express the view that a disabled life, even when good, is nonetheless a lesser life. At the end of chapter 5, as at
the end of chapter 4, I argue that the only good reason to permit selective reproductive procedures is to allow the woman to decide if and when she should bring
a fetus to term and raise the ensuing child. It must be the woman's decision as the
fetus is a part of her body, and when the child is born, she is the default caregiver.

3

The Limits of Choice

3.1 Planning a Trip to Italy...

In a now widely cited essay, Emily Perl Kingsley (1987) responds to questions she has received about what it is like to raise a child with Down syndrome, and she suggests that planning for a child is like planning a trip to some wonderful destination—in her example, Italy. She asks us to imagine the anticipation: searching out guidebooks, learning important sites to visit, anticipating the thrill of finally experiencing Michelangelo's David and other artistic wonders one has known only second-hand. But, when the plane lands, the stewardess announces, "Welcome to Holland." Surprise and disappointment—after all, this was to be a trip to sunny Italy, not cloud-covered Northern Europe.

The baby has Down syndrome. It is not the child you anticipated and dreamt of throughout your life. Once the shock and disappointment are overcome, writes Kingsley, you discover that Holland has tulips, windmills, and even Rembrandts and Vermeers. Holland, as it happens, turns out to be a lovely place, even if all your friends have relished their visits to Italy. If you focus on Holland's charms rather than those of Italy, a trip to Holland, while unexpected, becomes a wonderful adventure.[1]

---

[1] Some have argued that Kingsley's experience with her Down syndrome child ought not to be generalized to the birth of all children with disabilities. Some disabled newborns and children present very significant hardships for both parent and child. Some have claimed that they landed not in Holland but in a war-torn Lebanon or Syria—with an inconsolable infant who cried constantly or tore at its own body. It's important to acknowledge the experiences of these parents. At the same time we should ask if such experiences of rearing a disabled child are inherent to the disability or a consequence of failure of supports and lack of adequate research into the source of the pain or discomfort and into the possibility of amelioration. Even in these difficult situations parents still speak of the love and joy their child brings into the family—especially if the parents have the emotional and material resources to deal with the difficulties. See Solomon (2012) for a wide array of stories of parenting children with significant disabilities.

When I started my journey I was just twenty-two, married to a man of twenty-five, and we were both brimming with health and vitality. My youth and the absence of any genetically linked diseases or disorders in our families would have made us unlikely candidates for genetic tests or prenatal screening in 1969, the year of Sesha's birth. Even by today's standards, this was a 'low-risk' pregnancy. The first use of amniocentesis for prenatal diagnosis occurred in 1960, but it took another fifteen years for it to be developed as a technology that was used with any regularity.[2] The first class of genetic counselors had not yet been graduated.[3] Most tests for genetic diseases were many years away, and routine early screening was not yet available. Testing was invasive, and abortion was hardly considered— Sesha's birth was four years before *Roe v. Wade*, which changed the legal landscape for abortion of any sort.[4]

To ensure that I would have the healthiest baby possible, I immediately gave up my pack-and-a-half habit of seven years; read all the pregnancy, natural childbirth, and nursing books on the market (which were a manageable number at the time); walked a lot and embarked on eating well and avoiding inhaling or ingesting any poisons, toxins, or questionable substances. (It was, after all, the sixties!) Following the pioneering health-food guru Adelle Davis, I even had daily drinks of awful-tasting yeast-fortified shakes that were supposed to assure the health of mother and child. My partner and I chose a medication-free childbirth method that depended on a form of self-hypnosis through breathing techniques developed by the French physician Ferdinand Lamaze. Neither "natural childbirth" nor breastfeeding were easily accommodated by hospitals at the time. Persistence and faith in the new methods and a belief that we were doing things that would be most beneficial for our child led us through the appointed journey to give birth to our marvelous baby who was—quite without my efforts—growing bigger and bigger. We were all set for our "Italian trip."

Pregnancy and childbirth perplexed me somewhat because it was a process that, while happening in my body, went on without my conscious control and was independent of my agency. If I couldn't fashion this child with clay or marble,

---

[2] See https://history.nih.gov/exhibits/thinblueline/timeline.html for a timeline of prenatal genetic testing. Also see Leong (2008). And see Cowan (1994) for a history of the development of amniocentesis and chorionic villi sampling.

[3] In 1971, two years after Sesha's birth, the first class of master's degree level genetic counselors graduated from my alma mater, Sarah Lawrence College, in Bronxville, New York. See Leong (2008).

[4] Colorado, in 1967, was the first state to pass a law permitting abortions in case of a child being born with "physical or mental defects." After that and prior to *Roe v. Wade*, seventeen states passed similar laws permitting abortions. But in 1969 in New York State, when I was pregnant, abortion was illegal, and it was not until 1970 that the state passed legislation making abortion permissible in such a case. Thus it is not even clear that it would have been possible to have a legal abortion should I have chosen testing and aborting had the results proved positive.

I could control the circumstances of her birth, and so I did. I exercised control and agency by determining my diet, avoiding poor habits, maintaining hygiene, eschewing risky activities, and carefully planning for the birth of the child. As I mentioned at the outset, the one item in the prenatal arsenal not available to us (would we have used it?) was prenatal testing. But the odds of having anything but a healthy, intelligent (maybe brilliant?), competent (maybe talented?), and joyful child was as likely to be as assured as possible by our situation and our efforts.

This baby was, moreover, a girl. A girl, one growing up in a feminist world that I, along with the nascent feminist movement, was helping to bring about. She would have options that I didn't have. I looked forward to raising a young woman who would have the strength and daring that I lacked—a girl with whom I could both recreate the closeness and best of my own relationship to my mother, and at the samed time avoid all the mistakes (of course!) of those tangled ties. So many dreams of Italy—of the accomplishments, of the relationships, of the aspirations—were all waiting to be realized in this child. This was the family we planned for, the dreams we dreamt, the trip we embarked on.

When the baby was born, we thought we landed—not in Italy, but in paradise. We fell in love immediately and madly with this sweet child. But we did not yet know that our love was in fact grounded not in our dreams, but in the reality of the small person who was entrusted to our care. This concrete individual, the love we bore her, the care she inspired, was our trip, and the destination was far less significant than we imagined it ever could be.

3.2   Landing in Holland

"Yes, the baby should be lifting its head by four months. Sesha is hypotonic. Her muscles are lax, and she lacks control over them. We have to find out why." It was an ominous sign, and the prognosis was not what we had hoped for. I tell my story now whenever I speak to people about genetic testing and prenatal diagnosis. One could read that story as an argument for prenatal testing—and I am not opposed to such testing, as I will explain later. But I tell the story only to remind people that plan as we may, we still lack veto power over the outcome. Still more important, I tell my story to underscore that love for one's child does not depend on our plans turning out as we had intended.

The Enlightenment brought with it the surety that reason—and its prized child, science—would improve the lives of human beings. The hope was that, as we learn more and understand better the universe we inhabit, we could control our destiny. Modern man is Faustus turning swamps into fertile farm fields. We could end hunger, disease, even wars. Among the most grandiose of these visions has been the ambition to "improve" the human stock and to allow us to control reproduction—both its timing and its results.

The very fact of choice is intoxicating, promising increased freedom and power. John A. Robertson captures this mood. "Until recently," he writes, "all human reproduction resulted from sexual intercourse, and couples had to be prepared for the luck of the natural lottery. Now powerful new technologies are changing the reproductive landscape and challenging basic notions about procreation, parenthood, family, and children" (Robertson 1994, 3). In stark contrast to this triumphalism, Sandel (2009) urges us to embrace the luck of the draw. Children need to be accepted as gifts, and parents need an attitude of humility regarding aspirations for their children. From a disability standpoint, there is much to applaud in Sandel's position. However, we need to acknowledge that modern reproductive technology is merely an extension of conscious reproductive decisions humans have always made.

The consequences of this changing reproductive landscape are dizzying, pitting many long-held intuitions against one another. Family choice offers feminists (also heirs to the promise of the Enlightenment) a cause for both celebration and concern. Feminists have also fought for women's ability to decide whether or not to have children, how many to have, with whom and when to have them. It is probable that women's achievements would not have advanced as far as they have without the right and the means to make these procreative choices.

Evolving *social technologies*, such as increased acceptance of divorce, non-traditional gender roles, gay marriage, and open adoption, have legitimated more varied sexual arrangements and family forms. Remarkable reproductive technologies (from birth-control pills and various contraception devices; to in-vitro fertilization; preimplantation selection; egg and sperm donations; cytoplasmic transfer; cryopreservation of sperm, oocytes, and embryos; embryo transfer; diagnostic ultrasound; gestational surrogacy; genetic screens and tests for a wide variety of conditions; in-utero surgical intervention; and most recently CRISPR interference)[5] have developed in tandem with new social arrangements to offer more reproductive choices and more ways of becoming families.

Arguably, our lives have been immensely improved by our growing knowledge and our openness to more family forms and more agency in reproductive decisions. Andrew Solomon (2012), in his extensive set of interviews with families where the children are very different than their parents, where the "apple falls far from the tree" and children have what he calls "horizontal identities,"

---

[5] See Liao et al (2015).

finds great richness in the acceptance of diversity within the family.[6] At the same time, he finds that parents want children to share in their "vertical identities," identities that are inherited from one's ancestors. Control over reproduction is key to the transmission and preservation of these vertical identities.[7]

Nonetheless, control of reproductive choices remains elusive. We need to address the triumphal response to the choices reproductive technologies present. We also need to confront a number of the more troubling questions raised by certain innovations that aim to eradicate forms of human diversity deemed inferior or undesirable. Lady Luck is still with us, and as we shall see later, there is reason to think that this may not be such a bad thing.

3.3 Choosing Children

The valorization of choice is an expression of the liberal values of autonomy and the freedom to live one's life by one's own lights. One mother interviewed by Solomon remarks that having considered the matter, she would not choose to abort a fetus because it shows indications of Down syndrome, but she was glad she had the choice (Solomon 2012). I am not interested here in arguing that we either should or should not choose against (or for) disability. In this chapter, I want only to argue for epistemic humility for whatever choices we make. This is required both because of the nature of choice itself and because we don't always know what we are choosing when we make choices. Whether the very fact of choice—and the way our choices are determined—serves the aim toward which it is directed is a matter worth exploring, especially in the context of procreative decisions.

We already noted that procreative choices are not due to technologies alone, and we can add that there is no such thing as a family that is not the product of someone's—a partner's, a couple's, or a family's—choice. The choice involved in the coupling reflects implicit (if not explicit) choices about the race, ethnicity,

---

[6] Solomon writes: "Such horizontal identities may reflect recessive genes, random mutations, prenatal influences, or values and preferences that a child does not share with his progenitors . . . Physical disability tends to be horizontal identity, as does genius . . . So are conditions such as autism and intellectual disability" (2).

[7] Solomon: "Many parents experience their child's horizontal identity as an affront. A child's marked difference from the rest of the family demands knowledge, competence, and actions that a typical mother and father are unqualified to supply, at least initially. The child is expressly different from most of his or her peers as well, and therefore broadly less understood or accepted. Abusive fathers visit less abuse on children who resemble them physically . . . Whereas families tend to reinforce vertical identities from earliest childhood, many will oppose horizontal ones. Vertical identities are usually respected as identities; horizontal ones are often treated as flaws" (2012, 4).

build, talents, and health of the child. Making no choice is often itself a choice. One may have a choice only in an attenuated sense, where none of the alternatives are viable options, but one must choose nonetheless. The family that emerges is shaped in large measure by who gets to decide, which is a matter of social norms.[8] Enlarging choices for those who have lacked much choice, such as women and sexual minorities, should be viewed as a positive thing;[9] and reproductive technologies, in tandem with changing social technologies, have given rise to a liberating and even dizzying array of choices to those previously excluded from reproductive decision-making.

Consider the situation of a young man I know who is gay. He married another man, and their child is genetically the product of one man's sister who donated her egg (she is Caucasian), and the man's partner, who donated his sperm (he is Asian). The embryo was implanted in a woman who was a surrogate birth mother. This interracial couple is now divorced, and the Caucasian "father," who is genetically the uncle (and Christian), is raising his son with his new (Jewish) boyfriend who has just adopted the child. These young men have overridden restrictions of gender, race, and religion that prevailed in more traditional settings and which determined who had children with whom. This, we can say, is a family of choice.

The example stands in stark contrast to the traditional trajectory of my own son, whose children are genetically the product of him and his spouse. In their case, conception and birth required little innovative technology, and they went through the pregnancy without genetic testing, prenatal screening, or anything other than the usual paraphernalia of birth today. Yet my son's family is as much a family of choice as our friend's family is: he and his bride chose one another, they chose to marry, they chose to have whatever child was born of their union, and while they eschewed genetic testing or prenatal

---

[8] This is also not to say that some of the events leading to a family may not genuinely be coerced—a pregnancy that results from a rape in a society where abortion is not available, for instance. Yet continuing the pregnancy, having the child, and creating a family with that child may be coerced in a far more attenuated sense. There is a radical sense of choice in which even what is coerced in these attenuated ways is chosen—chosen over other still less, or equally, unpalatable alternatives. Virginia Held has controversially, but I think correctly, reasoned in her essay "Birth and Death" that while in some cases death may be the only alternative to becoming or remaining pregnant, it is nonetheless an alternative, for, as human beings, we are capable of taking our own lives (1993, 115). As such, she has argued, for a human being giving birth to a child is always, even in the most extreme cases, a choice, even if it is not a desired outcome. In this radical sense, then, every family is a family of choice.

[9] The television series *Mad Men* is set at the dawn of the feminist era in the United States, when women were beginning to openly confront their limited ability to make choices, to make decisions. "Well, aren't *you* lucky to have *decisions*," says Peggy Olsen, the proto-feminist of the series, to her married lover as he walks out the door, having told her that one day she will be glad he made the decision to do so.

screening, they chose many of the circumstances of the pregnancy—the expectant mother abstained from all alcohol, drugs, and tobacco, and she carefully monitored her diet. The youg man I refer to above would not have realized a family he would choose in this way. The expansion of choice has been hard-won and is still not easily accessible to many.[10] However, the expansion of choice comes with costs.

3.4 The Problem with Choice

> Remember that not getting what you want is sometimes a wonderful stroke of luck.
>
> —attributed to the Dalai Lama XIV

We began this section with the sense that reproductive technology is increasingly sophisticated enough for us to have a choice about the sort of child we have, a view celebrated by a number of philosophers and bioethicists. Yet there are reasons pertaining to the process of choice itself—not its potential outcome—that suggest that such triumphalism is not fully warranted. When we make choices, when we decide among alternatives, we believe that the choice will accord with our aims.

Choice, however, for the reasons listed here, is not always what it seems and too often promises what it cannot deliver:

First, the opportunity for choice itself paradoxically can lead us away from what we actually want.

Second, we frequently over- or underestimate the desirability of that which we choose. There are potent psychological mechanisms at work that make such errors in judgment part and parcel of decision-making.

Third, we are regularly influenced by the framing of a given choice. Given two slightly different framings of a situation in which the alternatives are presented, we may make opposing decisions. Our preference for one alternative over another will be deeply influenced by the framing of the problem.

Fourth, we assume that making one choice rather than another will bring about a desired outcome in circumstances where in fact our control over the outcome is minimal—factors about which we know little and have even less control over may turn out to be determinative.

---

[10] My only reservation is that gestational surrogacy presents moral hazards, ones that deserve a separate discussion.

The second and third factors are truly illusions, and just as in the case of optical illusions, we can do little to see past them. We know that a straight stick does not bend when placed in the water, yet we cannot but see it as bent. This persistence makes this an *illusion*. If however we would still act as if the stick were bent, while aware that we are witnessing an optical distortion, then we would be willingly *deluding* ourselves. The first and fourth are more precisely delusions in which we are complicit in the deception. We are complicit in taking something to be true that we know to be otherwise. I will explain these points in turn.

3.4.1 The Choice Too Many

First, how can the opportunity for choice itself lead us away from what we actually want? If a person tends to try to maximize the outcome of any decision, an increase of choices can have negative effects. For such a "maximizer," an increase in choice perversely introduces the possibility that the choice foregone would have better answered her needs. The person might end up foregoing an option that would have made her happy in the absence of alternatives—perhaps happier than the decision she makes in the presence of greater choice.

There are perverse results with "the lure of choice" (Bown, Read, and Summers 2002). A rat, for instance, will chose a route through a maze that will provide it with a second set of options, even when repeated experiences teach it that there is no greater reward to be discovered by taking the route with the additional choices. People behave in a similar fashion. Say someone would prefer to see the movie *The Imitation Game* rather than *American Sniper*, but *American Sniper* is playing in a multiplex theater while *The Imitation Game* is at a single-screen theater. A person often chooses to go to the multiplex theater because she thinks that the multiplex may offer the choice of a still more desirable movie and winds up seeing *American Sniper* rather than the movie she preferred. The fact that the multiplex offers a choice "lures" her into seeing a less preferred film (Bown, Read, and Summers 2002). This preference for choices appears to be simply irrational behavior, but some psychologists say that it may serve survival in natural settings (Bown, Read, and Summers 2002). Still, it can serve us poorly in reproductive choices.

When a wanted pregnancy comes, we tend to be content accepting whatever reproductive choices were made prior to conception. But when screening and diagnostic tests are introduced, we are drawn to optimize our choice, just as the rat in the maze is lured by choice. For some, these added options—more choices—are not welcome. To return to my son's case, he and his wife were offered and encouraged to undergo the maternal serum alfa feno-protein (AFP) blood test that is used to screen for a number of genetic disorders, along with other prenatal screens and diagnostic tests. My son has lived all of his life with a sister who has a very significant intellectual disability, cerebral palsy, and a seizure disorder, yet no genetic basis has been identified.[11] I believe that the doctors presumed that he and his wife would be anxious to undergo as many screenings and diagnostic procedures as are available—or at least that they would welcome having these offered—to maximize their chance of having a "perfect" baby.

However, these options were not welcomed. Having to consider whether to abort a very-much-wanted pregnancy on the possibility, or even the likelihood, that the fetus had an impairment was a most unwelcome intrusion into the expectations blossoming in their bosoms. The intrusion was not merely that of an undesired possibility: that this baby may not be all right. (While my son loves his sister very much, he wants his own children to have every capacity and every opportunity.) The intrusion was rather, to import Bernard Williams's phrase, "one thought too many" (1981, 18). What is that unwelcome thought? It is the thought that I will love and accept this child if and only if he or she possesses traits that I value—a view my son, in an exchange with me, dubbed "the family as an exclusive club" (see the discussion in chapter 4). Aside from the utter vulnerability of a child to the treatment at the hands of a parent, we can say that at the very least, children are entitled to an unconditional love, since it is *they* who are really the only ones in families who truly don't get to choose.

3.4.2 Hopes and Fears

Second, psychologists have found that we systematically overestimate the displeasure we will experience from negative outcomes and the pleasure we will derive from positive ones. One well-known study showed that paraplegics adapt far better than most people presume and that lottery winners are far less satisfied in the long run by their change in fortune (Brickman, Coates, and Janoff-Bulman 1978, also cited in Kahneman and Tversky 2000, 765).

In account after account, the literature on disability testifies that it is not the impairment itself that is the primary source of the disadvantages experienced by disabled people. Instead it is the social responses to the impairment and the discrimination experienced that are the major problems. Many insist that if there was a single thing in their lives that they could alter, it would be some lack or circumstance entirely

---

[11] When I wrote this, no genetic basis was known. In 2018, at age forty-eight, my daughter has been diagnosed with a random, de novo mutation on the PURA gene—a mutation only first discovered in 2014. As this is not hereditary, there is no greater chance that my son or any of my descendents will encounter this mutation than exists for anyone else. Would this knowledge have changed my son's decision not to have genetic testing? It is unclear, but I suspect that it would not have.

unrelated to the disability. In memoirs and interviews, many prospective parents speak of having underestimated the pleasure and overestimated the disappointment of raising a disabled child.[12]

Two psychological features are largely responsible for this inability to accurately predict responses. One is adaptation (although, as I explain in chapter 5, I would rather speak of "adjustment"). The other is that pleasure depends as much on contrasts as on a state's specific "endowment of utility" (i.e., the actual pleasurable moment). This holds as well for our expectations. If we assume that a lottery win will solve our problems and it fails to do so, then we are even more disappointed by the winning than we would have been had we never won. With respect to our prospective children, we proleptically experience the prodigious talents: "I am musical. I choose to marry a man who is musical. My children will inherent our musical gifts." To such a woman, the idea of having a child that is tone deaf may be unbearable. And yet along comes a child with whom you fall in love and who turns out to be deaf. You come to appreciate many other wonderful qualities, and you adjust remarkably well.[13] You find you have overestimated the negative effects of a hearing-impaired child and underestimated the positive effects.

3.4.3 Choices Are Framed

Third, we are notoriously influenced by the framing of decision problems, as the responses to these two problems presented by Daniel Kahneman and Amos Tversky illustrate:

Problem 1: Assume yourself richer by $300 than you are today. You have to choose between:
A. A sure gain of $100
B. A fifty percent chance to gain $200 and a fifty percent chance to gain nothing

Most people will choose A, which makes you richer by $400 than you are today.

Problem 2: Assume yourself richer by $500 than you are today. You have to choose between:
A. A sure loss of $100
B. A fifty percent chance to lose nothing and a fifty percent chance to lose $200

---

[12] See a further discussion of these points in Chapter 5.

[13] Solomon, for example, reports one parent as saying: "In the beginning, it's all sadness and woe and horror. My mother said, 'He'll end up in an asylum.' In her generation, you were deaf and dumb, you were sent away. But I had this gorgeous, blue-eyed son who just beamed at me. It didn't take long for me to say, 'Who has the problem here?' Because he was perfectly fine to me" (2012, 80).

Most people will choose B. Yet in both problems, the first choice, A, makes you $400 richer than you are today (Kahneman and Tversky 2000, 762). Similarly, in both problems, the second choice, B, offers you a 50 percent chance of being $500 dollars richer and a 50 percent chance of being $300 richer. What accounts for the difference in choice is the framing of the problem. In the first problem, choice A is a sure gain; in the second, choice A is a sure loss. This changed frame alters one's perception of the outcome and the risks one is willing to take. Again, not the final value but the possible gain or loss tends to determine the choice. Similarly, we begin with expectations of the family we wish to have. To ensure that those expectations are realized, we will take risks overestimating the real probabilities that a gain (or the realization of the favorable expectation) will be the result. Where we think that there may be a loss, we will avoid risks, often overestimating the probabilities of a loss.

These framing effects are important to consider when we think about offering prenatal screening and diagnostic tests. Consider how probabilities and risks involved in genetic screening and diagnostic tests are presented. Consider the AFP blood test that is used early in the pregnancy to screen for a number of genetic disorders. It is a relatively noninvasive screen, but in 95 percent of cases, a positive result is inaccurate. The large probability that a positive result will be incorrect is discounted in favor of the small probability that an actual problem will be detected. For those seeking to avoid giving birth to a child with a disability, a risk-averse strategy will be to take the test and perhaps abort, overestimating the likelihood that the positive result is accurate. Taking the risk of aborting an unimpaired fetus may not be warranted by the degree of the test's accuracy. But one is tempted to justify it because of the perceived gain of a healthy child in a future pregnancy.

One also has a choice to not abort early but to do more accurate testing later. Yet later tests may have significant risks of miscarriage—risks that we might well underestimate given our psychological propensities—and the later tests come at a time when a strong attachment has already been made with the developing fetus, making the decision to abort, while not necessarily less likely, much more painful.

There is a feature of how we undergo pregnancy that is tangentially related to framing, namely experiencing pregnancy under the assumption that all is well. When tests with poor predictive ability are on offer, they do little to enhance the possibility that we give birth to a nondisabled child, while they destroy the joyful anticipation and preparation for parenthood. If one decides to abort on the basis of nondefinitive early tests, one may regret the possibility that one has aborted a fetus that was unaffected. We may also regret our choice when we reflect that, had the fetus been affected, it would

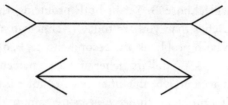

The top line appears longer than the bottom one but is
actually the same length.

Figure 3.1 Illusion: two lines that appear different, but actually are equal, in length.

have developed into a baby we would have loved nonetheless. It is conceivable that such regrets come to cloud the relationship we have to the present child. As women give birth later in their lives, into periods where their fertility diminishes, aborting a wanted pregnancy can result in not being able to birth a child at all.

This application of the dilemmas of choice involved in prenatal testing and selective abortion, however, is soon likely to be outdated because of the development and increasing availability of MaterniT21, a new DNA-based test that requires only a maternal blood sample as early as ten weeks into the pregnancy. The test boasts of correctly identifying Down syndrome in 99.1 percent of cases and correctly identifying the absence in 99.9 percent of cases.[14] The influence of these framing effects will, however, continue to be relevant for conditions for which MaterniT21 does not test.

Framing effects operate not just in subtle ways, but on a grosser level as well. In Kingsley's story, her framing of the birth of the Down syndrome child as analogous to arriving in Holland, which is a place different, not necessarily worse than, the one she intended, allowed her to appreciate what was so wonderful about the child to whom she gave birth—a child she may not have chosen, and perhaps a child she would not have chosen to keep once born had she not provided herself with an appropriate frame. These behaviors in the psychology of choice, as Kahneman and Tversky show, are persistent even when we have knowledge of the framing effects. In this they are just like perceptual illusions, as in Figure 3.1.

In contrast, the fourth source of error concerning the reality of choice-making more closely resembles a delusion than an illusion.

---

[14] See Kaposy (2013) for an analysis of the likely impact of such an early, noninvasive, and accurate test on the moral question of whether we should select against Down syndrome.

3.4.4 Do We Know What We Choose?

Fourth, for most of us, our families—whether traditional or not—are among our deepest sources of joy and misery. We desire as much control as we can hope to exert, control that can at best be partial. Upon such a thin thread hangs our happiness. We cling to the delusion that we, not fate, are at the helm. In fact we know that no set of behaviors and no tests will assure us a healthy baby, one with no impairments; no assurance of genetic normalcy will ensure a life lived to its full potential, nor will any amount of genetic enhancement guarantee the realization of our fondest hopes. This much is certain.

Even when genetic tests do detect an anomaly, they can only rarely give us an indication of the expressivity—that is, the degree of severity of the anomalous condition.[15] If we develop tests for autism, we most likely will be unable to determine what features of autism will affect the child. While we can detect Down syndrome with great accuracy in amniocentesis, with a high degree of accuracy in the sonographic prenatal screening scan and the nuchal scan, and with still greater early accuracy with MaterniT21, the tests, if positive, do not tell us whether the child will be highly dependent on care or be able to graduate high school, even attend college, and perhaps marry. Early detection of spina bifida will not tell us whether the resulting person will have very significant impairments or just have persistent lower back pain.

Furthermore, social acceptance, educational advances, and medical interventions can profoundly change the prognosis in many disorders. Children with Down syndrome today have a vastly different life than they did a mere forty years ago. Except in the case of a few disorders, even when the test is positive, we scarcely know what we are choosing for or against. We make our choice of marriage or sexual partner sometimes with those features that we want to see in our offspring in the back of our minds. We may choose to be impregnated with the sperm of a Harvard valedictorian, but regression to the mean ensures that there are no guarantees that the child's potential matches that of the parent. Nonetheless, most people persist in trying to reproduce themselves when they want a family, rather than adopt a child that needs a home. We want to believe that the apple does not fall far from the tree. But the process of shaping one's child in one's own image is nearly as uncertain as a lottery.

All the conditions around my daughter's birth were optimal, and yet this did not secure the expected outcome. Like Kingsley, I planned for Italy but wound up somewhere else. And, like Kingsley, the strange and foreign land, with few

---

[15] For a discussion of variable expressivity and reduced penetrance, see Andrews et al. (1994); also NIH (2016).

interpreters and fewer signposts, is the land I have occupied with my partner and my deeply loved disabled child—a land her fully able brother joined later. It is not one I would have willed, and yet, as it lay before me, I chose to stay. The choice I never thought to make presented me with the most cherished choice I have ever made, which was to stay by this child, give her all the love I had to give, shepherd her through this world—as I would any child of mine—and fight for her continued well-being.

3.5 So What Does "Choice" Mean?

When I question the evident desirability of choice, do I mean that we ought not to try to take charge of that which we can control? Ought I not to have given up my pack-and-a-half-a-day smoking habit when I was pregnant—because, after all, the child may be impaired in any case? Of course not. But I do mean to caution humility in the face of the vast uncertainty that choosing a family— any family, traditional or wildly untraditional—involves. A danger, or trap per- haps, of prenatal testing and selective abortion is the false assurance that, as a result of the choice, everything will be as we wish it (or think we wish it). Having exercised what we took to be control of our fate, we feel bewildered and betrayed when we nonetheless find ourselves subject to the luck of the draw.

What we *can* determine is the way we frame the options before us. Rather than see the birth of a child with Down syndrome (or with another disability, or even with properties different from those we hoped for) as landing in a place of pestilence and misery, we can frame the situation as arriving in Holland, a place replete with tulips, delicious herring, and lousy weather perhaps, but great Rembrandts and Vermeers.

4

The Ethics of Prenatal Testing and Selection

> Eugenic logic . . . tells us that we can avoid disability and even elimi-
> nate it from the human condition. This understanding of disability as
> somehow detachable from human life rather than essential to it fosters
> the idea that disability does not have much to do with us unless we have
> the misfortune of having it descend upon us.
> —Rosemarie Garland-Thomson (2012, 342)

4.1 The Question

Thus far we have considered only psychological and epistemological questions related to the idea that we can participate in choosing features of the children we have. Do these considerations necessarily lead us either to refuse selection or to refuse selection based on disability? I do not believe so. In the previous chapter I have argued only that we must be humble as we decide—aware of how little we know and the many conceptual and emotional traps that await us.[1]

At the same time, there are important moral considerations. Many bioethical arguments have been made that suggest that we have a moral obligation to select for the best child possible. We will contend with these arguments in the chapter that follows. In this chapter, I want to look at the opposing view, usually presented by many members of the disability community who have argued that questions of prenatal testing and selection are moral questions because they constitute forms of discrimination against people with disabilities (Asch and Parens 2000). They argue that accepting the idea that we should prevent certain conditions from occurring comes with a moral hazard: the failure to accept people currently living with these disabilities.

---

[1] This chapter is based in part on Kittay and Kittay (2000).

4.1.1 To Select or Not to Select, That Is
the Question—Or Is It?

Before we work through the many arguments made on all sides of the debate, it is worth laying out the conceptual map of the terrain that the discussion in this chapter and the next will cover. In the face of the reproductive possibilities opened by new technologies, we encounter opposing moral intuitions and correlate claims. The opposing views can be summarized as follows:

	Impermissible		Permissible		Obligatory
1	Selection tout court	vs	Selection tout court		
2	Selection against disabling traits	vs	Selection against disabling traits	vs	Selection against disabling traits
3	Selection for disabling traits	vs	Selection for disabling traits		
4	Selection for enhancing traits	vs	Selection for enhancing traits	vs	Selection for enhancing traits

Line 1 lays out the opposing positions on the morality of selection, *tout court.* Those who oppose selection *tout court* argue that we ought to welcome whatever child we might bring into the family, while others claim that there are no moral objections to selection. Debates concerning the morality of selecting *against disabling* traits are represented in line 2. While some argue that it is impermissible to select against disabling traits, others argue that it is not only permissible but morally obligatory to do so. Line 3 reflects the competing intuitions concerning the permissibility of selecting *for disabling* traits, as some deaf couples have wanted to do. (No one argues that we are morally obliged to select for disabling traits.) Finally, line 4 sets forth different intuitions concerning the morality of selecting for enhancing traits. This last debate is postponed for discussions treated in *Who is Truly Human?*

There are two sets of concerns that are distinguishable but are often conflated. One is whether it is morally acceptable to permit or prevent the birth of a child who will be disabled (line 1). The other is whether it is morally acceptable to select features of a prospective child (line 2). One argument against selection is that parents should unconditionally welcome whatever child comes into their family. A variant is that parents should be open to the unbidden and not try to determine what features a child might have. Another argument focuses on the idea that a family should be a place of unconditional love and acceptance, whereas selection indicates that only children with certain features would be loved and accepted.

The debates in lines 3 and 4 are reflected in the following arguments. The view that selecting for disability per se is impermissible may allow for selecting for traits that are disabling but that are also ones that situate a person within the community valued by the prospective parents. A major argument opposed to selecting against disability maintains that such selection expresses the view that a disabled life is not worth living or is an inferior life. This is known as the expressivist argument. Another adds that selecting against disabling traits is a form of eugenics; this applies the standard arguments against eugenics.

Arguments that selection against disability is morally permissible (or even obligatory) will insist that we ought to select for a child who will have a fully flourishing life, and that disabilities make such a life less likely. Another argument points out that, since a disabled child can have a negative impact on other members of a family, one may (or ought to) select against disability for the sake of those others. One argument that we will examine in detail maintains that while disability is a lesser harm to a child than not being born—as being alive is such an immense gain—a disabled child brings less good into the world than an able child would. Therefore, we should try to bring more good into the world and opt to select for an able rather than a disabled child. In these arguments, not only is not selecting against disability morally questionable, but selecting for given features is also thought permissible, or even obligatory. Generally this view holds that selection against disability is morally obligatory, and selecting for enhancing features is morally permissible. Still others insist that we are morally obliged to have the best child we can have, and that means that enhancement is not only permissible but morally obligatory whenever possible.

Another position argues for the moral permissibility of selecting against disability, but only under certain constraining conditions: It is permissible to select against a given disability only if we could justify to the child that would have been born, why we choose to abort him or her. We will directly address only a few of these various arguments, but many that are on offer overlap or are variants of each other. Still, it is worthwhile to see at the outset that the question of *selection* is one thing, while the question of the *permissibility of bringing a child into the world who will be disabled* is another.

Addressing questions of reproductive selection requires still more discernment, for there are at least four distinct perspectives from which these concerns may be viewed. There is:

1. The perspective of the prospective child;
2. The perspective of the disability community (assuming, against fact, that there is a *unified disability community perspective*);
3. The perspective of the parent; and
4. An impartialist perspective, that is, a perspective from the society or the universe as a whole.

Each perspective identifies a stakeholder in these debates, although of course, there is no single child, parent, or community perspective. While I will try to represent divergent views within a given perspective, in general I will try to represent what one might call a loose consensus.

Rosemarie Garland-Thomson (2012) has called the unifying view of arguments that permit or oblige us to select against disability "eugenic logic." However, it may be just as appropriate to claim that eugenic logic stands behind all pro selection arguments, especially if one cleanses the term *eugenics* of its negative associations with the compulsory eugenics that dominated discussions and policy prior to the Second World War. My own quest in the chapters that follow will be to avoid a eugenic logic and yet allow women to maintain control of the reproductive capabilities of their own bodies. It may not be possible to walk this fine line, but I believe we must try.

4.2 First Encounters with the Prenatal Testing Debates

My first forays in writing professionally about disability came from an invitation to participate in a Hastings Center two-year workshop on prenatal testing and selective abortion. From the letter of invitation, I gathered that I was expected to oppose prenatal testing and selective abortion in the spirit of solidarity with my disabled child and the disability community. But in that expectation, I would have to disappoint. After all the readings and discussions and reflections through which I have come to understand the position of those who oppose prenatal testing and selective abortion, I continue, by and large, to hold the view I held when I wrote my response to the letter of invitation. My reasons for not opposing prenatal testing and selection were:

1. In a society as unresponsive to the needs of the child and the family as ours, even a far less significant disability than that possessed by my daughter can be devastating. In the face of this reality, we celebrate the rights and dignity of people with disabilities, and the joy and goodness possible in the lives of people with even very significant disability, but we must respect the right of a parent either to undertake what can be an emotionally, physically, and economically difficult journey, or to refuse it. To deny parents the ability to opt out when that possibility exists prior to the birth of the child is an unwarranted imposition, unacceptable in a liberal society.

2. While some argue that giving a child up for adoption is an option that is available, for many women (and men) the idea that they abandon the child to the care of strangers is wrenching—a sorrow that they carry throughout their lives. Adoption may be a choice for some, but its costs are so great that these ought never to be imposed on someone.[2]

3. Ultimately, the argument comes down to this: as long as we believe that abortion is permissible for any reason, and we believe that a woman has the right to make her own reproductive decisions, we must grant the permissibility of abortion (or prenatal selection in whatever form) in this instance as well.

My stance did not deter the organizers from insisting that I participate in the workshop, and so with some trepidation, I did. After the first meeting, I returned home shaken. There were other parents there, none of whom felt as I did. But they each had stories of how their physicians had originally given them prognostications that underestimated what their children were able to accomplish. The early prognosis for Sesha was not far from the mark. If anything, they overestimated what she might be able to do. The parents at the workshop could speak of their children's "independence." Not so in our case. One of the well-known disability scholars in that meeting chastised me for speaking of the "burdens" involved in raising a child like Sesha. She, who did not have children of her own, insisted that it was no extra burden to raise a child with severe disabilities and that I was just angling to be congratulated on my "sacrifices."

I was truly rattled. Moreover, dredging up memories of Sesha's early childhood was difficult. It roiled what were by then still waters and reactivated the early trauma. As I came home and related the day's events to my husband Jeffrey and my son Leo, I explained the opposition to prenatal diagnosis and selective abortion based on disability, and especially the expressivist argument. The expressivist argument holds that choosing to be tested for the possibility of the fetus's impairments and choosing to

---

[2] See The Factsheet on the Impact of Adoption on Birth Parent (Child Welfare 2013) at https://www.childwelfare.gov/pubPDFs/f_impact.pdf) for studies that document the emotional cost of adoption on the birth parents.

abort in the face of positive results expresses a view that is disrespectful to disabled people. It purportedly sends a message that either a disabled life is not worth living, that a disabled life does not have the value of a life without disability, or that the disabled are not welcome in this world. Thus, its impact on people with disabilities, the very "message sent," is discriminatory and injurious to disabled people who already exist. Hence selective abortion or approval of such selection against disability is unethical, even if abortion itself is not subject to ethical opprobrium.

Given my own experience, I believed then (and continue to believe) that the expressivist objection to selection against disability could not be right. I fiercely believed that my daughter's life was worth living, but I could imagine being tested and choosing to abort an impaired fetus. This was so because I believed I could not raise still another child with the additional needs a disability might bring and still give my already existing disabled child what I thought she needed to have a good life. To my surprise, my son did not agree with me, but with the opponents.

I asked if he really believed that were I to have become pregnant and chose to abort if there was a likelihood that the fetus was impaired, these actions would belie everything our life with Sesha made apparent. How, I asked, could he have gotten a message that I believed that a disabled life was not worth living when our life with Sesha made it evident that we cherished our disabled daughter every bit as much as our able son, that her life was as precious to us as his? But he did not waiver. My son, with his newly minted bachelor's degree in philosophy, and I pursued this conversation in a series of emails that became the paper in the volume issuing from the two-year workshop.

My daughter has not been my only teacher in matters of disability. Her sibling, my nondisabled son, had lessons of his own to offer. My son and I initiated the correspondence with the letter I had sent to the workshop organizers. In Leo's reply to my opening letter, he voiced three compelling arguments against genetic selection, which I will call the "extinction or 'something would be lost' objection," the "all children are burdens objection," and the "a family is not a club objection."

There has been a growing literature on the topic over the many years since the Hastings Project, but in revisiting the question of prenatal testing and selective abortion, I will use our correspondence—in particular, the objections that Leo raises to my contentions—to frame the discussion for the issues.

4.3 "Something Would Be Lost"— The Extinction Objection

The first objection Leo raises to my views is what I will call the extinction objection. The worry is that selection could lead to the extinction of the populations of people with cognitive disabilities and that something invaluable would be therefore be lost.[3] Leo writes:

> People must be made aware that [raising a child with cognitive impairments] . . . is just as fulfilling as raising a normal child, albeit differently fulfilling. If it ever feels more fulfilling . . . it is probably because we just expect it to be less so. (Kittay and Kittay 2000, 169)

Leo supposes that many women will abort precisely because they anticipate that the experience of raising a disabled child would not be fulfilling or as fulfilling as raising an able child.[4] If this goes uncontested, the result would be the extinction or significant reduction in number of people with certain forms of cognitive disability, making it impossible for people to experience just what would have prevented the elimination of those people in the first place. A reply to this objection has two prongs. One questions whether extinction or severe reduction of populations with certain sorts of disabilities is possible or likely. The other tries to discern what would be lost in the eventuality that some sorts of disabled people are no longer born or if all disability could be eliminated by preventing births of disabled people (Kittay and Kittay 2000, 169).

The extinction objection raises worries about eugenics. In responding to my son, I evinced skepticism concerning the possibility that cognitive disability would be entirely eliminated. In light of recent developments in genetic and prenatal diagnosis, I have to acknowledge that there is some truth to Leo's concern. With respect to the worry that something is lost, I concede that something would be lost. The challenge is whether we can articulate what of value is lost and whether the loss can be accommodated or justified.

4.3.1 Eugenics and the Elimination of (Certain) Disabilities

Eugenics, by and large, retains the moral opprobrium it gained from practices in the United States, Scandinavia, and most especially Nazi Germany to reduce the number of "unfit" people in the world and so, presumably, improve the stock of the species. Some have tried to save the term "eugenics" from the damnation it received when it was marked by enforced sterilizations and genocide. Two critical distinctions separate the negative eugenics associated with American racism and Nazi genocide from a putatively benign eugenics. Negative eugenics uses

---

[3] What I am calling the "extinction objection" is squarely addressed more recently in Garland-Thomson (2012).

[4] In a study of women in the Netherlands cited in Kaposy (2013), 61 percent of women who underwent testing for Down syndrome reported: "I thought I would be unhappy with having this child."

violence and coercive practices, while "positive eugenics" relies on procedures sought out by parents themselves. Negative eugenics aims to eliminate "undesirable" traits or people while positive eugenics works to promulgate positive traits thought to improve current and future populations. Yet the more benign forms of eugenics are, according to some, still morally suspect. The "freely" made individual decisions, motivated by a variety of reasons, can have the same result of eliminating whole populations that have genetically transmitted conditions. Philip Kitcher (1997) calls this "laissez-faire" eugenics, and Tom Shakespeare (Shakespeare 2006) refers to it as "emergent" eugenics. Eliminating whole populations with certain genetic features, the opponents of such selection argue, is itself morally objectionable whether or not coercion is used. Could "positive eugenics" effectively eliminate cognitive disability, and if so why would this be objectionable?

Laissez-faire eugenics might conceivably succeed in rendering extinct forms of chromosomal atypicality such as Down syndrome. It is the case that genetic testing and prenatal diagnosis have already greatly reduced the incidence of babies born with infantile Tay-Sachs, severe cystic fibrosis, and other serious genetically related conditions (Mansfield, Hopfer, and Marteau 1999). Perhaps most will agree that infantile Tay-Sachs is one disorder that the world is better off without, as the infant has a relatively short and painful existence (although one may not want to say this in the case of adult-onset Tay-Sachs, which, although debilitating, is not fatal and has a more varied outcome).[5]

Given current trends it seems possible, perhaps even likely, that Down syndrome will also be eliminated. Even when using technologies that generally involve a second-term abortion, the abortion rate was as high as 85 to 90 percent of those diagnosed (Mansfield, Hopfer, and Marteau 1999). The women who are tested are generally over thirty-five and are viewed as being "at risk" of giving birth to a child with DS. Today most Down syndrome children are the children of younger women, generally because these are women

---

[5] Most assume that Tay-Sachs affects only infants, but in the 1970s the first cases of the late-onset varieties (juvenile and adult-onset) were diagnosed. In late-onset Tay-Sachs, the disease progresses slowly and can be very debilitating, but it is usually nonfatal. Tay-Sachs is the result of a mutation of the HEXA gene, which regulates the production of the enzyme hexosaminidase A. Infantile Tay-Sachs is marked by a complete absence of the enzyme, while late-onset forms are a result of varying degrees of deficiencies of the enzyme. Hence the late-onset forms vary in symptoms and severity depending on the level of enzyme activity. I thank Phillip J. Nelson for alerting me to the difference between adult-onset Tay-Sachs and infant Tay-Sachs. For more information about this disease, see the webpage for the Late Onset Tay-Sachs Research and Education Foundation: http://www.lateonsettay-sachs.org/index.php?p=ct&pgid=7 and http://rarediseases.org/rare-diseases/tay-sachs-disease.

who are not tested. The fact that today highly accurate diagnosis that will allow for first-semester terminations is available,[6] and that women under thirty-five are being encouraged to get tested,[7] lends credence to the view that Down syndrome eventually could be eliminated. What we see today is a great irony, one that is being repeated for many other disabilities. Namely, as we have increasing reason to believe that the people with Down will be significantly reduced, if not entirely eliminated, the longevity of people with Down syndrome has reached into the fifties, and people with DS lead increasingly rich lives. As Solomon (2012) writes: "Social progress is making disabling conditions easier to live with just as medical progress is eliminating them. There is something tragic about this confluence, like those operas in which the hero realizes he loves the heroine just as she expires" (20–1).

Yet for this very reason—that the lives of people with Down syndrome have been so improved—we should be cautious in making prognoses. It is useful to remember that the figures on abortions tell us only about those women who have availed themselves of the testing, often having already concluded that they would abort if the results reveal that the child has a severe disability. These figures do not include those who chose not to be tested, either because they were young or because they decided that they would not abort if the fetus had DS. Indeed, it appears as if current rates of abortion based on prenatal diagnosis have dropped in the United States. The most recent evidence suggests that the 67 percent of women abort as opposed to the earlier figure reported by Mansfield, Hopfer, and Marteau (1999) of 92 percent (Natoli et al. 2012). It is conceivable that as more Down syndrome children and adults participate in all walks of life, including TV and movies, more women will refuse prenatal tests or will refuse to abort even in the face of a positive test.[8]

One reason that people become concerned about the possible reduction in the number of children with Down syndrome born is because they worry that in smaller numbers there will be less political clout to make the changes that have so dramatically increased DS people's longevity and participation. However,

---

[6] These technologies include the blood test MaterniT21 and ultrasound, which is routinely used to determine the likely age of the fetus and can be used to assess the thickness of the fetus's neck, an indicator of Down syndrome. These methods are far less invasive than amniocentesis, pose less risk to the fetus, and give a more certain and earlier result.

[7] In January 2007, the American College of Obstetricians and Gynecologists (2007) "revised its guidelines that now recommend offering fetal chromosomal screening to all pregnant women, regardless of age."

[8] See Kaposy (2013), who takes a more pessimistic view of the future.

there is little indication that the diminished numbers, thus far, have resulted in worse outcomes for those who are not aborted. On the other hand, increases in the diagnoses of autism have garnered more attention and poured significant financial resources into improving the lives of people on the autism spectrum. The high incidence of autism (1 in 110 children are diagnosed as autistic), doubtless helped along by autists who have been able to speak out, may be diminishing the stigma attached to this rather than other types of developmental and cognitive disabilities. However, it is not clear that all the funding is really a sign that autism is more accepted than other cognitive disabilities. It is worth noting that the largest amount of funding has been allocated for prevention or "cure."[9] It appears that the bulk of funds raised for the cause of autism is going to eliminate autists, not to care for them or to offer them greater opportunities for a full life.

Reproductive biomedical technologies are not the final word in whether there will be an effort to eliminate a form of disability. In the case of the orthodox Jewish community in which arranged marriages are still the rule, matchmakers ask for genetic information and do not match couples who are both carriers of Tay-Sachs.[10] This has led to a nearly total eradication of Tay-Sachs in the orthodox Jewish Community using only minimal diagnostic procedures.

The elimination of certain diseases and disabilities is greatly assisted by medical technologies, and the eugenic urge arguably is expressed in the *routinization* of screening and testing procedures. But the eugenic urge and the negative views of disability express themselves very forcefully without medical technologies and routinized diagnoses. For example when we as a society do little to support disabled people and their families, leaving parents to bear the full brunt of the

---

[9] Health and Human Services funding for autism falls under the Combating Autism Act, with the purpose of "fighting autism" through research, screening, treatment, and education. Sixty-eight percent of the $693 million is allocated to research. See the Association of University Centers on Disability's publication on the "Combating Autism Reauthorization Act of 2011" at http://www.aucd.org/. Disability rights activist Ari Ne'eman has spoken out against funding efforts aimed largely at curing and preventing autism rather than improving the lives of autistic people. In an interview with Wired.com, he says: "Obviously, funding autism research is very important. There's a lot that could be done to significantly improve autistic people's quality of life. But instead, groups like Autism Speaks have been prioritizing things like developing prenatal tests to detect autism in the womb. That doesn't help the millions of autistic people who have already been born. Very few of us wake up in the morning and think, 'Have they developed a proper mouse model for autism yet?' Instead, autistic people and their parents worry about finding the educational and support services that they need" (Silberman 2010).

[10] The program is known as Dor Yoshorim. See http://doryeshorim.org/ for information on how the program is carried out. There is little objection raised to the program, perhaps because abortion is not involved and they are mostly concerned with devastating and fatal recessive genetic conditions such as Tay-Sachs.

additional costs and responsibilities of raising a child with the disability. Such policies do little to welcome disabled people into the world.

4.3.1.1 A Fool's Errand

Thomas Shakespeare (2011) writes:

> While the proportion of prospective parents opting for termination remains constant, at just over 90%, there has been a 71% increase in diagnoses of Down syndrome over the last 20 years in Britain. Despite screening, over the last 15 years there has been an increase of 25% of babies with Down syndrome being born. (Buckley and Buckley 2008, 42)

To account for this, he points to the later age at which women give birth as a major factor, which, together with decreased rates of fertility resulting in more assisted reproductive techniques, have "necessitated increasing technologisation of conception and pregnancy." That the total population of people with Down syndrome has still grown indicates that these technologies are less effective in eliminating a disability than we imagine. Similarly, as Jeffrey Brosco (2010) has found,[11] our ability to save very young neonates, and to save the lives of people who have suffered massive brain injuries, have added enough people with intellectual and developmental disabilities to keep the incidence of cognitive disability constant. As Brosco's and Shakespeare's observations indicate, prenatal testing, for better or worse, may be able reduce the incidence of a particular disability, but the quest to eliminate all disability is a fool's errand not only because it is foolish to desire this, but it is foolish to think it possible. Developments of this sort, along with the inherent fragility of the human body (including, of course, the brain), give us myriad reasons for saying that the attempt to eliminate all cognitive disability is a fool's errand: it is impossible even if it were desirable.[12]

[11] Brosco (2010) conducted an extensive epidemiological study to determine if all the preventive measures that have been taken since the late 1960s to reduce the incidence of intellectual and development disabilities (IDD) have resulted in a lower rate of IDD in the population. He concluded that the rate of serious cases of IDD have remained constant, even when we take into consideration the controversial means of measuring IDD and the frequent changes in labeling.

[12] Furthermore, most cases of cognitive disability have not been shown to be genetically determined, nor are the various consequences of chromosomal or development abnormalities all detectable in utero (Acharya 2011; American College 2007). According to the NIH 30 to 40 percent of

4.3.1.2 What Will Be Lost?

But is it desirable? Why should we not give in to "eugenic logic" by "laissez-faire" means? The objection voiced by my son in our exchange was that something of value would be lost. In chapter 2, I argued that able parents' seemingly self-evident wish to have a "normal" child is partly explained when we see that normal already refers to what is valued and thereby desirable. But as we also saw in chapter 2, while intertwined, the concepts of desirability and normalcy are not equivalent. A vital humanity needs to imagine many ways to be in the world, and, in this respect at least, eliminating disability would constitute a loss.

The question that my son raises—"what would be lost?"—supposes more than simply a loss of diversity. He claims (and I agree) that the world would be a poorer place without people such as my daughter or Michael Bérubé's (1998) son Jamie, or Donna Thomson's (2010) son Nick. If there is a value to each one of these individuals, to whom are Sesha, Jaime, or Nick valuable? To start, we can say that first of all, the person is of value to herself. I hope to have indicated in chapter 2 how and why a good life can be had even in conditions of very significant disability. Again, this is a theme that will be evident throughout this book. Every expression of joy is an argument for the importance of Sesha's life *for her*. The value of a child is also very much a value to the parent. Like all the parents who have first-hand experience with a son or daughter whose intellectual development is "not normal," my experience has forced me to think more profoundly about what it is to be human, what our obligations are to each other, what the source of these obligations are, what gives rise to sorrow and what permits joy, and what gives life its meaning. Without a child such as Sesha, these reflections take a different, and arguably a much shallower, course.

Leo suggests that raising such a child may be more gratifying than the normal experience of childrearing precisely because we expect it to be less so. Perhaps. I cannot expect to get a report card with As, but I can see the appreciation for my child in a teacher speaking of my child's unique qualities. I cannot expect worldly accomplishments, but I can take pleasure and pride in small accomplishments acquired with much effort. I cannot have the sorts of discussions I have with my other child, but I can sit and enjoy the breeze with her, enjoy music with her. The delights and thrill of the connection, of the expansion of selfhood, of the love and care directed toward another—these are still present and sometime more intense for being so hard-won.

children with special needs do not have a diagnosis (National Human Genome Research Institute 2018). Technologies, at least, will not detect or eliminate all cases of intellectual or developmental disabilities—although genetic anomalies that result in cognitive disabilities are being discovered at an astonishing rate. Our increased longevity now means that many develop late-onset cognitive loss.

In the correspondence with my son, I wrote that Sesha and others similarly disabled have so much to teach us not because

> Sesha is so different from us, or . . . [that] she is so much like us, but that at the very core, we are so much like her.[13] We understand so much more about who we are and what moves us, when we see what moves Sesha. (2000, 172)

Addressing my son, I added: "I understand so much more of what it is to be a parent and love a child like you, when I know what it is to love Sesha" (2000, 172–73). For example, we learned that a parent's love has little to do with children's achievements, even as we hope for and relish them. When I spoke in chapter 2 of the components of a good life as consisting in "love, joy, and the ability to appreciate the gift of just being," it is a lesson I could perhaps have learned elsewhere, but nowhere could I have learned it better.

The cognitively disabled person has a value as a member of her society. Anita Silvers and Leslie Francis (2005; 2010) have proposed that having people like Sesha in our midst allows us to see what sorts of people are trustworthy, and so help to make a society more cohesive. (They have even suggested that this may have evolutionary advantages.) Christie Hartley, who argues that all individuals can contribute to social cooperation, has suggested that the social value of intellectually disabled people lies in their ability to "contribute to the family and civil society more generally by helping others develop values that are important for fair cooperation" (Hartley 2009, 29). But we should also be able to consider the value of people with severe cognitive disabilities to the larger community apart from whatever beneficial features they may bring out in others.

People with disabilities will often have what Andrew Solomon (2012) called a "horizontal" identity. Because of such a horizontal identity, disabled people have a value to other disabled people, for without them such a horizontal identity cannot emerge. Some may want to argue that the very properties that are targeted for elimination bring something very important into the world— something more than the totality of individuals with that disability. The argument made by the deaf is of this sort. Deaf people are keenly aware of the value deaf people have to other people with the same disability. Deaf culture has produced full-fledged languages, as well as developed cultures expressed in and through sign language. They report experiencing their world richly without all the distractions of sound, and sharing that experience with others who are

---

[13] See Elizabeth Spelman (1988), who speaks of the practice of saying about some people who are viewed as Other "but they are just like us" as "boomerang perception," one in which we can see the other only as "just like us" and never see ourselves as "just like them."

hearing impaired. For the rest of us, simply knowing that this is a possibility makes the world more interesting.

I do not think that there is a cognitive disability culture, although there is no doubt that there are important and valuable understandings among cognitively disabled people. There may also be something unique and wonderful when people meet the world without an abstractive reasoning that can distract from the fullness of concrete, felt experience. Moreover, it seems clear to me and to the people who work in Sesha's house that disabled people have a real sense of comradeship with each other. I cannot say if Sesha feels a bit less lonely in her disability being around others who share her disability, but if the experience of other disabled people is also her experience, then it is safe to surmise she does. That is, disabled people are of special value to each other.

In the end, however, the value of people like Sesha exceeds whatever their value may be to their parents, society, or community of disabled people—just as the value of any person exceeds such instrumental or relational considerations. Sesha's value is in her singular embodied subjectivity, an intrinsic value just as the value of each human being (and not only human beings) is intrinsic. It is a unique and irreplaceable human life, and the textures of our lives are enmeshed in the uniqueness of each other. Disability makes it no less so and no more so.

To exclude people with a certain disability from the realm of intrinsic value is as if we were to say all artworks are valuable except those sketched in charcoal. If we eliminated these, what would be lost? What is lost is simply all the artworks that might have been sketched in charcoal. We don't need to specify it any more than that. The same should be said of people with disabilities. What is lost are just those persons. If we think artworks are of value, then there is a real loss of value. If we think persons are of value, then there is a real loss of value. I still believe what I said those many years ago: "Whenever something that is valuable in and of itself vanishes, the world is diminished." I would modify Wittgenstein's (1921) statement "The world is the totality of facts," and say instead: "The world is the totality of intrinsic values."

Is this response to the question of what is lost merely an evasion, as evasive as saying simply that one loses diversity? A distinctive individual may be a suffering one for whom nothing can be done to alleviate a life of pain and affliction. If a distinctive way of being in the world is a life that cannot be a flourishing life, then perhaps the only thing that is lost is misery, and we certainly can do with a lot less of that. But if a life lived with even severe disability can still be a good life, then the distinctiveness of that goodness is lost.[14]

---

[14] In the next chapter, we will see that there are those who argue that this disadvantage puts a moral obligation on the woman to give birth to a nondisabled child when there is a choice to do so. This claim is based on a hypothetical comparison between a disabled life and the same person's life

To those who do not live with disability, either in their own person or in the person of a loved one, the claim that a disabled life can be very much worth living is somewhat paradoxical. For doesn't disability involve some form of disadvantage,[15] and why would we want to insist on the goodness of disadvantage? This question is especially apparent in the case of the sorts of disability that Sesha has. Although some of the disadvantage is a consequence of social attitudes, manmade structures, and failures to accommodate the disability, Sesha is surely disadvantaged when it comes to surviving on her own because of her intellectual limitations. Yet even a seemingly devastating cognitive impairment such as my daughter's may allow for an intensity in enjoyment that most of us miss. The world is poorer without her joy.

While Leo's question presumes that something has been lost if intellectually disabled people are not born, this presumption runs counter to the more usual presumption that something valuable is lost when a child with such a disability is born. Some philosophers, among them Jonathan Glover (2006a), have argued that not only should we choose to have a child that can flourish; whenever possible we should choose the child that has the better chance at flourishing. Daniel Brock (2004; 1995) has made the even stronger argument that if we fail to intervene in preventing the birth of a child with disabilities when we have the opportunity to do so, we have violated a version of the harm principle. I will consider these arguments in chapter 5.

Although I want to defend the right of a parent to select against disability, I find myself in agreement with Leo's challenge that something valuable would be lost if we were to succeed in eliminating all forms of cognitive disability. But just as surely as we are human, we are vulnerable to disability, and just as surely, there will never be a world without cognitive disability. We should therefore instead be concerned that measures are taken that will allow a disabled life, like the life without a disability, to be a life filled with opportunities for flourishing.

4.4 "All Children Are Burdens"

Leo's second objection can be stated thus: To argue from the premise that there is a greater burden placed on families raising children with cognitive disabilities gives rise to a slippery slope, as there is no clear demarcation of when the normal

---

with a disability. In chapter 5, I question the validity of such a comparison and the conclusions one can draw from it.

[15] To say that disability can involve some sort of disadvantage is not the same as to say that disability is inherently disadvantageous. For an excellent discussion of this point see Barnes (2016).

burdens of raising a child become burdens too onerous to expect parents to undertake.

It is at once a moment of pride and embarrassment when your son responds to your speaking of the "burden" of raising a child with disabilities with: "But beware the slippery slope, Mom. Are not all children a burden?" "Yes," you say, "all children are burdens, even you," but you add that it is a burden borne with gladness. And perhaps that is the real point: it is not *how* burdensome a task may be, but how willing one is to assume it, given the help and support available to lighten the load when it is too heavy to bear alone.

The willingness of others to share a burden helps assure that a decision to assume a responsibility does not turn into resentment and bitterness. If parents are denied supports, they are all the more likely to make decisions that, as more accurate and less invasive technologies become available, may render some sorts of people with disabilities extinct. At the same time, the question arises: "Why should the larger society bear the costs and burdens of an eliminable or avoidable disability? If parents choose to give birth to a child with disabilities, why should they not bear the brunt of the additional costs and responsibilities the child imposes?" A full reply requires that we raise questions of justice. But the poignant question my son posed—"Aren't all children burdens?"—is certainly a partial reply. All children are burdens, and we do acknowledge that children deserve the resources that their parents can provide. Nonetheless all, except perhaps recalcitrant conservative libertarians, will recognize that some costs for children ought to be shared by the society at large.

The question remains: Should the parents' decision whether or not to bring a pregnancy to term depend, in part at least, on the burdens posed by the potential child's disability? The first thing to notice is that women are already free to abort any fetus for any reason, including the reason that having a child at this time or at any time is too much of a burden (Shakespeare 2006; 2014; 2013). Why should we say that disability cannot be a reason? A fifth child will impose too much of a burden on many, but others will embrace it. A second child may be the backbreaking straw for some, and for still others just one child is one child too many.[16] The second thing to note is that, burdensome as they are, children are never only burdens. As long as we agree that it is morally acceptable for women to determine what is or is not a burden for her in childbearing and childrearing, we must allow them to decide whether disability is as well. But we must add that women need access to information and to families who have raised children with comparable disabilities.

---

[16] See James Nelson (2000), "The Meaning of the Act: Reflections on the Expressive Force of Reproductive Decision-Making and Policies."

4.4.1 Aborting *This* Prospective Child or *Any* Prospective Child

Is there a distinction to be made between aborting for all the various reasons women choose to terminate a pregnancy and the one reason that the resulting child will have a disability?[17] Feminist disability rights activists have claimed that it is one thing to determine that you do not want to have a child (that is, abortion *simpliciter*, "aborting *any* fetus"), and another to say that you do not want to give birth to *this* fetus who manifests such and such a trait (that is, selective abortion, "aborting *this* fetus").[18] However, at least in some sense, every abortion is a selective one. The trait that defines the choice may not be disability, but 'being the offspring of this man,' or 'being a third child,' or 'being the child I have conceived at this infelicitous time in my life.'[19] Whatever reason women choose (unless they have determined that they do not want to have a child at all) is a choice about *this* fetus. The objection to this defense is that selecting against disability selects on the basis of an intrinsic trait (i.e., the impairment), not a relational one (e.g., being a third child). This distinction, however, cuts against the claim most disability advocates endorse: namely, that disability is a relational trait. Disability, that is to say, is a relation (in particular, a misfit) between one's body (or mind) and the physical and social environment.

Another way to defend the "any child versus this child" argument would appeal to discrimination: Selecting against a potentially disabling trait selects against a group that is already the object of systematic discriminatory behavior. The social, economic, and political indicators all substantiate the claim that the disabled all suffer extensive discrimination. The expressivist argument maintains that in the context of this socially prevalent discrimination selecting against fetuses with disabling conditions expresses a message that a disabled life is not worth living. That selecting against an impaired fetus expresses a derogatory message about disabled lives is surely an argument worth taking seriously.

---

[17] This question arises for selection via abortion only because embryo selection only takes place when the decision to carry a child to term has already been made. It is conceivable, although highly unlikely, that all the embryos will have the same impairment. In that unlikely case, the equivalent question would be whether to start the process of in-vitro fertilization anew.

[18] This is a position that has been elaborated by the disability scholars and bioethicists Adrienne Asch and David Wasserman (2005). See also Marsha Saxton, "Why Members of the Disability Community Oppose Prenatal Screening and Selective Abortion," in Asch and Parens (2000), and Adrienne Asch and Gail Geller, "Feminism, Bioethics, and Genetics," in Wolf (1996).

[19] For a more complete argument of the same point see Nelson (2000).

It applies to all forms of genetic testing and prenatal diagnosis as well as to selective abortion.

Asch and Wasserman (2005) write that their objection to selective procedures opposes the underlying presumption that a single feature is sufficient to characterize everything about an individual. Synecdoche is the trope by which we signify the whole by a single trait. It is also typical of discrimination, as when we take a person's color as indicative of an entire set of characteristics. They claim that when we abort a fetus based on a disabling trait, we commit the "sin of synecdoche," just as we do when we discriminate against a disabled person based on the individual's impairment.

But what is happening in the case of reproductive selection may be subtler. A being in utero may be infirmed, but it is not yet disabled if disability is construed on the social model. An impairment pertains to an individual as such, and in principle may be alterable. This is different than other intrinsic properties that become the basis of discrimination, such as race—which is an unalterable characteristic of a person (and is not an impairment of the human organism either). It might be possible that there is a medical procedure that could repair an impairment. Therefore, if the impairment could be remedied in utero, the same person who would choose abortion would happily have *this* child. The point is that synecdoche is not at work here in the same way as it is in discrimination by race or even discrimination against born individuals with disabilities.[20] It is true that it is the *trait* that is targeted, and the targeting means that this individual fetus is not born. But it isn't that the trait is taken as standing for the individual—for if the trait could be altered or eliminated, the individual would be accepted. It is rather the effects of the trait—the disability that ensues when the baby is born—that are unwanted.[21] The rigid designation of *this* child is not what fuels a woman's rejection of this pregnancy, even though it means that this child will not come into being as a consequence of her choice.

---

[20] One might claim that some pathogenic genetic mutations and chromosomal anomalies are more akin to race since such anomalies pervade the organism in a way that other anomalies do not. But if the effects of such pathologies or anomalies could be altered in utero—perhaps at an early stage in the pregnancy—the same argument I use in the section above would pertain.

[21] Contrast this with the rejection of a fetus because of its paternity. One could rightly say that the fetus is rejected because of the property of being the offspring of a certain man—and that is not an alterable property. You cannot have the same baby if the father is different. While it is generally difficult, if not impossible, to imagine what a person might have been like without her disability, the situation of a fetus in utero is different. Arguably, one becomes a someone with recognizable traits only after birth. One can therefore conceive of the possibility of this same fetus but without the impairment.

4.4.2　Children Are Not Only Burdens

Choosing to have or not to have a child is, of course, not only a matter of burden, since, while all children are burdens, all children are so much more. This is how I put the point in my response to Leo:

> Burden though they are, even under the harshest conditions, even in slavery, many women had their babies and raised them. Harriet Jacobs, a young slave woman, wrote that when she "pressed her own infants to her heart," she had "the feeling that even in fetters there was something to live for" (1861, 427). I can add that even where a child is as profoundly disabled as Sesha, there is so much to treasure.

Perhaps it is best to place both the burden argument and the "*this* versus *any* child" argument on their heads. To the extent that we have a choice, each procreative decision is a determination to take on one burden, not another, to bank on one set of hopes and expectations and not another. We make each choice aware, if only dimly, that we may not get what we signed up for. We may land in Holland and not in Italy; in Timbuktu, not in Hawaii; even in Syria in the midst of a civil war, not in the Promised Land.

This means that if the option to choose against having *this* impaired fetus is to be a genuine choice, two issues have to be squarely faced. One is the lack of material resources, the other is stigma. As long as these constraints serve as thumbs on the scale, a decision to bring a pregnancy to term is not free. Each makes it far more burdensome to raise a child with disabilities than the actual impairment might otherwise demand. The material resources available in many parts of the world are far from adequate. Among wealthy nations, the United States fares rather poorly.

The social failure to provide adequate assistance and support to people with cognitive disabilities and their families is linked to the persistence of the stigma of the disability. The stigma of disability lies ultimately in our difficulty in facing our own vulnerability. Dan Goodley (2013) puts the point this way: "we disavow our vulnerability in the many forms that stigma takes." Cognitive disability remains among the most stigmatized forms of disability. Even though one group of cognitively disabled people, people with DS, have become more visible in the media,[22] such exposure has not in itself been sufficient to ensure that a diagnosis

---

[22] By 1996 when my son and I wrote our article, the TV show *Life Goes On*, which featured a young man with Down syndrome, had already aired. Since then images of the person with DS have featured adults as well as children. Benetton has had a series of ads; a striking Target ad has been much acclaimed for including, but not highlighting, a young model with Down syndrome; and we have seen a (small) number of models with DS, including the Australian model Madeline Stuart,

of Down syndrome will not result in abortion.[23] In a world where cognition is highly valued, it is hard for people to see intellectual ability as only one among many valuable traits. Two recent stories show that even as people with Down syndrome are more accepted, they also continue to be abused. In one story, a waiter asks an individual who has made rude remarks about a Down syndrome child who is at the restaurant to leave. He is heralded as a hero.[24] In the second story, a policeman seriously manhandles and kills a man with Down syndrome who will not leave a movie theater when ordered to do so by a theater employee.[25] Despite advances made in the past twenty-five years, "retard" today remains a common form of abuse.

There is still another resource question that needs to be addressed. This one concerns the individual and familial emotional resources. Having to raise a child with serious disabilities may be a source of much joy, but, as I already remarked, beyond the additional burdens of care, there is also a great deal of pain. These children are so vulnerable, and many are prone to illness as well. Many of the disabilities that result in intellectual and developmental disabilities are accompanied by medical fragilities. In my daughter's case, her inability to communicate through language means that it is much more difficult to catch an illness in its early stages. It is difficult not to think about the experiences that your child will miss, to worry about her neediness for you or others to survive, much less thrive, to dread dying before she does. Parents—and I suspect, people with disabilities—must frequently call on emotional resources others rarely need. The emotional resources to deal with the many difficulties that are par for the course in the case of serious disabilities, and which cannot easily be mitigated by the diminishment of stigma or material supports provided by the larger society, are among the considerations that make me loath to to attach any moral opprobrium to selecting against disability and to make me strongly oppose any policies that might constrain women from making their own choice, when there is a choice to be made.

In speaking to my son, I wrote:

Perhaps some people shouldn't be parents at all, and some shouldn't be parents to disabled children, at least when that situation can be

who has walked the runway at New York Fashion Week. More people with Down syndrome today are attending their local elementary, middle, and high schools. A vice-presidential nominee brought her DS baby on the campaign trail.

[23] Rayna Rapp (1998), in her study of why pregnant women chose to abort or keep a fetus with a positive diagnosis for DS, recounts how two women went to a group home to help them decide. One then decided to abort, while the other visitor chose to carry the fetus to term.

[24] See Estreich (2013), also Flam (2013).

[25] See Downes (2013). Also see *New York Times* Editorial Board (2013) and Vargas (2013).

foreseen. . . . I have heard parents say that their love for a child was diminished because the child wasn't as smart as they wanted their child
to be. How sad for that child, I think. How much more devastating for
a child not to get the love and the special care that she needs to sustain the illnesses, the pain, the loneliness that . . . [may] accompany a
disability. People who come into our house say Sesha is lucky to have
parents who love her so much. And our standard response is that we are
lucky to have Sesha whom we can love so much. But, in truth, they are
right. . . . To be able to love her so, to find it hard to imagine that anyone
couldn't love her so, is to be touched by a bit of grace, and it has been
our good fortune to be granted that grace. But what would her life be
like if she didn't have people to love her as we do? (2000, 181)

Having said this, I come to a point that may most test our emotional resources:

That, my dear, is the most painful thought—the thought of what
happens to her when we are no longer around. No, these are things
no one has any right to tell a family—no one has a right to say to a
family: You must take this on and if you don't you are immoral, you
don't value a life that is disabled. (2000, 181)

4.5 With Reproductive Selection, "Families Become Like Exclusive Clubs"

Leo's third objection may be stated as follows: When a parent makes a decision
to have an abortion based on certain properties of the fetus, the idea that the
family is a site of unconditional love is thrown into question. In this objection
the expressivist thesis is interpreted not as the message sent to disabled people
nor to society at large, but what would be expressed to existing or future siblings.
   Leo argues that one of two different messages might be received by siblings:

a) The love my parents have for me is a condition of my being mentally and physically sound, not just of being a child of theirs. . . . b) My
parents wouldn't just love any child they might have; they love me because I possess the desirable properties or characteristics that make me
who I am. (2000, 169)

   In either case the choice itself throws into doubt the surety of parental unconditional love: "The family starts to seem more like a club, and less like a family."

In a club, membership is based on meeting certain criteria of selection. If one comes to fall below that mark, membership may be withdrawn, and with it the acceptance that membership brought with it.

Adrienne Asch's critique of prenatal selection directs our attention to a similar sort of message (Asch and Parens 2000). She argues the pernicious message that these technologies send is that some children are not welcome in this world. It is the failure of families to welcome any child that is born that sends such a damaging message to disabled people. For Michael Sandel (2009) it is a failure to be open to the unbidden, to accept a birth of a child as a gift.

Elaborating the idea that "the family starts to seem more like a club, and less like a family," Leo provides two possible messages that he himself might have received if I, his mother, had chosen to abort an impaired fetus. One is a clearly negative message.

1. Had I, while a fetus, been impaired, I would not have seen the light of day. Therefore, I must be wary of losing my intellectual and physical capacities for I might then be rejected as was the impaired fetus.

The second message is more positive, but contains a poison pill that leaves the parent–child relationship feeling equally tenuous:

2. My parents chose me. My intellectual and physical potential and capacities have earned me the love of my parents. But with this affirmation comes the spoiler: Should I have the misfortune to be unable to fulfill this potential or to lose these capacities, I will lose my parents' love.

If we believe that a family ought to be a place where a child feels unconditioned love, then for a child to receive the message that love is conditioned by the possession of certain traits undermines what the parental relationship is at its best. As selective technologies aim to prevent the birth of a child because of certain traits that are targeted, they disturb the notion that when we give birth to a child it is that child we value, and not its particular traits or properties. This is so even when we try to think the traits apart from the child. Therefore Leo's objection—that selective abortion sends a message that the value of a child is conditional upon the possession of certain inherent traits—is impossible to dismiss.

To address the point that selection has a bearing on the constitution and meaning of a family, we need to tackle the broader expressivist objection. In both cases we have to suppose that *a message is sent*. Is there a message that is sent?

At first glance it may seem obvious that the answer is yes. If fetuses that have trisomy 21 are consistently aborted, what else are we to conclude but that Down syndrome is viewed as so undesirable a condition that one is better not to be born than to be alive with it? Yet who is sending a message? Certainly it is not the intention of many, or even most, to send such a message. Women have different motivations for their choices. Perhaps it is the mere availability of these technologies that "sends" the message. Yet even if some interpret the use of these technologies as "sending a message" we still have to ask if a message, an univocal message, has in fact been sent. After all, how one reads the actions or even the words of another is subject to misunderstanding, to misinterpretation. I may count your walking past me without acknowledging me as a sign of disrespect or dislike. But I may be wrong on either count. You may simply be distracted and have failed to see or recognize me. I took you to be sending me a message, but you were doing no such thing. If one wants to stop the "sending" of a putative message when no one has in fact sent such a message, then the remedy is to clear up a misunderstanding, and not necessarily to interdict the action that prompted the miscommunication.

Rayna Rapp's studies provide evidence of women who had experience with DS and even worked in the field of special education, but chose to abort. They understood the value of people with trisomy 21, but their experiences made them feel that they lacked either the material or emotional resources to undertake the job of parenting a child who required the sort of care these children needed. It is, however, more difficult to argue that the cumulative product of all the different and differently motivated decisions fails to have the effect of "sending a message." Still to have the effect of sending a message is different from the message having in fact been sent.

What does it mean to "send a message"? Presumably there needs to be a sender and a receiver, as well as the message communicated. The great linguist Roman Jakobson (1963) pointed out that even more is needed. In addition to a sender and an intended receiver, we need an open channel of communication through which the message is sent (for example the intended message needs to be heard or read), a common code or language that both sender and receiver share, and some context within which the message is understood (for example, knowing that an actor on stage, not an audience member, is shouting "fire"). Should any of these requirements be absent or have misfired, a message might be sent but not received, or received but not sent.

Surely women often decide to abort because they believe that a child with such and such impairment cannot live a good life, or that a life with such an impairment is not worth living. No doubt some women will abort or select against an impairment because they believe that having to raise a child with such a condition will make their own lives hard, and they do not wish to welcome a child who brings this hardship. These decisions can reflect an ignorance about a condition, alterable with better information, and they sometimes reflect a reality—also at times alterable, if for example better supports for families with disabled family members were available. The changed situations would have changed the calculus. The decisions likely reflect the prejudices of the larger society toward people with disabilities, but they do not necessarily "send a message" from individuals making these decisions to anyone at all. If the under-lying attitudes about life with disability were to change very significantly, and a person would choose to abort, say, a fetus with Down syndrome, we would not necessarily say that they didn't value a life with DS—rather we would be puzzled by the decision, or think that the decision to abort might have to do with other circumstances than the finding that the child had Down syndrome.

Rather than worrying about the message sent by selective procedures against disability, it seems to me that we should understand what lies behind these decisions—the attitudes or misconceptions or adverse realities they reflect, and what we need to do to address them. However, expressivists argue that selec-tive procedures do not merely reflect but also contribute to the oppression. But that is like saying that symptoms of a disease contribute to the misery of the disease. True, but it still doesn't mean that in treating the symptom we get at the underlying problem, and treating symptoms alone can sometimes aggravate a condition. Without giving people the means to be the best parents they can be, we should neither legislate nor shame people into having children they are un-willing to raise. Poor communication offers only a poor basis for making moral evaluations.

The effect of parental relationship to the nondisabled sibling is rarely discussed in conjunction with selective reproductive technologies. In my response to my son, the first thing I had to clarify was the difference between the commitment one has to a child already born and a commitment to a fetus. Granted, this is not a moral distinction everyone shares. But for those who insist on a woman's right to an abortion, this is a critical difference.[26] Beyond this, what I learned from my son's correspondence was how little effort our family had put into opening the channel for such an interchange. As I reflected on my son's concerns, I realized that we hadn't had more communication in part because I presumed that the message we were sending to him in raising up our daughter was unequivocal. In loving a daughter who evinced no possibility of achievement in normal terms, the unconditionality of our parental love for both children was, we thought, self-evident. But my son believed instead that he needed to compensate for Sesha's inability to achieve. When Leo was a child of four, he told us that he believed we loved him less because we were so much more affectionate to Sesha. We had

[26] It is a difference that diminishes with the progress of a pregnancy. At the point at which the fetus becomes "my child," the attachment forces upon us a moral commitment. We fail to honor such a moral call only at a very high cost to our emotional well-being and our self-understanding as morally worthy.

to make clear that while we had many ways of expressing our love for him, including engaging him in conversation and doing various things together, affection was the only form of language and one of few forms of interaction we had with Sesha. It appears that we presumed the line of communication was open, that we shared a common code, but we fell short, and messages got mixed.

Leo responded:

> Yes, the lines of communication must be open. And this is incredibly difficult. As open and honest as our family is, only in my twenty-first year have you and Dad and I discussed at any length many of the more painful, difficult aspects of having Sesha in the family. I have not even allowed a healthy dialogue to take place in my own head about Sesha until recently . . . You write that aborting a disabled fetus will convey a harmful message of conditional love to the sibling unless the following condition is met: "If we treat persons with disability with care and respect; if we attend to need when we see it and listen to the voices of those who wish to speak; if we treat all persons as moral equals, irrespective of ability or accomplishment; and if a household reflects this in all that it undertakes, then no child should think that it is valued only for having certain desirable traits." There is only one problem, Mom. No child is consistently under the impression that the above condition [is met]. In fact, no person for that matter thinks that his or her family is always treating him or her in such a way all the time. (2000, 189)

Leo then reveals that although we never aborted an impaired fetus, the very concerns he had about the message sent to the able sibling in the case of selection against disability nonetheless have plagued him in his dealings with us:

> Even though you did not abort Sesha, I remember experiencing every feeling that we have discussed a would-be sibling would go through as a result of a selective abortion. . . . I still managed to feel quite frequently and strongly throughout childhood, and even during many of my most formative moments, that Dad's and your love for me is a condition of my physical and mental abilities. Without these, I often felt, on some level, that I would not command your love and respect.

Our open discussion in these letters, he says, have helped him see wherein the problem lies.

> It was in those moments in my upbringing when I felt treated as more than equal, when I got more attention than Sesha, or alternatively when

I did not feel treated with the same care and respect as Sesha, that my young mind sometimes interpreted Sesha's nonequal treatment in terms of the inequalities and not the equalities. I thought I must have been getting more attention than her because I can do more, or that I was getting less because she needed more. I think to some extent this phenomenon exists between all siblings, even between a child and a parent's career, between a child and the other spouse whenever a parent's energies have to be distributed fairly. Anytime a child feels his status change, he is constantly searching for the cause of the change. Only a completely open line of communication continually sending a message of equally high value to all can truly do away with a mixed message. So, yes, Mom, I think you have hit on the secret of how not to send the wrong message to one's children when one decides to abort. I think it also happens to be a secret of parenting in general. (2000, 193)

4.6   Making the World a More Welcoming Place for People with Disabilities

Degraded messages are being received all the time, by others in our society, by the groups affected, by our children. Once again, I would say that the focus should be less on the message received and more on the conditions that bring us to make our inferences. Speaking of the decision by the North Dakota legislature to outlaw abortions based on disability, Alison Piepmeier, herself the mother of a daughter with Down syndrome and concerned with the high rates of abortion for DS fetuses, responded to parents of DS children who claimed it was a great day to see a state outlaw abortion based on disability. She wrote:

If North Dakota really does want it to be "a great day for babies in North Dakota"[27] and wants to prove that "a civil society does not discriminate against people . . . for their sex or for disability,"[28] it should make the state a welcoming place for people with disabilities . . . The state could take the cash reserves it has put aside for legal challenges to its laws and use those funds to train public schools to be meaningfully inclusive . . . [to] provide easily accessible medical care and early intervention. . . . develop independent—but supported—housing for adults with intellectual disabilities . . . improve criminal justice responses to

[27] See Eligon and Eckholm (2013).
[28] See Ertelt (2013).

rape. . . . Let women have abortions for whatever reason they choose but make it a world they would like to bring a child into—even a child with an intellectual disability. (Piepmeier 2013)

Does this mean that if all were fully informed and if social supports were plentiful and generous, no one would choose to make use of selective technologies?[29] I believe it would not. Some potential parents still would want to avoid all foreseeable hardships, cling to the idea of a "perfect baby," or be incapable of accepting the idea that a life with a significant impairment can be a good life. Some families do view themselves as exclusive clubs and cannot imagine things to be otherwise. Like my son, I view such an attitude to parenting as unfortunate and believe children and society as a whole are better off welcoming whatever children they have. To be able to do so, I believe, makes us more likely to be able to cope with all that is unexpected and untoward as we make our way through parenting's minefields.

---

[29] For a poignant and beautiful account of the reasoning behind such decisions, see Kaposy (2018).

5

How Not to Argue for Selective Reproductive Procedures

The arguments addressed in the previous chapter come from those in the disability community who are wary of selective procedures.[1] As we saw, the most prominent objections are versions of the expressivist objection (EO). To recap, we can say that the EO in its strongest form says that:

> EO (strong): To prevent the birth of a disabled child is to express the view that a disabled life is not worth living.

In its weaker form, it says that:

> EO (weak): To prevent the birth of a disabled child is to perpetuate the stigma of disability or send the message that disabled people are not welcome in this world. (Asch and Parens 2000)

The disabilities that have been at the heart of the controversy we are discussing here are ones that are diagnosed and prevented by technologies such as genetic testing, embryo selection, prenatal testing, and selective abortion. While those arguing from the disability community generally presume the moral questionability of selecting against disability, arguments leveled against not selecting against disability or selecting for ability claim that choosing for disability is morally problematic.

A number of bioethicists who support procreative selection to avoid serious cases of disability have tried to fashion their arguments to be responsive to the

---

[1] This chapter first appeared as an article published in the *Kennedy Institute of Ethics Journal* 27, no. 2, June 2017, 185–215. I owe a major debt of gratitude to Steve Campbell for his tireless attention to this chapter.

expressivist objection.[2] Their arguments acknowledge that the EO has merit and that one ought not to increase the stigma against people with disabilities. Furthermore, they have read the literature demonstrating that people with disabilities believe that their own life is good, and they take the point. They insist that their views do not imply that a disabled life is not worth living and consequently that their views are not subject to the EO. Nonetheless, they insist that prospective parents are obliged to avoid giving birth to a child with a disability when they might have given birth to an able child instead. Their arguments propose that prospective parents ought to select for the best possible child or the child with the better life chances, where "better" or "best" is understood in terms of the child's well-being, although the authors have somewhat different conceptions of what the best child or the better possible life may be. For most, the obligation is a moral one.[3]

I mean to contest the claim that there is a moral obligation on the prospective parent to select *against* disability (or *for* the child that is "the best" among the possible outcomes), *and* that one can make this argument without further stigmatizing disability, that is, without running afoul of the EO, even in its weaker formulation. Among those who promote a version of this claim, Daniel Brock (1995; 2004; 2005) focuses on the sort of harm that results when a prospective parent does not choose against disability, especially "serious disability,"[4] that is, when a prospective parent fails to fulfill a moral obligation to select against serious disability. By aiming his inquiry on the harm, Brock provides the sharpest lens by which to examine whether the moral obligation he claims prospective parents have skirts the objections of the EO. Therefore, I have chosen to focus my critique on Brock's position.

My argument means to show that the objections to selection against disability voiced in various versions of the EO and the views that Brock, in particular, holds with respect to selection against disability are incompatible. The arguments favoring the moral obligation to select against disability make the very assumptions about disability that motivate the EO. This is apparent in Brock's arguments, which already incorporate views that many disabled people reject as false or misleading and are expressive of conscious and unconscious biases that make their lives less good. These include the view that a life with a

[2] The bioethicists include Brock (1995; 2004; 2005); Savulescu (2001); Buchanan (2000); Glover (2006a); Savulescu and Kahane (2009).

[3] However, none, to my knowledge, propose coercive methods to get prospective parents to comply. Instead, they believe that persuasion and argument ought to be employed.

[4] Brock limits himself to what he calls "serious" disabilities, those in which life can still be good but that involve the absence of important capacities. His paradigm cases are blindness and significant intellectual disability.

disability is, ceteris paribus, one with less well-being than a life without this disability, that more capacities necessarily lead to more opportunities for well-being, and the conclusion that prospective parents have a moral obligation to opt for nondisabled over disabled children.

Disabled people, as has repeatedly been shown, do not necessarily regard their lives as bad, and do not see the goodness of their lives as a feature of how many intact capacities they have. Instead they view the goodness of their lives as a function of what they can do and be with the capacities they have, given an environment that is accommodating. Many see measures to avoid giving birth to children with disabilities as sending a message that disabled people are not welcome in this world. Instead they urge us to appreciate how the diversity of bodies and minds adds to the world's richness (Asch and Parens 2000; Garland-Thomson 2012). Insofar as he depends on assumptions many disabled people reject, Brock cannot both argue that there is a moral obligation on the part of the parents to prevent the birth of a disabled child so that an able child might be born in its stead, and claim that he is doing so without running afoul of the EO.

5.1 The Nonperson-Affecting Harm Principle

Brock, though claiming to appreciate the EO and to recognize that a disabled person can have a good life, nonetheless wants us to see that the fact that a child is likely to be disabled, when the disability is a serious one, is a moral reason to prevent its birth if we can give birth to an able child instead. To appeal to our intuitions that a wrong is done when a prospective parent fails to prevent an avoidable birth of a child with a disability (when a "normal child" could be born instead), Brock (2005) presents the following hypothetical example, originally introduced by Derek Parfit (1984, 367). In Brock's telling:

> [A] woman is told by her physician that she should not attempt to become pregnant now because she has a condition that is highly likely to result in serious mental retardation [sic] in her child. Her condition is easily and fully treatable if she takes a quite safe medication for one month. If she takes the medication and delays becoming pregnant for a month, the risk to her child will be eliminated and there is every reason to expect that she will have a normal child. Because the delay would interfere with her vacation travel plans, however, she does not take the medication, gets pregnant now, and gives birth to a child who is seriously retarded [sic]. (2005, 80)

Brock presumes that we can agree that the woman acts wrongly. It is, no doubt, difficult to sympathize with the choice of a woman who prefers to take her vacation rather than attend to her future child's well-being. Brock grants that in more realistic cases a woman might not be morally required to prevent the birth of the disabled child, as there might be morally relevant facts.[5] Nonetheless, he insists that "the question is whether the disability that the child will have constitutes any moral reason at all to prevent it, even if preventing it or not doing so would both be morally permissible," and that the answer, he maintains, is clear: the disability in fact does constitute such a reason. If such a reason exists in this case, then in those cases where there are morally relevant facts that might not require the woman to prevent a preventable disability, the disability will nonetheless constitute a moral reason for doing so.[6]

Brock assumes that a life lived with a serious disability has less opportunity and well-being than one lived without a serious disability, all things considered. I will refer to this as the ceteris paribus assumption. With that assumption in mind, giving birth to the disabled child might appear to wrong the child that was born. But this cannot be right. The reason is found in what Parfit called the nonidentity problem. The nonidentity problem arises because the child who might have been born without the disability is not identical to the child who would be born with the disability—each child would be the product of the unique fusion of two different sets of gametes. Since the child born with the disability was not first a nondisabled child, but a child altogether different than one who would have been born instead, there is no one individual whose situation was made worse by the woman's actions. Since birth bestows on the child a gift of life, and so gives it a far greater good than whatever disadvantage results from a disability (save one that results in early death or is full of unbearable suffering),[7] it appears as if no one was wronged by the actions of the woman in the example. If it is not a wrong suffered by the child that was born, we are left with a conundrum: if no one is wronged, why do we have the strong intuition that the woman has not acted morally? Brock suggests that what is needed to explain the wrong is not a person-affecting harm principle, but a *non*person-affecting

---

[5] A more realistic case presents itself in the face of the Zika virus, which is believed to cause microencephalitis and other effects on the growing brain of the fetus. Consider a woman in her early forties, who believes that now is her last best chance to have a child. She might choose to get pregnant even though she lives in an area infested by a Zika-carrying mosquito. Given her age, and the uncertainty that the infestation will be cleared or a vaccine will be discovered, she has a morally valid reason to try to get pregnant. Many women in Brazil, where the Zika virus has taken hold and where contraception and abortion remain illegal, face just this decision.

[6] Note that Brock insists on claiming that the likely disability of the child constitutes a moral reason, not a prudential or pragmatic reason.

[7] This presumption is not necessarily shared by women who chose to abort based on a diagnosis of an impaired fetus.

harm principle. To explain, he characterizes a nonperson-affecting harm principle (NPA) as follows:

> Individuals are morally required (or have a moral reason) not to let any
> child or other dependent person for whose welfare they are responsible
> experience serious and inadequately compensated harm or loss of ben-
> efit, if they can act so that, without affecting the number of persons who
> will exist and without imposing substantial burdens or costs or loss of
> benefits on themselves or others, no child or other dependent person
> for whose welfare they are responsible will experience serious and inad-
> equately compensated harm or loss of benefit. (2005, 89)

One could be forgiven for finding this statement opaque. It means to say: while
the disabled child who would be born is not harmed (in the sense of being made
worse off by being born),[8] the child with the disability will have a life with less
opportunity and diminished well-being compared to a child that would be born
without the disability.[9] The opacity of the definition may result from the desire
to say at once that bringing into the world another child who does not have the
disability is morally superior, without at the same time implying that there is any
person who would be wronged if the disabled child is born instead—a tricky
position to take, because we still suppose that there must be someone for *whose*
sake the disability should be prevented. But Brock states that the point of the
principle is to establish that we do not need to ask for *whose* sake we should
prevent a harm. Instead he says, we ask, and can answer, for *what* sake the disability should be prevented. The answer, he avers, is that it is "for the sake of
a world with less diminishment of well-being or limitation in opportunity that
the woman should take the medication and wait a month before conceiving"
(2005, 87).[10]

---

[8] There is an ambiguity here: the phrasing of the NPA indicates that he does think that giving
birth to a child with a serious disability would bring into the world someone who will experience "serious and inadequately compensated harm or loss of benefit," although the child is not thereby worse
off. That is because the gift of life is a greater benefit than the serious and inadequately compensated
harm or loss of benefit that results from the disability.

[9] Brock acknowledges that some will argue that "the world would nevertheless be a worse place
without people with disabilities in it" (2005, 88), but he says he believes that even though people
with disabilities have achieved much that is of value to themselves and others, "it remains true that
for the entire class of people who suffer a serious disability it is, on balance, a burden" (2005, 88).

[10] Brock writes:

> Such [NPA] principles reject the assumption or principle that for an action to be wrong,
> it must wrong someone, or that for it to be bad, it must be bad for someone. . . . While
> nonperson-affecting principles in effect reject the need for an answer to the question for

5.2 The Structure of Brock's Argument

Insofar as the claim he makes is not that the *person* born with a disability is worse off by being born (that is, by employing a nonperson-affecting harm principle instead of a person-affecting harm principle), Brock intends to account for the wrong that the woman did without running afoul of the expressivist objections of the disability community. As he puts it:

> As the nonperson-affecting principle stated here makes clear, the action should be done for the sake of less diminishment of well-being or opportunity in the world; our action is aimed at the disease and its bad effects, not at the person who will experience them if it is not prevented. (2005, 87)

One must concede that Brock's argument avoids the strong version of the EO. He avoids saying outright or implying that it is better never to have been born than to have been born disabled, or, stated otherwise, that a disabled life is not worth living. But it is not the case that he avoids weaker versions of the EO. The use of the NPA does not avoid stigmatizing the disabled. Let us now examine the argument in detail. His argument invokes several explicit assumptions and implicit presumptions. The explicit supposition is apparent in his dependence, in one of his premises, on a ceteris paribus clause. We can call this the lesser well-being supposition (LWS):

> LWS: If everything else is equal (that is, ceteris paribus), there are more opportunities and less diminishment of well-being in a life without disabilities than in a life with disabilities.

The importance of more opportunities for what Brock believes to be a better quality of life in turn rests on what we can call additive suppositions (AS). Concerning the lives of individuals, we have:

> i. IAS (for individuals): People have more well-being when they have more capacities to take advantage of opportunities.[11]

whose sake should a disability in cases [such as the example] be prevented, we can answer for *what* sake or reason the disability should be prevented by not creating the child with the disability when a nondisabled child could be created instead. It is for the sake of a world with less diminishment of well-being or limitation in opportunity that the woman should take the medication and wait a month before conceiving. (2005, 88)

[11] He does acknowledge that how we count capacities may perhaps require some adjustments when we consider disability. He appears to accept the argument by Asch and Wasserman that a

And a second supposition aggregates the additive supposition (AAS) for the world:

> ii. AAS (for the world): The world is a better place when there are more opportunities and less diminishment of well-being in it.

We then have two premises:

> (P1) There is less diminishment and there are more opportunities and benefits to be had in a life without disabilities than in a life with disabilities, ceteris paribus (by LWS and AS).

> (P2) The world is better when people have less diminishment of well-being and more opportunities (AAS).

From these we draw the first conclusion of Brock's argument.

> Conclusion 1. The world is a better place when an able child is born than when a disabled child is born.

We need to determine not only if Brock avoids the EO, but also if conclusion 1 is right. When we add the nonperson-affecting harm principle we get premise 3:

> (P3) A wrong is done even if no person is harmed but the universe itself is a worse place (that is, there is "a diminishment of well-being or opportunity in the world") because of this action (by NPA).

P3 in conjunction with P1 and P2 gives us conclusion 2:

> Conclusion 2. Our intuition that the woman in the hypothetical case has done wrong is explained by P1, P2, and P3.

We need to ask if there are any other explanations for our intuitions that the woman does wrong. In conclusion 2, we can see why Brock believes that he skirts the EO. His argument does not hinge on the undesirability of disability *tout court* (that is, he is willing to accept that a disabled life can be a good life), nor is he claiming that the child who would have been born with the disability

---

capacity that *appears* intrinsically good may *in truth* have mostly an instrumental value, a value that can be accessed through other capacities. The aesthetic experience that sight provides may be satisfied through other modalities (Brock 2005).

would have been made worse off by being born. Therefore, Brock believes he can claim that his argument does not add to the stigma of disability, nor stigmatize disabled people per se. Hence Brock's third conclusion:

> Conclusion 3: Using the nonperson-affecting harm principle, one can argue that one ought to prevent the birth of a child with disabilities when a child without the disability could be born instead without running afoul of the expressivist objection.

I have conceded that Brock's argument does avoid the strong version of the EO, but we need to see if it succeeds in avoiding the criticisms of the weaker versions.

Let us then examine his premises. I will only indirectly speak to the NPA. There are cases, as we will see later on in the chapter, where it may be appropriate. Our focus will be on the three premises that speak directly to the question of preventing the birth of children with a disability if a nondisabled child could have been born instead. We will begin with P1 and ask: is it the case that, ceteris paribus, a life without a disability is one that has more well-being in it than a life with a disability, or is this just a prejudice that contributes to the stigmatization of disability? We will then turn to P2 and P3. We ask if we are warranted to claim that *the world is a better place when an able child is born than when a disabled child is born* and that it is a moral wrong if we fail to act according. Or is it the case that we are expressing and reinforcing a mere prejudice against what Elizabeth Barnes (2016) has called "the minority body"? If so, then it seems that we are rehearsing the view that a disabled child is not as welcome in the world as an able child.

5.2.1 The Relative Badness of Disability for a Person Who Would Be Affected (P1)

Brock takes it to be indisputable that disability limits a person in his or her ability to pursue certain important life activities, and that such constraints can be the source of physical and sometimes mental pain or anguish. Relying on the definition of disability that is used in the Americans with Disabilities Act as a "physical or mental impairment that substantially limits at least one major life activity," he writes:

> On this account, a disability is bad for a person, other things being equal, because it reduces the person's abilities or opportunities to pursue major life activities as compared to what they otherwise would

have been, and because it reduces the person's well-being to the extent that it consists in part of successful pursuit of such activities. Serious disabilities tend to make the achievement of some life goals more difficult or less successful. (2005, 72)

The upshot is that disability is "bad for a person, other things being equal." While the nonidentity problem means that we cannot argue that disability is a reason not to bring a child into the world because of the harm to the child herself, we can still pose the counterfactual, asking if that child would have been better off had she been born without the disability. The assertion that this is so is the first premise of the argument, the lesser well-being assumption. There are two aspects to this claim since well-being involves both a subjective feeling of well-being and an objective measure of one's quality of life.

Let us first consider subjective well-being. Since a person who is born with a disability is unable to compare her life with and without the disability (unless of course a "cure" is found), it may be easier to consider the case of an acquired disability. The comedian Richard Pryor developed multiple sclerosis in midlife and was compelled to end his career as one of the most sought-after comics. Yet he remarked in an interview that getting MS "has been a blessing. . . . Because it really made me slow down and think about things," describing his situation as one where "you can't walk the way you're used to, and you have to depend on someone to walk. You have to trust someone to depend on them. To depend on someone—that's been the hardest thing to learn to do" (Gross 2000). He goes on to explain that his life was one where he never trusted, and to learn to trust was what was so wonderful for him. One could respond that the MS was only an instrumental good.[12] Had he learned to trust but not had the MS he would have been better off, and so Brock might be correct, in this instance at least, when he says that disability is "bad for a person, other things being equal." Nonetheless, Pryor viewed himself as being better off with MS than he had been without it, contrary to what a third-person perspective might lead us to believe. Pryor's own description is not just about learning a particular skill that is separable from the whole experience. The trust that he valued came from the very experience of being dependent, a dependency that few other experiences would supply. He talks about himself as someone who has had a transformation.

Laurie Paul speaks of transformative experiences as being epistemologically transformative or personally transformative or both. The epistemic transformation comes from an "experience that gives you new abilities to imagine, recognize and cognitively model future possible experiences of that kind." Pryor's

---

[12] Also see Barnes (2014).

learning to trust and depend on another is just such an epistemic transformation. Furthermore, Paul writes: "A personally transformative experience changes you in some deep and personally fundamental way, for example, by changing your core personal preferences or by changing the way you understand your desires, your defining intrinsic properties or your self-perspective" (2015). After the advent of Pryor's MS, what we see is not the brash, hard-edged comedian, but a softer, more reflective person who is no longer out for fame and fortune, and happy for that very transformation—a transformation of his desires and preferences. This is a profound transformative experience that goes far beyond the learning of a particular skill or bit of knowledge gleaned from an illness that would be of instrumental value only.

Pryor's is but one anecdote. Within the disability community, there are different views about the impact of disability on how well a person's life goes. Ari Ne'eman of the Autistic Self-Advocacy Network (Ne'eman 2013) and Deborah Kent (2000), a woman with congenital blindness, are individuals who insist that their disability is a different, albeit equally good, way of experiencing the world. They and others do not see their disability as a mere lack of capacity, a mere absence (Albrecht and Devlieger 1999; McBryde-Johnson 2003 and 2005; Barnes 2014).

Disability can prompt one to use the capacities they possess for the enjoyment of the same or similar goods and to intensify the experiences we can have.[13] When disability is viewed not as a lack but as an atypicality, it is no longer self-evident that even "serious disabilities" will result in a significant reduction in well-being.

As Brock allows, there is substantial evidence, both quantitative and anecdotal, to suggest that having an impairment is frequently not an obstacle, *in a subjective sense*, to living a satisfying and worthwhile life. But, as well-being has objective measures of a good quality of life as well, Brock believes that these subjective reports should be challenged. We should worry about "the happy slave." This concern is about what is often referred to as "adaptive preference formation," or deformed preferences: preferences that appear to be self-undermining, and which prompt a person to be satisfied with an otherwise unsatisfactory condition. For example, a person may accept poverty and limited opportunities because she believes it is her fate or because she thinks she doesn't deserve anything more. A classic case is the poverty-stricken wife who receives a subpar diet because she eats only when the rest of the family has had its fill. She may herself come to believe she is satisfied while, objectively speaking, she is malnourished.

---

[13] See, for example, Hull (1997).

Disabled people too may be subject to adaptive preference formation. Hence the need for objective criteria of well-being.[14]

Among the objective criteria, Brock lists "accomplishments, personal relations, and self-determination, including having the reasonable set of opportunities that self-determination requires" (2005, 70). These "objective components" are not easy to quantify. Nonetheless, there is no reason to suppose that they are not among the determinants that lead people with disabilities (even the significant disabilities of which Brock speaks) to claim that they have a high quality of life. People with even significant disabilities can—and have—claimed accomplishments, personal relations, and self-determination as part of their own well-lived lives. Still, the opportunities needed for self-determination, personal relations, and accomplishments are very much affected by other objective measures of well-being on which people with disabilities fare poorly.

It is undeniable that the disabled are more likely to live in poverty, to be unemployed, to have fewer marriage opportunities, and to die at an earlier age. But many of the same things may be said of oppressed minority groups. As Brock readily agrees, we cannot claim that we do a wrong by bringing into the world a life that is subject to injustice rather than a life that is one of privilege. Unjust conditions will be reflected in these statistics. Yet we have no sure way of unpacking the injustices from the inherent disadvantages while the injustices remain. Thus, pointing to the higher probability that a nondisabled life will go better than a disabled life, even pointing to a parent's efforts to protect their child from acquiring a disability, cannot easily be untangled from all the issues of injustice to which disabled people are subject and which contribute to the objective measures that we cited.[15]

While a subjective sense of well-being *might* be suspect when one lives under conditions of injustice,[16] having a self-interested preference to live with an impairment even when that impairment is lived in circumstances that are unjust need be no more a form of deformed preferences than my own preference to be a woman even while living under conditions of sexism. We all live our lives knowing about both external constraints and internal limitations. We form our

[14] Steve Campbell has suggested an alternative explanation of disabled people's attitudes: perhaps they (along with many able people) simply disagree with Brock's controversial views about what the objective features of well-being are. There are many people, disabled or abled, who are open to acknowledging a wide range of objective goods but nonetheless reject Brock's view that opportunity is a basic welfare good (Personal communication, January 25, 2017).

[15] Another way one might think through the disadvantage of disability in the absence of ableism is to conceive of other possible worlds where the impairment exists but ableism is vanquished. Cf. Barnes (2014; 2016), who pursues this strategy and concludes that disability is, all things considered, neutral, that is neither an advantage nor a disadvantage.

[16] See Khader (2011b), Sen (1990; 2002), and Nussbaum (2000).

preferences according to these. Although we should not be quiescent about injustice when we can detect it, accepting limitations need not be suspect per se, and there is no reason to doubt the consistent claims of people with disabilities when they express satisfaction with their lives. Disability can involve a reorientation toward life that can be neutral or positive. As such, it can provide benefits that are both subjectively and objectively as good as those made possible using more capacities.

One can go further and remark that to refuse to accept the self-reports of people with disabilities leaves them without a voice. To dismiss these expressions of life satisfaction can be understood as a form of epistemic injustice, namely "testimonial injustice." Testimonial injustice "occurs when prejudice causes a hearer to give a deflated level of credulity to a speaker's word" (Fricker 2007, 9). It appears that it may not be possible to maintain the assumption in the LWS without additionally contributing to the oppressive conditions under which disabled people already live.

One could object that people with a congenital disability lack a basis of comparison, and so questioning the reliability of their subjective evaluation is not a case of testimonial injustice. How are they to know how much better off they would be without their disability? Yet claims of well-being by the people with congenital impairments are often shared by those who have become disabled, and so can compare past and current states. People will at first rue their lost abilities, but not uncommonly will adjust to their new circumstances, and develop different aspirations and abilities.

Brock speculates that the positive evaluations can be explained by three psychological mechanisms: adaptation, coping, and accommodation.[17] What Brock implies here is that this schema can *explain away* the self-reports of life satisfaction. Surely there are psychological alterations we need to make upon losing an ability if we want to live our lives rather than rue our losses. But these psychological mechanisms (or perhaps the nomenclature) do not do the explanatory work he thinks it does, since negative assumptions about disability are already built into the vocabulary. We *adapt* to a worse situation rather than a better one; we *cope* with difficulties, not with new possibilities; we *accommodate* when we must forego what we would have preferred. One could speak instead of "readjusting," "recalibrating," "learning new skills." I doubt there is any way of speaking of serious disability as inherently undesirable without missing the socially constituted disadvantages of a disabling condition, that is, without ignoring unjust circumstances. And, Brock admits,

---

[17] Here he cites Murray (1996).

injustice ought not to constitute a moral reason for not bringing a disabled person into the world.[18]

From the "horizon of ability," it is difficult to imagine an objective state in which a person's disability does not in fact impede the ability to live a good life, and in which a life without that disability would not be better. The difficulty that Brock (and many others) have believing that a person with a disability is genuinely not preoccupied with "the misfortune of being disabled" may be a consequence of systematic predictive errors (Kahneman and Tversky 2000).[19] Predictive errors of this sort can result from either overestimating how much goodness a gain entails, or overestimating the badness that a loss entails. That is, it involves misjudging the objective goodness or badness of both the prior and subsequent states. Thus, an able person is likely to overestimate how bad the loss of a capacity would feel. Even if self-reports of disabled people are accepted as subjective evidence, the able person assumes that the objective badness must still be there and that the disabled person deludes him- or herself about its presence. But the deluded one is more likely the nondisabled person who is in the grip of a common predictive error.

Such a failure of imagination extends beyond the goodness or badness of life with a disability. Although it is a difficult place to go, I will on occasion try to imagine my daughter Sesha, without her disabilities—but my imagination quickly falters.[20] I have no way of knowing which aspects of her personality, appearance, emotional makeup, and so on are ones that she would have without the disability. My child's is a disability she has had since birth. But even in the case of an acquired disability, it is often the case that the disability so shapes an individual's

---

[18] Note that the claim is not that all disadvantages a person might experience from a disability are a consequence of social injustice. It is rather that the entanglement of conditions of impairment and disability with social forms of discrimination and exclusion are such that we cannot isolate any particular disadvantage without also invoking social norms and expectations that impinge on a person's quality of life. An exception is unremitting pain. Shortened life is also an exception. However, life spans for people with many forms of disability have increased, suggesting that not only are medical interventions better, but also that as discrimination lessens, people with disabilities are given more access to medical treatment and forms of care that extend life.

[19] These are also discussed in chapter 3.

[20] Some would reject this thought experiment on the grounds that the disabled person would be a wholly different person—that they not only cannot sort out what aspects of the disabled person would remain in the alternate world, but that that person would simply be a different person. I am disinclined to say this because I believe that a part of a person's identity is relational. So were *my daughter* born without her disabilities or were her disabilities such that shortly after birth the impairments would be repaired, and she would not be disabled, she would in both cases be *the self-same daughter*. However, that element of identity bears but little on either who she would become in the two scenarios or how we might compare how well her life goes.

trajectory that it becomes an integral part of who she is. To imagine what a life like that would be otherwise would be a vain and futile exercise.

This imaginative exercise, however, gives us a clue as to why the thought experiment in which we imagine the same person with and without a disability is problematic. When a person sees their disability as an integral part of their identity, one without which they cannot imagine themselves as themselves, the ceteris paribus clause is not just abstract, it is without content. The proposition "If I were not disabled, I would likely have a better life (all other things being equal)" means nothing if the *I* of the antecedent is distinct from the *I* of the consequent.

One might respond that the sentence "If I hadn't been disabled, then I* (the person I would have been) would have been better off than I am now" is a meaningful sentence. It is true that there may be a possible world in which I* am not disabled and that my life is better than it is now. But there may be many possible worlds in which I* am not better off than I am in the actual world. So, while this gives some meaning to the ceteris paribus condition, it does not decide the question in favor of the supposition (LWS) that a nondisabled life is better than a disabled life, ceteris paribus. The ceteris paribus condition is too abstract to be definitive. Life is so strewn with contingencies that the presence or absence of a disability in an individual's life is still a poor predictor of what would be a better life for that person. The child who is without significant impairments may be born into a family that is not quite as loving, not quite as resourceful, not quite as accepting, as a person with severe impairments. A significantly impaired child blessed with loving parents and a supportive environment, and undaunted by the challenges of her impairment, may flourish and have a wonderful life. Even in case of identical twins, where one develops an impairment in utero or early in life—this is about as close as one gets to the ceteris paribus condition—there is little assurance that the nonimpaired twin will fare better. The nonimpaired twin may marry an abusive spouse while the impaired one has a wonderful happy marriage. As their lives diverge, the impairment is only one of many determinants of life's opportunities for happiness and fulfillment (Wade 2005). The ceteris paribus clause leaves us with an empty abstraction, an idealized condition with little relevance to our nonidealized world. It cannot support the claim that a disabled life, all things considered, is a worse life than an able one.

5.2.2   What About the Additive Suppositions?

If we cannot say that, all things considered, an able life is better than a disabled one, then the claim that a prospective parent has *a moral obligation* to avoid giving birth to a disabled child, when a choice to give birth to an able child exists, loses much of its force. It looks less like a moral imperative and more like a view that has bought into the stigma of disability. But the view that we have such a moral obligation also makes another supposition that, on the face of it, seems undeniable: that *people have more well-being when they have more capacities to take advantage of opportunities* (what I have called IAS).

We can hold on to the view that avoiding the birth of a disabled child is morally preferable if we insist that having more opportunities depends on more capacities, and that therefore more capacities are better than fewer. But the claim that more capacities rather than fewer make a life go better has an empirical component, and the claim has little evidence to support it. If we simply postulate that more is better, then the claim reduces to a tautology. To say that we want as much of a desirable trait as can be had is foolish. Height is desirable, but being 10 feet tall has few advantages that can compensate for the disadvantages. Even great intelligence is desirable only within an acceptable range and when complemented by other capacities. A great intellect devoid of the pro-social attitudes that could keep it in check could devastate humankind along with all living creatures. Prodigious musical gifts can seem more like curses than blessings to the prodigy. Of prodigies, Solomon (2012, 405) writes that "These people have differences so evident as to resemble a birth defect." He cites the pianist Lorin Hollander, who says:

> The giftedness comes equipped with this hell. No one tells you this. The music starts racing faster and faster and faster, and you can't hold on to it. I'd hide after performances. I'd leave stages at the end of a concert with the audience standing and cheering. I'd go out a back door to drown in my shame. (429)

Solomon concludes: "Anyone who has worked with prodigies has seen the wreckage that can ensue when someone is asynchronous, which is the condition of having intellectual, emotional, and physical ages that do not align" (426). Similarly, having many talents can leave one unfocused, so that one doesn't develop any of them fully. Having only one talent can give one a direction in life. One advantage to studying disability is the insight that what is better and worse is not as self-evident as we often think it is.

The outcome of these considerations is that it is not nearly as self-evident as Brock presumes that a life without a disability is, ceteris paribus, a better life than one with a disability. In maintaining the LWS, we fail to give credence to the testimony by disabled people about the goodness of their lives and may perpetuate the prejudicial attitudes toward the disabled that are the target of the EO. Thus far, we see that by incorporating both the IAS and the LWS, Brock utilizes assumptions that run afoul of the EO and contribute to the injustice that disabled people experience.

5.2.3 Preventing Disability for the Sake of a Better World

Recall, however, that Brock does not want to say that we should avoid giving birth to a disabled child because we do that child a wrong. It is for the sake of a better world that Brock believes we have the moral obligation. This is because he thinks it is indisputable that (AAS), a world with more opportunity and less diminishment of well-being is a better world, and that (P1), a world with more disability results in less opportunity and greater diminishment of well-being. Although we have disputed it, let us suppose that P1 is correct. Would it then be the case that a world with more opportunity and less diminishment of well-being, because there is less disability, is a better world?

How should we understand the proposition that the world is a worse place if y rather than x happens, if no one is made worse off by y, as would be the case if P1 were true and a disabled person instead of an able person were born? At least in the case of disability, it is difficult to get one's mind around the idea of a nonperson-affecting harm principle.

To fix our ideas, let us consider the worldwide attempt to eradicate polio. No one believes that the world would be better off with, rather than without, polio; that consensus accounts for part of the success of the program. Polio survivors were active in the disability rights movement's fight for accessibility and inclusion. Yet they have not, as far as I know, protested the worldwide eradication campaign. Nor have they argued that the eradication effort diminishes their worth, nor protested that the diminished number of future survivors will lessen their political clout.[21] With respect to diseases such as polio (as well as other diseases such as smallpox or typhus), the fact that future societies will have fewer victims of these illnesses is not lamented, but celebrated. In these sorts of cases, it is clear what it means to say that the world would be better off without polio (or smallpox or typhus).[22]

But such consensus does not apply to all conditions. People who do not subscribe to what Tobin Siebers (2008) has called "ability ideology" do not think that the world would be a better place without people with Down syndrome. What accounts for the controversy in one case and not in the other?

---

[21] According to the World Health Organization, polio survivors are the largest group of disabled people.

[22] The same may be said for the Zika virus, which attacks the fetus in utero, more or less the same way polio attacks a child sometime after birth. The fetus is an entity prior to, or independent of, the Zika virus.

One response is that ridding the world of future cases of polio does not entail preventing the birth of an individual with polio. It is eradicating a disease, not persons. Brock states that the effect of the NPA allows one to make the distinction between the disease and the person in the same way in other cases of disability, ones that cause "serious disabilities" such as blindness or intellectual disabilities. But it does no such thing. Unlike polio, where one can distinguish the disease that caused it from the person who lives with its disabling effects, this is not in general the case. For example, how is one to distinguish between the condition of a doubling of chromosome 21 (Down syndrome) and the child born with this anomaly? To rid the world of DS means to prevent the birth of DS people or, more drastically, to kill or allow to die those who are born with DS. The case of spina bifida stands midway between the two cases, as it is a congenital condition, and yet it also can be prevented—when women take folic acid during their pregnancy—without preventing the birth of people with the condition. Taking folic acid before and during pregnancy is also beneficial in other ways, helping to reduce the incidence of conditions other than spina bifida. Thus one can at once protest the abortion of a fetus with spina bifida, and yet have no objection to prenatal care that includes folic acid.[23]

The difference in the cases presented is sometimes said to revolve around the reduction of an individual to a singular trait, namely the disabling one (Asch and Wasserman 2005). Selection involving in vitro fertilization (IVF) demonstrates the point more starkly. Excess embryos are routinely discarded in reproduction by IVF, as they cannot all be implanted. Those who oppose selection because it reduces an individual to a single trait are wary of selecting embryos by identifying traits to select against.

But this argument supposes that all disabled people resist identifying themselves via a trait (or cluster of traits). Some couples, such as the lesbian couple Sharon Duchesneau and Candace McCullough (Mundy 2002), have sought out a deaf sperm donor to increase the likelihood that their child would share their genetically based deafness. The case has generated much controversy precisely because the couple wished to select *for* disability. Is the objection to selection based on the view that an individual is reduced to a trait, or that the individual is reduced to a trait that is viewed as undesirable? If that disabling trait serves as a desirable identity, rather than as a misfortune, then those who assume that identity generally do not believe that we benefit the world by preventing the birth of a child with (or because of) such a disability. Many in the deaf community worry about a world in which deafness would be eradicated, seeing such a world as a far

---

[23] Other useful discussions of these points can be found in various writings by disability scholars, especially Asch and Parens (2000), Asch and Wasserman (2005), and Barnes (2014; 2016).

less desirable one, even though most hearing people believe that we should try to eliminate causes of deafness.

Autism is another contested area. Many parents of autistic children would prefer if their children were not autistic and would want to see a world in which autism disappears. But many autists do not share this view. They are not interested in finding "cures" for existing cases of autism, or preventive measures whose sole target is autism, and they would not endorse the view that the world would be a better one if autism were eliminated (Ne'eman 2013).

Insofar as a disability is understood *only* as the occasion for suffering, just as if we think of disability *only* in terms of limitations or an absence of abilities, even those who are not constrained by an ableist ideology might concede that the world would be better without the source of that suffering and limitation. An incapacity or trait that is the source of unremitting severe pain may be such a limiting trait, although this is not the sort of disability that is in question in any of these discussions about the morality of selection.

Are the sorts of *serious* disabilities Brock wants to consider merely sources of suffering and limitations? The two paradigms Brock uses are blindness and cognitive disability.[24] Stephen Kuusisto (2015), author of the blog *Planet of the Blind*, represents his blindness as anything but an absence of capacity. He writes:

> There are landscapes inside us. Introverts know it. Artists see them. When you're blind these lands are persistent and strange: where you've been and where you might go become fanciful. I see the meadow where a little girl played a flute for me when I was four years old. We were in Finland. I was the blind kid who saw only colors and shapes. The meadow was the girl's music; music was sky. I whirled around birches in buttercup light. Whenever I hear a penny whistle I think of yellow air and a yellow girl. Many of my blind friends report the same thing: the spaces before us and the spaces behind are rich and alive within. We navigate by memory and creativity.

Even a seemingly devastating cognitive impairment, such as my daughter's, may allow for an intensity in enjoyment that most of us miss. My daughter's appreciation of music is such that at times she can hardly contain her joy. Would she enjoy it more if she had the intellectual ability to understand exactly how the music is constructed, the form of a sonata, the distinctive lines of a fugue? Perhaps. Or perhaps not. Perhaps that is a different and not inherently superior way of enjoying music. When it comes to the role of music in a flourishing

---

[24] Brock uses the term "mental retardation."

life, as far as I can conceive of a flourishing life, she has at least one element of it in spades. The caveat is that without the appropriate social environment, that capacity might not be recognized or encouraged. She needs me to turn the music on for her. Her flourishing may therefore be more precarious, but it is no less fulsome. The reorientation toward life that so many people with disabilities point to suggests that Brock is wrong to view disability as a mere lack, a mere diminishment of well-being and reduction of opportunities. When the disability is regarded as primarily social, those exempt from the ableist ideology celebrate the diversity that the anomalous condition introduces, and they do not accept that a world with this diversity is a less desirable world.

One can hear the person with the disability in question ask: "Why, if you value me as much as the next person, would you say that one should welcome the nondisabled person instead of me for the sake of a better world?" This is particularly so, because the claim is that what is at stake is a *moral* wrong, even if there is no *person* who would be wronged. This raises an important question, the question of *for whom* is the world a better place if we believe that we ought to select against disability. That world may be preferable for the able, but not for the disabled if they are made to feel unwelcome in it.

The reader may wonder whether I think the world would be better without the disability my daughter has. There is no question in my mind that the world is a better place, a richer place because my daughter inhabits it. Is it a better or worse place than a world in which the child that might have been born in my daughter's place would have been—or a better world than it would have been if the very individual who is my daughter existed but did not have had the impairments she has? The question addles the brain. It might have been better; it might have been worse; it might have been just as good but in different ways. By what criteria is one to judge? Brock asks us to consider well-being and opportunities. But opportunities for what? More opportunities for mischief does not make the world a better place. The opportunities my daughter offers for love, beauty, and delight are as great as any benefits life has to offer. More well-being? If well-being is modeled on the life and capacities of an abstract nondisabled person, then *by definition* the answer is that she has less well-being. But if well-being is determined by the joy one has in life, the extent to which one can appreciate the gifts of life, love, and community, rather than the exercise of more capacities, then my daughter has more well-being (and enhances the well-being of others more) than many with much higher intellectual capabilities and achievements.

Does this mean that I would refuse to opt for a life without intellectual disabilities for my child rather than a life with such disabilities? The best answer I can give is that I would opt for my child, with or without the disabilities, even if her having disabilities would in some way make the world a worse place. Once I make the commitment to a fetus, once this being becomes *my child*, my obligation is to give her the possibility of having the best life she can have with the abilities, talents, interests, and disposition she has. (It is the same obligation any parent has vis-à-vis any child she might have.) The moral grounding of this response derives from a belief that the parental relationship that makes a child *my* child also makes my relationship morally prior to any obligations that might arise because of the child's intrinsic traits or capacities.[25]

Where does this leave us with respect to the question of whether or not we act for the sake of the world when we prevent the birth of a child with a serious disability? The conclusion we can draw is that there are some disabling diseases that the world is better off without. But generally, we cannot separate the disability from the people who have the disability. Thus, to rid the world of the disability we would also have to rid the world of people who might be born with the disability, and we cannot affirm that proposition in the same way we can affirm that the world is better off without disabling diseases such as polio. Nor can we endorse the view that a (potential) parent has a responsibility to the world (rather than to her child) to assure that the world does not have one more child born with a serious disability. And while there may be some diseases that disable (e.g., polio, smallpox) that the inhabitants of the world are better off without, there are other disabilities whose existence introduces important goods and different valuable ways of being that may otherwise be unavailable (Garland-Thomson 2012). Still other disabilities may not make the world a better or a worse place to inhabit. This would suggest that except for the first category of disabilities and diseases (and I do not believe that these track Brock's categories, and then only qualifiedly), Brock is wrong in arguing that the mere fact that a child would be born with a serious disability constitutes a *moral* reason for a parent to act to prevent that birth. Not only is Brock wrong about this claim, but the argument for the claim is such that it makes disabled people feel unwelcome in the world, which is one version of the EO. Once again, the argument has not only not skirted the EO, it has committed the very offense that the EO identifies.

5.2.4 The Woman Who Does Wrong

The arguments so far have cast doubt on the idea that prospective parents have an obligation to select against disability if they can give birth to another able child instead. If that is the case, we throw into doubt conclusion 2, which is an attempt to explain the intuition that the woman in the hypothetical case does

---

[25] There are surely limits to this general proposition. Protecting a child that has committed heinous crimes would be one instance. But meeting the obligations of a disabled child, except in the direst circumstances, would not have such an ill effect on society that it would be morally warranted to put our obligations to society above those that we have to our disabled child.

wrong. It appears that she has not caused the nonperson-affecting harm that Brock attributes to her, because if choosing to avoid the birth of a disabled child rather than an able child is not a person-affecting-harm (as Brock concedes at the start of his argument), then neither is it a nonperson-affecting-harm. Only if the birth of the disabled child brings with it intolerable pain, suffering, and a short life is a harm done, and it is a harm because the child who is born has suffered a harm greater than what is compensated by the gift of life.

If there is no wrong, then how *do* we explain the strong intuition that the woman does wrong? We can note that even if giving birth to a disabled child results in a burden on society, this is not enough to insist that the woman has a moral obligation to avoid the birth of the child. As Hallvard Lillehammer says:

> Individual couples are not normally subject to ethical criticism for not considering the interests of all citizens equally when deciding whether to have children, with whom to have children, how many children to have, and so on. (2009)

Why should a choice to give birth to a child who is likely to be disabled be any different? Censure surrounding procreative decisions is normally directed at a person in her role as a parent, not her role as a citizen. This suggests that the most natural way to understand the intuition is that we believe the woman does wrong by her child. This opprobrium, however, does not withstand the counter from the nonidentity problem. Might it apply to her role as a prospective parent who, we believe, should want the-individual-who-will-be-her-child, *whomever the definite description refers to*, to have the best possibility to live a flourishing life? We can note that the woman seems not only indifferent to how disability will affect the child's life, but she is also oblivious to how her own future as a parent will be affected by her child's disability—a consideration that plays no part in Brock's argument.

The last point directs us to another reason why we think the woman commits a wrong: this woman acts thoughtlessly concerning a matter of much consequence. If a person acts wantonly with respect to weighty matters—procreative decisions, matters impacting the health and welfare of one's child, the special responsibilities of raising a child who will need added care and attention—she fails to act in a virtuous manner and is blameworthy, whether we are concerned about disability or any other condition.[26] Her disregard signifies a lack of respect and consideration for the well-being of all involved, including herself. Our intuitions that there is a moral failure in the case presented does not require

---

[26] Barnes (2014) makes a similar point.

that a harm has been done, but only that someone has failed to act virtuously.[27] Hurrying to an important appointment, I recklessly drive through a red light. As no pedestrian or vehicle crossed my path, I harmed no one. On the contrary, had I waited for the light to turn green, someone might have suffered due to my lateness, and I consequently would have caused more suffering in the world. Nor is it a nonperson-affecting harm. The world was not made worse by my traffic infraction. Yet in recklessly driving through a red light, I failed to act virtuously—as a responsible driver, I ought to have waited for the green light, because if everyone drove recklessly through a stoplight, we would have many more accidents.

Consider the difference in our moral intuitions if the prospective mother (in the example presented at the beginning of this paper) made a conscious decision not to take the medicine, not because she wanted to go on vacation, but because she objected to measures intended to prevent the birth of intellectually disabled children. Imagine that this prospective mother has worked around people with disabilities, including intellectual disabilities, and she has been convinced by the disability critique of selection. She knows that she *could* take the medication, delay the birth, and most likely have a child with normal intelligence. But she also knows what is involved in caring for a child with intellectual disabilities, and the prospect does not frighten her. She has garnered much love and value in her interactions with cognitively disabled people, thinks she has a gift for these relationships, and believes that people with cognitive disabilities add immeasurable worth to the world. She feels that by taking the medication and delaying the birth of a child so that she can avoid giving birth to a child with intellectual disability, she betrays her own repeated and deeply held conviction that all people are equally valuable. She knows not only that a person with intellectual disability is capable of a great deal of well-being, but also that she can promote as much or more well-being for such a child than many others can for a child without this disability.

This prospective mother is aware that most people believe that a life with intellectual disability means a life with limited opportunity. But she reasons that if what is at issue is opportunity, it is opportunity for flourishing that matters. She believes that as long as she does her part and fights for the increased acceptance of intellectually disabled people, her child can have ample opportunity for flourishing. After much careful deliberation, she chooses to forego the treatment. I believe our intuitions that such an action is morally wrong are now significantly undermined. Having accounted for the intuition that the woman does wrong then we can not only conclusively reject conclusion 2, but also see the

---

[27] See Hull (2009) for a discussion of the role of character in making reproductive decisions.

many ways negative and prejudicial views of the lives of disabled people shape Brock's explanation of why the woman did wrong.

This alternative picture of our prospective mother's reasons for making the choice she made is unconventional because most thoughtful women—women who truly care about the well-being of their children—are not likely to forego a treatment that would forestall the likelihood that their child will have a serious disability. It is more demanding to raise a child with a serious disability, and some disabilities come with conditions that involve an increased vulnerability to disease and early death—suffering that is not socially induced. Furthermore, when we think about having and raising a child, we imagine the experiences we valued in our own life or those we wished we had. Indeed, many disabled people who experience their lives as good prefer a child with their own disability, but not a different one. They have normalized their situation and see their own as a desirable way to experience life.

Let us dwell for a moment on the desire for normalcy that seems to underlie the conventional choice to avoid the birth of a disabled child, when an able child could be born in its stead, because this will help us in assessing Brock's third conclusion, that is, whether the use of the NPA skirts the expressivist objection. When Brock argues that making this choice is the moral thing to do, he argues for this claim because he believes that it is better to choose in favor of the child that has the best chance of having a good quality of life. This, in turn, he defines as a life with the most well-being. But he is interested only in avoiding the birth of a disabled child whom he presumes is comparatively disadvantaged compared to a nondisabled child. That is, he places a cap on the aspirations for a better child (a child with a better chance for well-being) at normalcy.[28] On Brock's view, intentionally giving birth to a disabled child—that is, one who falls below "normal," when the alternative for an able child is available—triggers the suspicion that a harm has been done. But optimizing the able child's chances carries no moral obligation. "Normal" as a floor may have many uses, especially when morbidity and mortality are concerned, but to insist on such a norm as a condition for birth, on the grounds of a nonperson-affecting harm principle, is highly problematic. As Savulescu and Kahane (2009) point out, the norm reinstates the prejudicial attitude that Brock is attempting to avoid.[29] It is one

---

[28] The point remains unchanged whether we think of normalcy as the species norm or a statistical norm.

[29] Savulescu and Kahane (2009) also believe that people have a moral obligation to avoid giving birth to a disabled child when an able child can be born in its stead. But they invoke what they call a principle of procreative beneficence, which maintains that prospective parents have a moral obligation to have the best child possible. Unlike Brock, they do not cap the aspiration at the level of normalcy, for the reasons given here.

thing to say of any individual that she is better off, ceteris paribus, if resources are directed to restore her "normal functioning" or "normal health"—although what counts as "normal" and the extent to which "normal" is necessary or desirable are all contested questions. But it is quite another thing to say that producing an individual who would not meet a standard of normalcy is a harm and that his or her place in the universe should be taken by another who meets the norm. If that is not effectively to say that the disabled do not have a right to be in the world, it is surely to say that their right is subordinate to the right of a nondisabled person to be in the world. If we hold on to that view, we can support a lot of policies that subordinate the rights of disabled people to those of the able, particularly when we are making arguments from the perspective of scarcity. This is not a conclusion that Brock wants to endorse, and it surely is a worry of those who object to procreative selection against disability, that is, to those who have put forward the expressivist objection. It now looks like one cannot make a claim that the NPA principle allows one to argue for procreative selection against disability (even in the restrictive way that Brock does) without running afoul of the expressivist objection, if only in its weaker formulations.

5.3　How Not to Argue: Hypotheticals, Idealizations, and Thought Experiments

In constructing his arguments, Brock makes ample use of a favorite philosophical tool, the hypothetical case. What are hypotheticals meant to accomplish? They are meant to single out a conundrum under discussion (e.g., the nonidentity problem). They are constructed to ignore the messy nature of real-life questions. And they are used to test our intuitions and root out prejudice by presenting the problem in an unfamiliar context. That, at least, is the intent, and sometimes their use can be illuminating. Hypotheticals strip down the problem to features that we think require our consideration. While doing so, we may omit those features that offer better or truer insights. In the thought experiment that Brock borrows from Parfit, we conclude that giving birth to a disabled child is bad when the problem is that the woman is being thoughtless about a matter of great importance. The prejudices that the cases are meant to root out get reinscribed surreptitiously either because we omit aspects of the problem that would direct our intuitions differently—omissions we make because our prejudices limit what we think is relevant—or because they enter as presuppositions we fail to notice. In the example at issue, rather than test our intuitions about the wrongness of not preventing disability, the narrative portrays the person who makes this decision in a decidedly negative light by *already* supposing the badness of disability.

Another form of the hypothetical that plays a big role in the argument is the comparison of the hypothetical of a life lived without disability and the life (actual or hypothetical) lived with a disability. These are arguments using the ceteris paribus condition. When hypotheticals create idealizations bearing no resemblance to reality, they can confound our intuitions, rather than sharpen them. In the comparison of a hypothetical of a life lived with and without a disability, we are meant to judge two outcomes as if everything but the disability could be held constant. The absurdity of the comparison is that in reality, the outcome of a life is determined less by the capacities one has than by what one does with those one has. And what one can do with the capacities one has depends very much on the availability of needed social supports and material resources. That is, the different outcomes of the disabled and nondisabled life have less to do with the number of capacities one has and more to do with concrete social, political, and economic conditions. These idealizations give us no purchase on the different outcomes.[30]

What can we learn from the "what if" comparisons in the face of unknown and unrealized capacities, uncertain circumstances in any life, and the many ways people develop these capacities in situations in which they find themselves? Given an idealized comparison of a future child about whom we know that she will have a disability (with its putative disadvantages) and another child about whom we cannot predict what disadvantages are in her future, the nondisabled child will win out every time. The very unreality and abstract nature of the hypothetical comparison, just as in the case of the underdescribed thought experiment, is supposed to sharpen our intuitions. But, as Alfred North Whitehead wrote: "An abstraction is nothing else than the omission of part of the truth. The abstraction is well-founded when the conclusions drawn from it are not vitiated by the omitted truth" (1938, 138). The information that would be necessary to weigh the desirability of the two possible lives is omitted and the conclusions of the hypothetical comparisons and the thought experiments are "vitiated by the omitted truth." Clarity and truth have come apart. Worse still, they reinforce preexisting prejudices. With the hypotheticals, we weave spider webs to follow the

[30] Donald Davidson, the premier analytic philosopher of our time and himself the author of a very famous thought experiment (the Swamp Man who is created out of the chemical reactions of the swamp and emerges a fully formed adult), said, at a talk much later in his life, that he thought that we should abandon the use of such hypotheticals, that we can't explore our intuitions based on them because we actually don't know what the examples mean. I grant that the examples and hypotheticals used in these discussions are not as outlandish as the Swamp Man example. The fact is that although there are many disabled and able people in the world, which makes us think we know what we are talking about when we make the ceteris paribus comparisons, I hope I have shown how the ceteris paribus comparisons are in fact not reliable ways of testing our intuitions.

threads of our arguments. But the threads are too delicate to bear the weight of the numerous and contingent realities that are givens in the real world.

5.4 Conclusion

One need not deny that disability can make the possibility of flourishing more precarious, that disability makes one especially dependent on conditions being amenable to one's flourishing. But such added precariousness comes not only from disability. A child born to a despised minority, a female child born in a highly sexist society, a child born during difficult economic times, and so many additional circumstances contribute to such precariousness. That such difficulties exist, and that the life of someone with disabilities is more precarious, does not give us a moral reason to prevent bringing a disabled child into the world. We would not say that we are morally obliged not to bring a daughter into a sexist world or a child from a despised minority into a world where the child is likely to endure discrimination.

A parent might reasonably select *against* disability, or *for* disability, or refuse to select *at all*. There are reasons one can give for any of these choices. *How* one argues for one's position, however, can be morally fraught.

Brock's third conclusion is unwarranted. His argument that disability can serve as a moral reason for selecting against disability runs afoul of the expressivist objection when it accepts the view that disability is inherently bad for a person, when it fails to give full credence to the view held by people with disabilities that their lives are not worse because of the impairment itself, and when it holds that bringing a disabled child into the world results in a world that is a worse place than one where an able child is born instead. Writers sensitive to the expressivist objection should abandon this way of arguing in favor of selecting against disability. These views are backed up neither by empirical evidence nor by sound argument. What they do is express the view that disabled lives are lesser lives and that disabled people are less welcome into the world.

Addendum: Mother's Choice

The conclusion I have argued for in chapter 5 is not that it is either permissible or impermissible to select against disability, only that there are some ways that we ought not to argue in favor of selection against disability. Arguments favoring giving birth to a baby without a disabling impairment because this child will have a better life than a child with the disability are problematic, because in the end they amount to the view that the lives of disabled people are inherently suboptimal. Such claims are unacceptable to most all disabled people and should be unacceptable to all of us whether or not we are disabled.

The position I argued for in chapter 4, that is, in my letters to my son, is the position I continue to hold after these many years. The argument against selection is compelling, but it starts at a point that is too early in the procreative process. If we accept a woman's right to choose whether or not to continue a pregnancy, then what matters is accepting the child that is born, not the embryo or fetus that is conceived.

Those who affirm the liberal value of equality have to affirm that people of all varieties have an equal right to be in the world. What is at issue in the case of reproductive selection, however, is whether all have an equal right to *come into* the world. Any right to come into the world rubs up against the right of the prospective mother to decide if she wants to bear, much less rear, this individual— an enormous commitment that lasts a lifetime. In a liberal society we generally believe that short of egregious behavior (and we allow all people, including those who are convicted of felonies, to reproduce), people have a right to procreate or not. Such procreative autonomy is expansive but is not absolute. As we know all too well from abortion debates, once we argue that the fetus is a person endowed with the same fundamental rights as the woman carrying the fetus, the determination of rights is no longer simply the question of the sole right of the prospective mother to decide. The question of abortion then becomes the question of what rights take priority. Judith Jarvis Thomson attempted to settle this question by arguing that even if the fetus is a person, the pregnant woman is not obliged to accept the burden of subjecting her body to a nine-month pregnancy.[1]

But procreative decisions are essentially relational. Onora O'Neill wisely states that "ideals of individual or personal autonomy . . . are unpromising starting points for thinking about reproduction" (2002, 61), because in the case of reproduction a third party is brought into existence.[2] O'Neill is surely right that there ought to be limits to procreative freedom. However, the third party is not simply an individual in his or her own right (which he or she certainly is) but one also utterly dependent on a parental relationship. If one takes the relationship itself as another stance from which to examine the procreative decisions, then procreative autonomy is not so much limited as it is enlarged to include consideration of that relationship. One could say that what I am arguing for is procreative *relational* autonomy.

I think that the real import of the Thomson thought experiment, however, is that without a relationship to a second person who needs to use your body for their ends, that second individual has no claim to the use of your body. Once there is a relationship and once a relationship is acknowledged, the moral landscape shifts. The relationship depends on the woman's will, on her body, and on her affectional, caring labor. Therefore, the first question for the pregnant mother is whether she is willing to acknowledge and affirm a relationship to an incipient being.

If we take into account the relationship, there are then three rather than two standpoints to consider (setting aside an impartialist benevolence emphasized by utilitarians): the parents' (especially the mother's) procreative rights, the rights of the resulting child, and the relationship between the parent (especially the mother) to the child-to-be, with all its attendant responsibilities. To discount the relationship of the mother to the child does violence to the relationship upon which all other relationships are based. In matters of reproduction, respecting a woman's right to determine the uses to which she lends her body includes respecting the presence or absence of a relationship between the woman and the fetus. It must be the woman's decision to endorse or reject that relationship. Are the arguments for or against procreative selection sufficiently morally decisive that coercion in either direction is justified? Given the extensive debates we have surveyed, the answer is "no." There is no socially effective, noncoercive, and morally sanctioned way in which to insist that a mother select for or against a child

---

[1] Her famous example envisions a person who is kidnapped and hooked up to a dying violinist for nine months so that the violinist might live. The analogy depends on the fact that the person who is hooked up did not consent to the arrangement and was even unconscious when attached. The analogy with a pregnant woman and the fetus is not only that the pregnancy was unintended, but also that the woman did nothing that would lead her to believe that a pregnancy was a possible outcome.

[2] This, she argues, puts a constraint on the autonomy of adults in procreation (O'Neill 2002).

depending on the likelihood of a disability. To do so positions the procreating woman as lesser than others; she is deprived of the status of a moral equal. Thus, in the end, either choice, when a choice is possible, must be hers.

What I have argued for does not preclude the need of society to offer education that will inform a prospective mother's choices. Furthermore, insisting on the right of the mother to choose does not preclude discerning the moral propriety of one choice rather than another—but it will depend on why and how the woman makes her decisions, how thoughtfully and wisely she reflects, given the circumstances in which she finds herself. A couple who chooses to abort a fetus likely to be born with Down syndrome because they already have a disabled child and cannot see their way to having multiple children with disabilities, and a deaf couple who wishes to choose to preimplant an embryo likely to produce a deaf child so that their child may be part of a rich community and culture—these are two examples that will irk people with different attitudes toward disability and selective procedures. But I believe all will agree that procreative freedom does not include the right of a woman to purposely take a medication to have a disabled child—say because she thinks she can use the child as a beggar to bring in heftier handouts than a "normal" child[3]—or, in a different scenario, to get a sympathetic response if she chooses to abort the fetus. Such instrumental attitudes toward the outcome of a pregnancy are always morally reprehensible.[4]

There is reason enough to believe that people with disabilities can have fully flourishing lives, lives no less flourishing than those without disabilities. However, people with disabilities may encounter medical or social conditions

[3] See Mistry (1996), where he describes the actions of some adults who have children in their care whom they maim so that the children can be more profitable as beggars. The movie *Slum Dog Millionaire* portrays a similar situation.

[4] This last point introduces a consideration raised by Lawrence Becker in a personal communication. He writes: "In deciding whether such selection is permissible, we should consider whether having (or adopting) an infant without the disability (for example, deafness), and then deliberately giving him that disability would—or would not—be a case of child abuse—criminal child abuse. If we do that thought experiment, surely we will reject selecting *for* disability. This is not a science fiction hypothetical. People have deliberately crippled children so that they could become better beggars." My response is that the thought experiment supposes that there is an obvious symmetry between the goodness or badness of having a disability and of causing a disability. That symmetry is not in fact obvious, as Barnes (2014) so astutely argues. Furthermore, I have argued not that one can *never* make a moral judgment about selection (*for* or *against* disability), but that such a judgment depends on the reasons a parent has for making that decision. No doubt, choosing an embryo that is likely to develop into a deaf child because such a child would make a better beggar than a hearing child is morally blameworthy. The decision was not made for the sake of that child, but reflects a fully instrumental attitude toward the child. Thus the thought experiment fails to capture the moral import of choosing for disability when, say, a deaf parent decides to choose a congenitally deaf procreative partner because she would welcome a child who will share her own valued identity as a member of the deaf community.

that make their flourishing rather precarious. Of course, the ability of anyone to achieve and sustain a flourishing life is precarious and contingent. For people with disabilities, however, some of these contingencies work against them with more regularity and greater force than for most nondisabled people. Hence the work that parents take on to foster the flourishing of one's child is more demanding when disabilities are in the picture.

Parents have an extraordinary responsibility when they choose to give birth to any child. They have a still greater responsibility to consider whether they are willing and able to meet the demands of fostering a flourishing life of a child with a disability. No one ought to shame, blame, or in any way coerce a woman into taking these responsibilities. Nor should anyone shame or blame the mother (or parent) who decides to give birth to a child that she has good reason to believe will be disabled, as long as she is committed to fostering that child's ability to flourish.

Although most who are engaged in the discussion argue whether or not one should give birth to a child who will have a disability, I have emphasized the concern with the difficulties and additional responsibilities that disability will frequently bring to the parent. A lucid assessment of these responsibilities is often most available to the disabled woman giving birth to a child with the same disability. Prospective parents must also assess their ability to be a good (enough) parent and live a good (enough) life together with their child and any other children they may have. One may think of this as akin to the question of whether one is prepared to adopt a child with disabilities if these are known beforehand. (Sarah Ruddick remarked once that all parents are effectively adoptive parents whether they adopt or give birth, since becoming a parent means affirming the choice to raise a child.)[5]

Some parents, even in the face of the option of prenatal diagnosis and selective abortion, have determined to bring a pregnancy to term regardless of the outcome of such testing or have chosen to forego the testing altogether. It was the choice my son and his wife made. I, however, did consider prenatal testing when I was pregnant with a third child. I worried that I might not have sufficient time to care and attend to the needs of two "special needs" children and devote myself to work that gives me an important measure of fulfillment. Needless to say, we may well underestimate our ability or willingness to deal with the fact that our child is born with a disability. It never occurred to me that I may be a good mother to a child with a significant disability, and yet I have cherished my life with Sesha. But I doubted whether I would have the wherewithal to raise two children with disabilities. Today I meet parents who have more than one disabled child, who

---

[5] In an interview recorded on disks available at http://rockethics.psu.edu/education/oral-history-feminist-philosophers.

have been as grateful to have these children in their lives as I have been to have my daughter. Nor have they have felt defeated or lost their zest for life. This may well have described me had I had two children with disabilities.

In many ways, none of us are able to properly assess our ability to parent a child with a disability, unless perhaps we ourselves possess the same disability. We may be wrong in our self-assessment, but it is as important to examine ourselves in this regard as it is with any other circumstance regarding parenthood. Would I want to parent without a partner? Are my current financial circumstances suitable for a family? Do I want a child with *this* partner? Do I want *another* child? Can I handle parenthood *now*? Needless to say, assess as we may, after the child is born our financial situation may change drastically, or the marriage fails, or we get pregnant again and can't bring ourselves to either abort or put the child up for adoption. Similarly, our child may *become* disabled, or we may learn of an unsuspected disability. As we remarked at the outset of part II, Lady Luck is still with us, and this is not always a bad thing. With the resilience to reassess and recalibrate, most can heed what Janet Lyons said to her bewildered husband, Michael Bérubé, upon the birth of their son Jamie: "We can handle this" (Bérubé 1998).

PART III

CARE IN PHILOSOPHY, DISABILITY, AND ETHICS

Man is a bundle of relations, a knot of roots, whose flower and fruitage is the world.

—Ralph Waldo Emerson

Overview: The Lessons of Care

Part II concluded that because each human infant is born utterly dependent and in need of the care of a mothering person, the individual who bears and who is principally responsible for the care of the child must be the one to decide about procreative matters. Care is central to the question of reproductive rights because the fate of dependent persons hangs on the question of care: who does the caring, how the caring is done, and how the ethical responsibilities and obligations inherent in taking on care are assigned and carried out. To the extent that the lives of people with disabilities are more precarious, they may be more dependent on care for more of their lives. It is particularly critical to have an ethics of care that meets the genuine needs and legitimate wants of people with disabilities in ways that preserve dignity and recognize the equal personhood of all engaged in the caring relationships.

In part III, I shall attempt to make the case that our human dependency demands that we have an ethics of care that is adequate to address dependency needs without diminishing carer or cared-for. What I present here is not to be understood as offering a complete ethic of care. Nor is it my intention to argue that an ethic of care is necessarily a complete ethics. Whether or not an ethic of care is a complete free-standing ethics or a part of a larger ethical theory remains, in my view, still undetermined. What I do believe is that an ethics of care introduces sui generis concerns, concepts, and values that are either absent or underdeveloped in current ethical theories. As such, it is a unique contribution to ethical theory. Moreover, it is a contribution that is of special relevance and importance in the lives of people with disabilities and their families. Still more important and pertinent to the goal of explicating what I have learned from my disabled daughter is that when we make an ethics of care accountable and relevant to people with disabilities, we strengthen and amplify the contribution of a feminist way to conceive of moral obligation.

It may appear obvious that care ought to have a place in the construction of a good and ethical life. Yet care is not a concept that has been much developed in philosophical thought. The idea that there is an ethics of care distinct from other ethical perspectives (especially those centered on the virtue of justice) was introduced by the psychologist Carol Gilligan (1982) as an account of a development trajectory exhibited mostly by girls and women. But an ethics of care is more than an ethic that describes the moral perspective of many women. I have come to see an ethics of care as exactly the moral philosophy needed to deal with inevitable dependency and to include disabled people, their families, and carers fully within the scope of ethical inquiry.

Scholars of disability do not always embrace issues of care, and sometimes prefer to speak of an ethics that centers instead on rights. Rights discourse, especially when focused on negative rights of liberty from interference, generally presupposes agents who are independent, fully functioning, and rational, that is, those who can make rights claims on each other. But rights included in lists of "human rights" need not be seen as the converse of care. The rights of many individuals (especially positive rights such as the right to food, shelter, and affinitive relationships, for example) are realized only through the caring work of others. Fully dependent human beings, such as my own daughter, realize their right to food only if there are caring others who provide food and assist with feeding. An adult quadriplegic can realize his rights to mobility and employment only if he is assisted by a personal care attendant. Since we all experience periods in our lives when we are dependent on the care of others, we all rely on care to realize our rights at some time in our lives.

Answering needs in a way that diminishes those who need care is rightly disparaged, as when persons, institutions, and the state answer what they take to be needs but run roughshod over the agency of dependent and disabled people. Such care, I argue, is not care in a fully normative sense. Care in the fully normative sense is care as it ought to be practiced if it is to do what care is supposed to do.[1] It is prescriptive, not merely descriptive of the way things are presently done. The point of care is not only to address needs. That is the means to an end. The end itself is to promote the flourishing of the cared-for.

If we take that end as an ultimate value, then it is a value for everyone, the carer as well as the cared for. Thus care, practiced in a way that conforms to the value care promotes, requires that the carer is able to care for the other without herself suffering neglect, exploitation, or abuse. Furthermore, care in a fully normative sense needs to be exercised in a way that it does not preclude others outside the caring dyad from receiving it. It may be impossible to ascertain if one's caring actions toward another avoid all negative ramifications for the care of another, but one can act so as to avoid that sort of harm to the extent that it is foreseeable.

I use the orthographic feature of small caps, CARE, to indicate this philosophical use of the term, and an ETHICS OF CARE, to distinguish this conception from the more general concept of an ethic of care.[2] This conception of care and an ethics of care will be developed in chapters 7 and 8. In these preliminary remarks, I want to propose that a fully normative conception of care is guided by regulative ideals, that is, ideals that we cannot fully realize but for which we should strive nonetheless. A fully normative conception of care, CARE, is grounded in the flourishing of all parties, carer and cared-for alike, and is commensurate with the flourishing of others outside the caring relation. One way to capture this notion is to say that CARE respects and addresses the *genuine needs* and *legitimate wants* of another, particularly when that other individual is someone who

---

[1] A recent book (Collins 2015) provides a different view of the normativity of care.

[2] I will at times want to use "care" in its more general sense. Sometimes that use comes very close to CARE. I will use the normal fonts for times when I would not specifically refer to care in its fully normative sense. I will reserve small caps only for the times I am using the term strictly in the philosophical use I give to it. I speak of an *ethics* of care or a care ethics when I am speaking of a theory that I, along with other feminist philosophers, am articulating. I speak of an *ethic* of care when I am not specifically speaking of a moral theory of care, but of a general orientation towards care in ethical encounters. I reserve the term an ETHICS OF CARE for the theory that employs the idea of a fully normative conception of care, CARE.

is permanently or temporarily inevitably dependent—that is, dependent due to biological facts that are not simply the outcome of social structures and prejudices.[3] I have said that care meets needs and wants, particularly of persons who must depend on others to meet these demands to survive and thrive. I speak of *genuine needs*, by which I mean those needs that, if not attended to, will cause harm or impede the flourishing of the one in need. Because I believe that care does and should address desires that may not be as urgent or pressing as needs, but are still important to allow a person to flourish, I include *wants*, specifically *legitimate wants*,[4] by which I mean wants that the cared-for should be able to satisfy without harming others.[5] To help another to flourish is, as I understand it, to promote an individual's good, as that good *is seen through the perspective of the one cared for*.[6] Here I summarize the definitions and principles that provide the regulative ideals characterizing the conception of care ethics that I will argue for in the chapters that follow:

[3] I speak of wants as well as needs to avoid limiting our understanding of care to the provision of a core set of goods that are minimally necessary for survival, or at best, a basic level of well-being. Needs are also often assumed to be objectively determined. Wants are more clearly subjective. They are things which persons believe or feel are important to them, or good for them, whether or not they are goods that others want. Those who are significantly dependent on care have as much call on the satisfaction of their wants as those who can satisfy important wants through their own efforts. I speak of needs and wants understood from the perspective of the cared-for, because the carer can have an understanding of the good for that individual, an understanding that may be rational but which fails to take account of what is most important to the cared-for (see discussion in chapter 8).

[4] I speak of *legitimate* wants because not all wants, or even felt needs when they are less than *genuine* needs, are compatible with living in a just and caring society. Perverse needs and extravagant wants that come at the expense of harming others are not morally acceptable in an ethic that cares about care. (See chapter 7, section 7.2.6, for a discussion of harm in an ETHICS OF CARE.) Notice that the constraints I am invoking are moral ones. What others might think are irrational wants can still be legitimate wants, as long as satisfying them will not involve harming others. Rawls imagines "someone whose only pleasure is to count blades of grass in various geometrically shaped areas such as park squares and well-trimmed lawns" (Rawls 1971, 432). We may view this as irrational, but as long as it does no harm, it can be a legitimate want for that individual.

[5] Except perhaps under a condition of very scarce resources and great hardships, genuine needs ought to be able to be satisfied without harming others and so are always already "legitimate." Some may claim to have felt "needs" that could lead to harm. For example, a person may claim that he "needs" a form of abusive sexual conduct. But such felt needs, despite their felt sense of urgency, are better thought of as *wants*. Therefore, the expression: "genuine needs and legitimate wants" seems to capture both the needed constraints and the important priorities of the cared-for to which carers ought to be responsive. I thank Richard Rubin for helping me find a phrase that is as concise as possible and still captures the concepts I want reflected in the phrase.

[6] On this understanding, flourishing has both an objective and a subjective component. For something to be a good, it may objectively be (or be commonly understood to be) a good, but

Definition 1. The *telos* of caring practices is the flourishing of those who are in need of care.

Definition 2. Those who are in need of care are those who will be harmed if care is not provided.

Principle 1. The *regulative ideals* of care are to provide care by assisting those who require care
 a. in meeting the genuine needs (that is, needs that have both an objective and a subjective basis).
 b. in meeting the legitimate wants (that is, wants that can be satisfied without thwarting another's possibility to receive the care another—including the carer—may require).

Principle 2. The flourishing of those in need of care has to be a flourishing *as endorsed (implicitly or explicitly) by the one cared for.*

My aim in part III is partially to envision a conception of care and an ethic that both people with disabilities and those who do caring labor can embrace. An ethic that is founded on CARE and the regulative ideals of an ETHIC OF CARE, I hope, will fit this bill. In the hope of accomplishing this mission, I develop my vision of an ethics of care in the following four chapters.

In the first of these, I call upon what I have come to understand of dependency from the years of living and caring for Sesha. Dependency, I now see, is not only a condition borne of her impairment, but an inevitable feature of the human condition. Most parents care for an utterly dependent being for a relatively short time. As the child develops skills and can move on, parents tend to forget that early period and revisit it only at times of illness, when a child or adult might need total care. I was able to live with my daughter's utter dependency over many, many years. That length of time gave me an opportunity to think about dependency and the role it plays in all of our lives. In chapter 6, I will discuss dependency, especially when considered in the context of disability.

---

it should also be good for the person concerned. While the idea of endorsement is often understood as a rational validation by the individual concerned, I mean it in a weaker sense. If one appears to others and to oneself as thriving when having this good, then one has implicitly endorsed it as one's own good. The question of whether something is a good for that individual is harder to answer if the good in question is not also understood as a good by seemingly objective criteria.

Although I believe that an ethic of care is or should infuse all aspects of life, it is *existentially* crucial in the care of someone as vulnerable and dependent as my daughter. Without care she would perish in a matter of days, just as a newborn infant would. Without good care she could not have a life in which she might thrive at all. Watching both skilled and less capable caregivers to whom I have entrusted the care of my daughter, I have come to what I believe to be critical characteristics of care that are the mark of CARE. Thus, in chapter 7, I put forward what I take to be the outlines of an ETHICS OF CARE as it has emerged both from feminist philosophy and from my experiences with my daughter.

Seeing how much care my daughter requires and the impact on her caregivers has led me not only to think of the obligations others have to caregivers but also to consider what can go wrong in the nested dependencies in which care is embedded. The person who does the work of care poorly may give preference to her own interests and desires, even when that is detrimental to her charge. She may be inattentive, unmindful, or neglectful, or she might exert her dominance over a vulnerable individual. Not only negligent or abusive behavior, but even good intentions borne of the carer's own needs and desires to be helpful, to do what she is sure is good for the cared-for even if the cared-for has good reason to reject these ministrations, can interfere with the care that is genuinely needed. The asymmetries in power between caregiver and cared-for easily, but not inevitably, lend themselves to abuses and failures of care. Such failures are "temptations" (Ruddick, 1989, 30) of care. Against these, the concept of CARE allows us to see that the question for a care ethic is how to prevent power from turning into domination, and instead make that power enriching to cared-for and carer alike.

My daughter's dependency, her evident incapacity to reciprocate in kind, and her inability to speak (and so express her response to our care verbally) allowed me to dismiss the idea that the reception of care is, as Bernice Fischer and Joan Tronto (1990) say, "a stage of care." Nel Noddings (1984) speaks of the completion of care in the other. When I had to care for my ailing elderly mother, who so often refused my care, I came to recognize that my daughter was in fact highly responsive to our care: that she did indeed complete our care. (In this case, I have come to see how easily one can draw the *wrong* lesson from the particularity of a caring experience, one that was corrected when observing other cases of care.) I have now come to believe that this completion is crucial to identifying a fully normative conception of care and, as such, inseparable from developing an ETHICS OF CARE. In my discussion of an ethic of care chapter 8, I incorporate the import of my daughter's tutoring on the completion of care.

In the final chapter, chapter 9, I put the ethics of care to work on a particular controversy surrounding a standard of care of people who are severely cognitively impaired and nonambulatory. The intervention has come to be known as "the Ashley treatment," after the combination of treatments used to keep Ashley X small so that she would be easier to care for, and so stay in the bosom of her family. I pose the question of whether the Ashley treatment is good care, understanding care as a value in an ETHICS OF CARE, for people with severe cognitive disabilities, and I answer in the negative. At the same time, the case illustrates the potential overreach in construing the self as relational and the need to understand the separation of individual selves as well as their connection.

Considerations of the Ashley treatment prompted me to think about the value and integrity of my daughter's body. Part III ends with a meditation that aspires to validate the importance of the body in coming to know another: its unique shape and form, its movements, its feel. Paradoxically perhaps, I come closest to an understanding of what a soul is when I am with the body of my daughter.

‖ 6 ‖

Dependency and Disability

6.1 Introduction: Dependency—Avoidable or Inevitable?

I first came to reflect on the question of dependency when I was thinking about equality.[1] The aspiration of equality has remained elusive for women. Early second-wave feminist work spoke disparagingly of women's dependency on men and women's quest for equality: liberation was freedom from such dependency. With the struggle for women's equality, many legal and social barriers have fallen. Even the emotional dependency, about which Simone de Beauvoir spoke so poignantly,[2] has ebbed as women's work and sexual opportunities have expanded. However, still today, women do not share the world with men in equality. The residual dependency, as I have argued elsewhere and as empirical studies bear out,[3] is largely due to the fact that women remain the caregivers to dependents. Having to address the needs of individuals who cannot fend for themselves leaves women *derivatively dependent,* unable to compete as equals in the workplace, and still dependent on the affections of a man, or the hard-to-come-by largesse of the state, for the resources necessary to support themselves and their dependents adequately.

Seeing dependency writ large through the extended and extreme dependency of my daughter, I have come to understand that while much dependency is socially constructed, independence is no less socially constructed. Moreover, Sesha's dependency has not been merely a burden or a problem; it has been the occasion for a particular sort of interaction, and a particular sort of closeness. This extreme dependency sheds light on the dependency we all experience

---

[1] Much of this chapter is included in Adams and Reuss (2015).
[2] See especially the chapter "The Woman in Love" (Beauvoir 1953).
[3] See Kittay (1999); ADAPT (2007).

at some time in our life. It ranks among the most cherished of my daughter's lessons.

Yet to conceive of dependency in these terms is to swim against the tides of the very social movements I embrace. Not only have women insisted on independence and rejected all forms of dependency, disabled people make independence a central demand in staking out their transformative social movement.[4] Writers such as Michael Oliver have maintained that dependency itself is central to the fact that disability is experienced "as a particular kind of social problem" (1989, 8). As such, it has shaped the social life of people with disabilities (Barton 1989). Against this position, other disability scholars have instead insisted that what undermines the ability of disabled people to flourish is insistence on self-sufficiency and self-reliance as not only a norm but also *the* desideratum for persons in a liberal society. These scholars have urged that acknowledging our dependency helps reshape our understanding and experience of both ability and disability (Shakespeare and Watson 2001; 2006; 2014; Weicht 2010).

The rejection of dependency by groups struggling for their full measure of rights is not entirely surprising given the stigmatized status that dependency has. This stigma is vividly on display in recent US history, especially with the rise of neoliberalism. The term is the anathema of the conservative right and is used as a battering ram to knock down the welfare state. Ronald Reagan coined the memorable term "welfare queen" as a way to discredit women who depend on government cash subsidies to support themselves and their children. But dependency is not beloved by liberals either: witness Senator Patrick Moynihan's description of dependency as "an incomplete state in life: normal in the child, abnormal in the adult." He wrote: "In a world where completed men and women stand on their own feet, persons who are dependent—as the buried imagery of the word denotes—hang" (Moynihan 1973, 17). The term "dependency" gained currency again in the 1997 debates on "welfare reform." "Welfare dependency" was the bugaboo of liberals and conservatives alike. Again in 2012, the failed presidential candidate Mitt Romney called 47 percent of the US population "dependent"—a remark widely perceived as sufficiently derisive of a vast swath of the electorate to have a decisive impact on his subsequently failed presidential bid.

If we step back, we well might ask why humans, who belong to a thoroughly social species, so despise dependency. Care, knowledge, culture, technology, and political, social, and economic goods—the sine qua non of human life in any era—are possible only because we can and must depend on others. None would be possible if humans were entirely self-sufficient and did not have

---

[4] See Kittay (2007) for a discussion of this tension.

organized systems that are based on our dependence on others. A reliance on government services counts as a primary advantage of a modern, relatively well-ordered state. We might as well decry our dependence on air.

6.2 The Registers of Dependency

There are historical, ideological, and structural reasons why we so often refuse to acknowledge our dependency. In a work on the keywords in the US welfare state, philosopher Nancy Fraser and historian Linda Gordon (1994) trace a "genealogy of dependence." Moynihan and Romney both suppose independence to be the natural state, at least for adults, and dependency to be evidence of a flawed character. Fraser and Gordon remind us that independence was once a status reserved for elites who could command the services of others, and only later became a status assumed by the many. With the emergence of wage labor, the spread of political enfranchisement, and the lessened importance of birth-based status, independence came with the ability to earn a living sufficient to support oneself and one's family. Women were precluded from economic independence by laws and conventions; paupers by their inability to become waged laborers; colonials by political constraints. Women's dependence on men, understood by feminists such as de Beauvoir to be a constraint that women internalized, needed to be overcome if women were to be liberated from male domination.

With the development of the welfare state in the United States, this internalized, now characterological feature of women was simultaneously encouraged and applauded in white middle-class women—who were *supposed to be* dependent on "their man"—and deplored in black women and other lower-status women, who were expected to labor no less than men (Solinger 2002). Women who depended on state welfare services were (and continue to be) thought to have a moral or psychological flaw, one shared by anyone in need of welfare services or otherwise excluded from independent status. Dependency itself now becomes stigmatized. Welfare dependency supposedly bespeaks laziness or deficient internalized cultural values; emotional dependency is thought to displays weakness; chemical dependency is seen as evidence of the lack of willpower.

Interestingly, disability as a source of dependency does not figure in Fraser and Gordon's account. In identifying four registers of dependency—economic, political, sociolegal, and characterological—Fraser and Gordon overlook situations in which dependence on another to obtain the necessities for life is tied to inevitable biologically based limitations. It is a fact that humans all have a period of extended dependency at the beginning of life, and during recurrent periods, such as when they are injured or ill or too frail to fend for themselves.

Therefore, to Fraser and Gordon's four registers, we add a fifth: *the register of inevitable human dependency*. While there are some sorts of inevitability we dread, such as death, most inevitable conditions we accept and meet with resilience. The need for food is inevitable, but we accept it as a condition of our lives. This inevitable need becomes the site of cultural identity, family warmth, artistry, and sociality. Dependency in the fifth register may not always be palatable. But neither must it always be undesirable. Nonetheless, we find a moral or psychological stigma attached to inevitable dependency no less than to other forms of dependency, with the possible exception of infancy.

No decent society fails to take some responsibility to meet (even if inadequately) needs of those who find themselves inevitably dependent. And just as inevitably, in each society there are others who must tend to these needs. These *dependency workers* may be family or paid caregivers or attendants. They may be privately provided, or state supplied. As their efforts and attention are used in the service of another's needs and wants, they are less able to attend to their own needs and to act as independent agents, becoming (as I pointed out earlier) *derivatively dependent* (Fineman 1995; Kittay 1999). This is especially so when they are unpaid family members.[5] Taking into account the fifth register reveals first of all that *dependency is not always socially constructed*. But it reveals more.

Meeting human needs arising from inevitable human dependency is a sufficiently complex undertaking, involving a good deal of time and material resources; when the dependency is very significant, it requires a division of labor. Those responsible for providing the resources to meet these needs, the *provisioners*, are often thought of as independent. Those who do the hands-on caring labor, the dependency workers, become derivatively dependent—dependent on someone who can provide the resources needed to sustain them and the dependent for whom they care. The caregivers have not only needs for their own sustenance, but they acquire a second set of needs, those of their dependents.[6] Some prefer to speak of the *interdependence* of all involved in the complex of dependency (Arneil 2009; Fine and Glendinning 2005). There is much to be said for emphasizing interdependence—especially what I want to call *inextricable* human interdependence. However, there remain some ways in which we are simply dependent and unable to respond to others' needs or to reciprocate another's care. And that dependency too is part of a normal human life lived intertwined with others.

---

[5] Data from the 1982–93 National Longitudinal Survey of Youth shows women experience a wage penalty of 7 percent per child (Budig and England 2001). For a more recent review of the literature see Glynn (2014).

[6] Katharine Wolfe (2016) calls these "second-person needs."

The paradigmatic occupant of the fifth register is the child. Young children's dependency is universal and a feature of the evolutionary process that has produced the particular species that we are. Children, especially when very young, are not stigmatized for their dependency, but because infancy and childhood serve as the paradigm for inevitable dependency, adults who are similarly dependent are seen as childlike. They are infantilized, viewed as incompetent, asexual, "cute," "in their second childhood," and presumed to be proper objects of paternalistic concern. These offensive responses to adult dependency can be traced to both emotional terror and conceptual error. We see adults in a dependent state and are reminded of our own vulnerability. We refuse to acknowledge that they are like us and we are like them, and that we, like them, can be thrown without a moment's notice into a state of dependency.

Beyond this common response to disability of any sort, there is a conceptual confusion at play. The mistake is related to the conceptual error in which we attribute to all members of a class the characteristics of the paradigm of that class. If the paradigm of dependency is the child, then all who are dependent are childlike. But taking all the features of the paradigm to be attributable to all members of a class is simply a mistake. Robins are paradigmatic birds, and penguins are also birds. Yet it would be a serious mistake to treat a penguin as if it were our red-breasted friend. Even features that the two species share can have different roles in the lives of the two birds. Both robins and penguins need their wings for mobility, but those of the robin are as useless in water as the penguin's wings are in air. Infants, people like my daughter, and patients with more advanced Alzheimer's disease are dependent on others to be fed, but what they eat, appropriate ways to feed them, and their response to being fed are as different as wings on robins and penguins.

Still, the conceptual confusion is persistent. In our modern industrial and postindustrial world, where independence is construed as the mark of adulthood, it is difficult for many to acknowledge that dependency may be a permanent feature of a life, and that dependency can recur (to various degrees and in different ways) throughout our lives, so that we are always vulnerable to once again becoming fully dependent.

Tobin Siebers remarked that "disability makes a scene."[7] In our unwillingness to embrace the inevitability of dependency and our vulnerability to disability, we either cloak these in invisibility, or stigmatize them by making them hyper-visible. The independence that modern society values in the "hale and hearty" worker comes at a cost. The underside of a society that places supreme

---

[7] This appeared in a description of a course offered at the University of Minnesota, called Disability and Design. He writes there: "Regardless of the model, disability makes a scene; it punctuates normative structures vividly." The point is also made in Siebers (2010).

value on the fully functioning, independent adult worker is the stigmatized and infantilized disabled individual.

6.3 The Construction of Independence

To counter both the image of the disabled person as an infantilized object of paternalistic concern and the supposition that dependency is necessarily and simply an inherent characteristic, disability scholars and activists countered the narrative of the *inevitability of dependency for disabled people* with a counternarrative (Lindemann 2001): people with impairments were *made dependent*, just as they were *dis*abled, by a social environment not accommodated to their bodies. With the appropriate accommodations and personal assistants who would be under their direction, disabled people could live *independently*. Judy Heumann, an early American champion of "independent living," promotes independence as "a mind process not contingent upon a normal body" (Heumann 1977).

The counternarrative depends on a shift from an understanding of independence as self-*sufficiency* to one of independence as self-*determination* (Young 2002, 45). This shift is found in the Independent Living Movement (ILM). In the United States, it culminated in the passage of the Americans with Disabilities Act (1990) and the Individuals with Disabilities Education Act (2004). The Independent Living Movement was founded in the late 1960s and early 1970s in the United States and then spread to other nations. Its early founders were relatively young, and their disabilities were physical (De Jong 1983). They called for accessibility in transportation, living arrangements, education, employment, and inclusion in social and familial life to allow them the measure of control over their circumstances comparable to those without physical disabilities.

Sorting out the different senses of independence promoted by the ILM has not always been easy, even for the disabled individual himself. As medical sociologist and disability rights activist Irving Zola writes:

> The important thing was that I got there under my own steam, physically independent and mainstreamed. But the price I paid was a high one . . . I, for far too long, contributed to the demise of my own social and psychological independence. (1988, 14–15)

Getting to some place under his "own steam" left him physically spent when he arrived, and so less able to perform the task that was important to him. Instead, he discovered, the independence to which he aspired was "the quality of life that [he] . . . could live *with help*" (De Jong 1983, 15; Zola 1988; emphasis mine).

Taking their cue from other civil rights movements, which fought against a privileged class that gained its material advantage by oppressing another group, the British Council of Disabled People, which identified itself as "the UK's national organisation of the worldwide Disabled People's Movement" or BCODP, wrote:

> However good passivity and the creation of dependency may be for the careers of service providers, it is bad news for disabled people and the public purse. It is a viewpoint which meets with strong resistance in our organization. (BCODP 1987, sect. 3.1, 5)

The rejection of dependency also hinges on the view that dependency set the disabled apart from the able population.

This counternarrative redefined independence as including "the vast networks of assistance and provision that make modern life possible" (Davis 2007, 4).[8] Then, as literary and disability scholar Lennard Davis says, "the seeming state of exception of disability turns out to be the unexceptional state of existence" (2007, 4). The call for independence has promoted the interests and improved the life prospects of people with physical and sensory disabilities, and it has successfully been expanded to include some with cognitive disabilities. Davis's attempt to assimilate the assistance disabled people need into the "networks of assistance and provision" of modern life has much to commend it. I believe, however, that there is still more to be said for unmasking the fiction of independence and self-reliance.

As long as we maintain the fiction, then those who are most disadvantaged when dependency needs go unmet will remain marginal members of society; public access to care and assistance will remain miserly, and the full participation and integration of people with disabilities will be hampered. Beyond this, the applicability of "independent living" may be limited. While the BCODP derides the idea that disabled people need to be "looked after," some people with disabilities and frailties do indeed require looking after. Surely we should give all people as much self-determination and control over their lives as possible. But some impairments affect the capacity for self-determination, just as some impairments affect mobility or sensory perception.

---

[8] One might say that these social dependencies, no less than the biologically based dependencies, are *inevitable*. The distinction I would make is to say that while the vast number of social dependencies are inevitable as a disjunctive set, it is unlikely that any particular one is inevitable. Even in an urban setting, it might be possible to grow our own food, for example. But as we add more needs and wants, it is increasingly unlikely that they all can be supported without our being dependent and interdependent.

Another problem with arguments for independence is that they are often tied to the idea that allowing disabled people to be independent ultimately saves public expenditures. The idea is that the provisions sought for independent living are less costly than residential placement. Moreover, with assistance, disabled people can become productive members of society, thus repaying the costs of the needed services and making important material contributions. While these utilitarian arguments strategically counter the image of disabled people as "burdens" on society, they feed the sentiment that the public should not have to be responsible for dependents who cannot pay their own way. Not only does this view disadvantage those least able to fend for themselves, shifting the cost and care to struggling families, but it also is liable to hurt those whose ability to be self-determining requires increased, not reduced, expenditures. Relatedly, arguments that bind independence to productivity are useful insofar as most people desire meaningful work. But for some, no amount of accommodation can make this possible. Where the expectation for work falls on those for whom it is impossible, meaningless tasks take the place of more fulfilling activity.[9] It is an especially punishing view for those whose capacities for productive labor diminish with age (Morris 2004; 2011).

Finally, the demand for independence for disabled people relies heavily on the availability and compliance of caregivers. But there is a danger in the claim that "independence" is achieved by engaging personal assistants. Might not the supposition that the disabled person is "independent" render the assistant invisible and effectively subordinate his (or more often her) status and interests to the disabled person she serves? These are questions I pursue in the sections that follow.

A consideration of dependency forces the question: can one still protect the benefits to be gained by disabled people's demands for independence without restigmatizing those who do not benefit? Can we accept the inevitability of dependency without denying the negative effects of an *imposed* dependency on the lives of many disabled people? And can we accept reliance on dependency workers without subordinating their interests to those of the disabled person?

---

[9] Also see Taylor (2004), who writes: "To ensure that employers are able to squeeze surplus value out of disabled workers, thousands are forced into dead-end and segregated jobs and legally paid below minimum wage (for example, in the case of 'sheltered workshops' for those with developmental disabilities). The condescension toward the workers in such environments is severe. Why should working be considered so essential that disabled people are allowed to be taken advantage of, and, moreover, expected to be grateful for such an 'opportunity'?"

6.4 The Cares of Dependency

Fraser and Gordon were interested in excavating the different registers of dependency that emerge in *historical* contexts, thereby revealing the extent to which dependency is socially constructed. Such a genealogical approach, *pace* Foucault, while valuable, misses the more transhistorical and biologically inevitable dependency of infancy, early childhood, disease, and significant impairment. Although inevitable dependencies are inflected by historical, economic, and cultural properties—for instance different cultural, historical, and economic systems mark the end of childhood dependency differently—they are not socially constructed through and through.

We need to come to grips with the ease with which dependency comes to be despised and stigmatized, particularly within an ideology shaped by the image of the independent citizen and amplified when other forms of dependency take on a characterological aspect. Recall Patrick Moynihan's warning that adults who are dependent "hang." The sense of dangling on a thread, of being at another's mercy, of a noose about to tighten, is what frightens us so at the thought of dependency, and no matter how forcefully we argue that dependency is inevitable and universal, unless we can address these worries, we will fail to move beyond the stigma and the terror.

What then are these concerns? When one is dependent, one cannot meet important needs and wants oneself. Those important needs, wants, and desires are the things that we have to have satisfied or we will fail to survive or thrive. They are the things we care about. As Harry Frankfurt convincingly points out, "the formation of a person's will is most fundamentally a matter of his coming to care about certain things" (1988, 91).

Departing somewhat from ordinary language (but not as much as first appears), I will call the things one cares about (including the things one requires in order to have the things one cares about) one's *cares*. Again, appealing to Frankfurt, we can, I believe, motivate this usage:

> A person who cares about something ... identifies himself with what he cares about in the sense that he makes himself vulnerable to losses and susceptible to benefits depending upon whether what he cares about is diminished or enhanced. He thus concerns himself with what concerns it, giving particular attention to such things and directing his behavior accordingly. (83)

As I have before, I will use an orthographic device to signal this usage: CARES. Using the term in this way helps us to see the inherent connection between an ethic of care and the fact of human dependency. The connection unfolds as follows: If I care *about* you, I have some concern for the things that are important to you, at least to the extent that these things are important for your flourishing. That is, *I care about your* CARES, and if you cannot attend to these yourself, I will do what I can to help you flourish.[10] That is, I will care *for* you. If I care *for* you, I attend to the things that you care about, or that are the conditions for you to engage in what you care about. Your cares become my second-person CARES.[11] When we cannot attend to our CARES on our own, we are dependent on others.[12]

6.4.1 Properties of the Relation of Dependency

Dependency is a relation, and relations have formal properties whose analysis can be very illuminating.[13] I should note here that when I speak of relations, I am speaking not of particular relationships. *Relationships* (as I am using the term) refer to specific connections of individuals that stand in relation to one another. *Relations* are the abstract roles or positions that individuals can occupy as *relata*. The analysis of the relation of dependency that I provide here is structural and abstract. What a *relationship* between actual individuals looks like is constrained, at least in part, by the structural features of the *relation*.

Dependency, as I have spoken of it, is a relation with at least three relata: the dependent individual (the *cared-for*), the assisting person (the *carer* or *caregiver*), and the things that the cared-for person cares about (the CARES). Often there are at least one or two more relata: *provisioners* and *goods*. *Goods* are provisions which are needed to address the CARES of the cared-for—that

---

[10] See definition 1 in part III, "Overview".

[11] The CARES that are of this sort are commensurate with what Katharine Wolfe calls second-person needs (2016), needs that we have because we care about another person having their needs met. It is tempting to adopt this terminology, but I want to hold on to the term CARES, which signifies not only needs but also important wants and desires. But it is helpful to adopt the attribution of a second-person relation to these CARES.

[12] Notice we may *choose* to engage another's help or assistance to meet needs or wants, and so become dependent on others. We may fail to learn the skills we need to meet our own needs, and the resulting dependency can become of vital importance for our survival or flourishing. Doing so is often the prerogative of the privileged. But these dependencies—although they pervade our lives—lack the force, and often the stigma, of inevitable dependency.

[13] The analysis of relations is explored in set theory. Relations have certain properties: they may or may not be symmetrical, reflexive (or self-identical), and transitive. For example, the property of "greater than" is asymmetrical, nonidentical, and transitive (if a>b and b>c then a>c), while the property of "equal to" is symmetrical, reflexive, and transitive. A reader who is less concerned with the fine points in the argument may wish to skip over the more technical parts of this section.

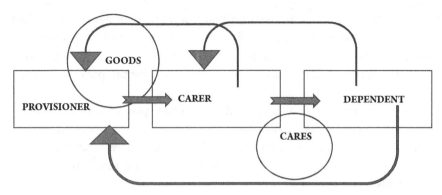

Figure 6.1 The Structure of Dependency: the thin lined arrows indicate the order of dependency, and the thick lined arrows indicate the direction of goods as they move to address the cares of dependents.

is, to meet the genuine needs and legitimate wants of the individual being cared for. They include provisions to meet the needs of the carers to sustain themselves and to care properly for those for whom they are responsible. *Provisioners* are those who are responsible for ensuring that the goods are made available. If the only obstacle to our tending to our CARES is an inability to obtain the goods we need for that purpose, then we are dependent only on a provisioner. (A child in her early teenage years is often in this position.) If we also need another to tend to our CARES—that is, one whose *caring labor* is required to makes use of the goods or services provided—then we are dependent on a carer. Carers cook the food for the elderly woman who can no longer prepare food for herself. They feed the disabled person who cannot feed herself. Many forms of inevitable dependency require both provisioner and carer. See Figure 6.1.

We need to remark that the discussion here is an abstraction of real caring relationships. We speak here as if the dependent, carer, provisioner are each a singular individual. In reality, a parent will often have many dependents; a dependent is often dependent on several caregivers; provisioners are often multiple, having tasks that are distinct or redundant. Real caring relationships need not be, and often are not, one-to-one. The abstraction is used only to extract some formal features of dependency relations.

If we collapse for the moment the relations the dependent bears to both provisioner and carer, and confine ourselves to the formal properties of the binary relation of dependency (the relation between the dependent and the provisioner/carer), we get an insight into some reasons that dependents find dependency to be a difficult condition to bear. The relation of dependency is *asymmetrical*, that is, the dependent depends on the carer/provisioner and the carer/

provisioner does not reciprocate the dependency; the relation is *nonidentical* (or *nonreflexive*), that is, the dependent is not the same individual as the carer/provisioner;[14] and it is *transitive*, that is, the dependent is not only dependent on the provisioner/carer, but is also dependent on whomever the provisioner/carer depends on.

As these formal relations are unfolded, we see the places where dependency is potentially oppressive. But we can also see how dependency can contrast with isolation rather than independence. Carol Gilligan,[15] citing studies in which high-school girls contrast dependence with isolation rather than with independence, writes:

> As the word "dependence" connotes the experience of relationship, this shift in the implied opposite of dependence indicates how the valence of relationship changes when connection with others is experienced as an impediment to autonomy or independence, and when it is experienced as a source of comfort and pleasure, and a protection against isolation. (1987, 14)

The nonreflexivity of dependency means that when dependent we need others; dependence stands in contrast to isolation. The asymmetry means that dependencies always involve us with others in relationships in which some have the ability to extend or withhold their assistance. The relationship has either the valence of connection or impediment to autonomy. The more powerful figure can either use that power to assist or to dominate. Furthermore, a willing carer may find herself incapable of providing the needed care because the provisioner on whom *she* must depend has not discharged her responsibilities (*transitivity*). A willing provisioner may fail to provide, because the others on whom *she* depends have failed *her* (transitivity). The properties of the dependency relation—that it is asymmetrical, nonidentical, and transitive—also mean that dependencies can be (and usually are) *nested* in other dependent relations. This sort of nesting reveals the chain of dependencies and interdependencies that allow societies to function and be well ordered. But the failures also mean that the dependent may be left with CARES that are not addressed. Note that these are *conceptual* and not historically conditioned features of dependency.

---

[14] Surely, we are all dependent on ourselves in some sense. But this sense of dependency is parasitic on the primary sense of dependency in a nonidentical relation.

[15] Gilligan cites two definitions of dependency offered by high-school girls she studied. One arises "from the opposition between dependence and independence, and the other from the opposition of dependence to isolation" (1987, 31–2).

When we seek independence, we try to assert a control over our fate, one that is always elusive. The more our relationships are symmetrical, the more power we have to constrain those with whom we are in an interdependent relationship, holding in check their ability or willingness either to harm us or to withhold what we need or desire. In an asymmetrical relationship, we are secure only as long as the other *chooses* to provide for us and to care about our CARES. And the asymmetry leaves us with a debt of gratitude that we may be unable to repay. Not only do we remain vulnerable, but the sense that we cannot repay a debt of gratitude gnaws at our pride and sense of equal worth.

Such asymmetry is also part of the human condition. We are not always equally situated and equally empowered. Our powerlessness in the face of the forces over which we have little control, and our need to unite with others who are willing to work in concert or provide asymmetrical care when necessary, re-quire humans to develop relationships of trust, to create systems of entitlements that make assistance and access predictable, and to form affective bonds that mo-tivate others to take our CARES as their own and that enjoin us to take another's CARES as ours. To say that we care about each other is to say that what matters to the other becomes our own CARES—our SECOND-PERSON CARES: we care that the other's CARES are addressed. The emotional connection or moral commit-ment we have to one needing care leads us to regard the other's CARES as legiti-mate demands on us. Nel Noddings puts it this way:

> When I look and think about how I am when I care, I realize that there
> is invariably this displacement of interest from my own reality to the re-
> ality of the other ... when the other's reality becomes a real possibility
> for me, I care. (1984, 13)

We hope to gain the trust of the dependent so that their sense of vulnera-bility is not overwhelming, and so that their indebtedness does not erode their self-esteem. For emotional bonding to take place, we need an emotional open-ness on the part of all parties. For trust to be instilled, we need trustworthy ac-tors. For a caring attitude to be present, we need parties that embody a robust ethic of care. And to give legitimacy to the CARES of the cared-for, for persons in need to not be diminished by their need, the cared-for and the carer require the backing and support of social institutions. Thus, while the vulnerabilities of the dependent in a relationship of dependency are multiple, unfortunate outcomes are not inevitable if the dependency is managed in the right ways, by the right individuals, with the right moral and emotional commitments, backed by appro-priate institutional supports.

6.4.2 Dependency as a Relationship

Dependency is not only a relation; it is also a relation*ship*. As a relationship it may be thicker or thinner. Thick relationships have value beyond the care (or goods) that the provisioner/carer provides. Such relationships are less fungible than thin relationships; that is, it is not only the care or assistance that matters, it also matters *who* provides that help. When relationships are thick and are successful, the dependency relationship *itself*, in excess of the assistance provided, is a reward for both parties. But with such thick relationships, a dependent has much to lose if a provisioner/carer disappoints: the dependent loses not only the needed assistance, but also a valued relationship. Similarly, the carer is especially vulnerable in a thick relationship when her efforts to care fall short or are rejected. Thicker relationships inspire greater trust, but eventuate in greater betrayal of trust when they fail.

One way to reduce the dependency and the threat of loss is to keep relations of dependency thin, so that if one person fails us, their role can be taken by another. When the provisioner/carer is fungible, the dependent has a greater sense of control and independence—but these come at the expense of the relationship, the full recognition of the labor and the value of the carer/provisioner, and the deepening of trust and trustworthiness. The trade-off is nonetheless preferable in some situations. Some in the disability community prefer more formalized relationships, preferring the term "personal assistant" rather than "caregiver" (which embodies the thick relational concept of a "gift" or "giving").

If we turn our attention to the needs and concerns in virtue of which the dependent is dependent (the CARES of the dependent), then we can understand another difficulty inherent in dependency. If we depend on another for something that has little importance to us, the deprivation doesn't count for much. It is when we *care* about things or people that we become truly vulnerable and dependent. It is important to keep in mind that a disability can bring in its wake a reordering of the things we care about. As I have stressed in previous chapters, we become aware of the malleability of human desire and capacities; we acquire the wisdom to explore new means of fulfillment. We need others who can take our new CARES to be significant; who will, at best, take the needs that arise from the new concerns and treat those needs as CARES they want to attend to, and who can (at the very least) regard these new concerns as worthy of their respect.

In part III's "Overview", I presented the idea of a fully normative conception of care, which I designated as CARE. What CARE requires is that carers/provisioners respect others' legitimate wants and genuine needs as CARES that need attention (Principle 1). Such care, then, will respect the viewpoint of the one needing care (Principle 2). The sort of care that was cited in the writings of Michael Oliver and the BCODP cannot be CARE. The complaints launched by Oliver and the BCODP indicate a failure of the provisioner, in this case the state, to take up the CARES of people with disabilities, *as the disabled understand them*. Instead, the provisioner's *own* view of what the provisions *ought to be* is substituted. The constructed dependency that disabled people decry is often of this sort.

In such constructed dependency, we can identify a "learned helplessness," the passivity that the BCODP decries. Learned helplessness is a psychological concept describing a passivity induced by an individual's repeated failure to control one's environment in aversive conditions (Nolen 2014). In the context of care, learned helplessness is the repeated failure of the provisioner/carer to be responsive to a person's CARES. Once again we see how a failure of genuine care in the face of dependency becomes the source of a loss—this time a loss of self-esteem. It is worth stressing that while the structure of dependency contains the possibility for such a miscarriage of care, such loss is not necessarily a consequence of dependency. Indeed, as I will shortly discuss, acknowledging one's need for care in some areas can allow one to better manage other needs.

6.5 Independence and the Personal Attendant

Because my daughter Sesha is totally dependent, and I have worked in academia all my adult life, my partner and I have been dependent as well. This dependence, which is on paid careworkers who worked in our home while Sesha lived with us, and at her residence where she now lives, is profound. I have come to appreciate the many "hidden skills" (Rollins 1987) of good caregiving. The skills of these carers exceed my own, and yet there are snares and contradictions lurking in such arrangements.[16]

As my life with a disabled person has led me to become more familiar with the developments in the larger disability community, I have also become aware of additional contradictions in care arrangements around disability. Just as I was coming to appreciate the importance and inevitability of dependency in our lives, the disability community was characterising the disadvantages of disability as neither natural nor inevitable. This *social model* of disability, so important in clarifying the sources of disability and countering the discrimination against people with disabilities, also brings to the fore contradictions that have much to do with our deeply distorted views about dependency and independence.

Michael Oliver, in his critique of social policy, contrasts the revised understanding of disability by the disability community with that of the "professionals"

---

[16] I (1999) write extensively about this in the chapter "Not *My* Way, Sesha, *Your* Way, Slowly."

who "tend to define independence in terms of self-care activities such as washing, dressing, toileting, cooking, and eating without assistance" (Oliver 1989, 14). Still, don't we have to ask: "What about those who do the washing, dressing, toileting?" Through the Independent Living Movement, disabled people have lobbied for—and partially succeeded in receiving—a right to a paid personal attendant. Although family members most often fill the role of paid attendant, the preferences of many disabled adults, interestingly, do not favor this arrangement. The sense of independence disabled people hope to attain is, according to some, best served by a paid stranger with whom one has a thin relationship of employer to employee instead of the thick relationships of family. In order to sustain a sense of independence—or as I will suggest, the illusion of independence—the personal attendant must become invisible. In the words of Lynn May Rivas, the carer needs to turn over "the authorship" of her work to the disabled person (2002, 77).

Rivas has written eloquently about her interviews with both people with disabilities and personal attendants. A daughter of a home caseworker, Rivas took over her mother's clients when her grandmother needed her mother's assistance. She opens her essay (tellingly titled "Invisible Labors: Caring for the Independent Person") by recounting her experience with a disabled man, Bill, who has quadriplegia and also dehydrates when he talks a lot during an interview. She describes the following situation:

> Twenty minutes into the interview, Bill coughs. . . . On a table next to him is a glass of water with a plastic top and a straw. Since he is unable to use his hands, I offer, "Um, do you want, would you like some water?" Bill raises his voice and calls, "Joe!" Then he explains, "I have an attendant." (2002, 70)

As his voice continues to deteriorate, he continues to call for his attendant who has gone outside to offer Bill privacy in his interview. Bill repeatedly refuses Rivas's offer to provide him with the water. Rivas writes:

> By this point, I feel frantic. I can't imagine why he won't let me give him water. "Do you want me to go outside and see if I can find him?" I ask in desperation, not sure what I should do. Bill responds, "Would you?" . . . I wonder what Joe will think when he gets to Bill's room. Will he think that I was unwilling to hold the glass of water? I want to tell Joe that I offered to give Bill the water, that I appreciate his giving us privacy, and that I am sorry to interrupt his break. I resist the impulse, however, saying nothing. I follow Joe back to Bill's room, and during the last twenty minutes of our interview he stands next

to Bill, offering him a sip of water every few minutes, seamlessly. (2002, 70–71)

Rivas uses this example to illustrate the extent to which the notion that the disabled person is independent requires the assistance (and the assistant) to be invisible.[17] Her help was not desired because, in this situation, she could not be invisible (and it may also be the case that Bill feared that her manner of assistance would not be sufficiently invisible, unobtrusive). Bill could accept the distanced help Rivas offered, when she suggested that she go out and find Joe, because that did not involve the bodily contact that he would accept only from his trained assistant. Rivas's own discomfort in how to speak with Joe needs some exploration. Did she feel constrained by the need to maintain the illusion that Joe was merely an appendage of Bill, not a person in his own right? Or did she believe that presuming that she could intervene in Joe's stead would be disrespectful of Joe's particular competence—implying that what he does could just as easily have been done by her?

Any answer requires us to see that *both* personal attendant and care 'consumer' had similar conceptions of what constitutes good care,[18] and that for both, invisibility of the carer was a requirement. One of the people with disabilities that Rivas interviewed stated:

Quality care is when that attendant has left, I feel good. I feel refreshed, clean, sitting in my chair correctly. I have everything I need for the day and I have an attendant who has come in and done it effortlessly. (2002, 77–78)

Rivas received similar responses from caregivers. One immigrant caseworker remarked:

---

[17] In addition to the reasons for invisibility discussed here, the attention that the caregiver provides the person she cares for is not reciprocated. Rivas remarks that not once in any of her interviews where the attendant was present was the attendant introduced. Beyond this, there is the invisibility of individuals in the demographic who are most likely to take on such difficult and ill-paying work. Ninety-one percent of home care aides are women. Fifty-six percent of these women rely on public assistance to meet their needs. One in four live in households below the federal poverty line. These are mainly immigrants (not infrequently ones who are in the country illegally) and working-class women, often from racial and ethnic groups who face additional discrimination and invisibility. Fifty-six percent of home care aides are nonwhite minorities. Twenty-four percent are foreign born. One in five are single mothers (PHI 2014).

[18] I introduce these terms insofar as some disability advocates want to promote the more impersonal understanding of the care relationships between the disabled person and the personal attendant.

It's being able to put yourself in a situation where you are almost not seen...where the recipient of care is so able to do what he wants...[It's] like you're there, but you're not there...[when they can do something] without even realizing that they're doing it because you're there, that's quality work right there. (2002, 75)

If this is the picture that the personal attendant and the disabled person both agree upon, is it right to say that the caseworker is oppressed? Rivas asks, "Must one feel oppressed to be oppressed?" She replies:

[This] transfer of authorship is a negative phenomenon... To be made invisible is the first step toward being considered nonhuman, which is why making another person invisible often precedes treating them inhumanely. To use Marxist terms, invisibility is the most extreme form of alienation—the ultimate manifestation of self-estrangement. (2002, 79)

If both attendants and disabled people are united in thinking that invisibility is called for in this position, they differ in their view of how the artful application of the ability to make oneself invisible should be viewed. While the washing, cleaning, dressing, providing sips of water, and so on are not actions that are clearly in view, the most difficult part of the work, the *emotional labor*, needs to be entirely invisible. There is emotional labor required in the vigilance and attentiveness to the other's need, in suppressing disgust in coming in contact with the bodily excretions of an adult, in maintaining good cheer in the face of another's sometimes harsh remarks. These must be really invisible and kept out of sight so that the transfer of "authorship" is "seamless." Such emotional labor is generally not seen at all by the cared-for, and yet it is the one that is most evident to the carer.

The fact that these aspects of the work are not visible as such results in two different versions of the work. On the one hand, says Rivas, "Ironically, handing over the authorship of caring labor may itself be the most caring part of care" (2002, 79). But then again, "How could something unseen be completely valued" (80)? The consumers wanted a "businesslike relationship," but the attendants valued the work insofar as it was a labor of love: "D'avian [an attendant] told me, 'It has to come from here.... You just got to have that love'" (81). This generosity of spirit went beyond the mere accomplishment of tasks.

Yet when the "consumers" were asked what the caregiver does over and beyond what is required, many interviewees answered the way this one did: "I can't think of a good answer to that. I don't know of anything that I ask of them that isn't what I consider to be part of that attendant's job" (82). As Rivas points out, such a seeming failure of sensitivity is a structural feature of the work. And yet the disabled person is as entitled to good care and assistance as the carer, in addition to receiving adequate compensation and respect, is entitled to having the full extent of her labor recognized. The logjam is, I believe, a feature of the overvalorization of independence and the stigma of dependency.

That the disabled person's reliance on assistance can constitute 'independence' requires more than the eye can see—or than the person assisted often can fully appreciate. Is it not better to recognize and to create conditions that foster relationships of dependency replete with the affective bonds and a sense that each participant has received her due; relationships which can transform otherwise unpleasant intimate tasks into times of trust and demonstrations of trustworthiness, gratifying and dignifying to both the caregiver and the recipient of care? A truly independent life—one in which we need no one and no one needs us—would be a very impoverished one, even if it were possible. The person with an impairment who requires the assistance of a caregiver is not the exception, but a person living out a frequent occurence in any human life, our inevitable dependency.

While most of us, disabled or not, can be self-determining to some degree, it is at best only *to that limited degree* that a self-determining life can be an independent life. But with self-determination comes a *presumption* of self-sufficiency, and such self-sufficiency is always a lie,[19] whether or not we are disabled. We are all better off when we refuse to live a lie. A life lived under such a false presumption involves us all in self-deception and self-distortion, as well as leaving us to the manipulation and exploitation of others. Disabled people and parents such as I will be able to live more authentic lives if we provide the appropriate recognition, appreciation, and support for caregivers.

We cannot rule out perverse people who take on care work precisely because they take pleasure in abusing and gaining a sense of power over vulnerable people in their charge. But the more attractive we make the position to those who truly have well-developed caring skills and dispositions, the less room there is for the abuser; the more respect, in the form of recognition and compensation we offer the caregiver, the more likely they are to use the power of their position to assist rather than dominate (Kittay 2000). Aside from such prudential considerations, it is a moral imperative to treat the caregiver or attendant in a caring and respectful manner and to recognize the value of their work. The moral imperative can be derived from the Kantian prescription to never treat another as a means only, but it also derives from an ETHICS OF CARE.

---

[19] See Young (2002) for a discussion of independence as self-determination.

An ETHICS OF CARE takes CARE as a supreme value, and while the scope of CARE is restricted by contextual considerations in any one deliberation, it aims at a regulative ideal that everyone is cared about and receives the care they need. That is, that everyone is enfolded into the circle of care. It may well be the case that the next step to liberation and progress for the disabled person and the caregiver alike (each of whom are members of oppressed and marginalized groups) is to expose the lie in the ideal of independence. The care will be more—not less—respectful, job turnover will be less as the gracious reception of care offers rewards and makes the work less alienating, and the disabled person will gain the dignity of living more authentically.

6.5.1 Managed Dependency

If absolute independence is a lie, but dependency remains wrought with difficulty, might we aim for an understanding of independence as *relative*? Even a relative independence will be at someone's expense if we do not weave dependency needs into the fabric of society—needs that are at the heart of the inextricable interdependencies that characterize all societies.[20] I propose that we take the occasion of disability to find a better way to *manage* dependency. Rather than joining the "abled" on a quixotic quest for a nonexistent independence, I suggest that we aim for a *relative* independence through the appropriate *management* of dependency.

In a particularly insightful article on managing dependency in frail old age, psychologist and gerontologist Margret Baltes (1995) distinguishes learned helplessness from what she calls "learned dependency" in the context of supported-living environments such as nursing homes and assisted living residences. In contrast to "learned helplessness," where people become passive and stop trying to be efficacious because their efforts do not produce predictable outcomes, "learned dependency" results in circumstances where an individual's *dependent* behaviors succeed in initiating social contact, but the individual's *independent* behavior elicits little response from others. In such environments, striving for "independence" is not rewarding. Baltes notes that some of the elderly in her study allowed themselves to receive assistance in areas where they could meet their own needs, but with great effort. They managed their dependency by choosing instead to reserve energy for areas of life that provided more satisfaction. Rather than battling the loss of capacities when the exercise of these interfered with more important activities, these elderly were capable of richer and more efficacious lives. They displayed "the virtue of acknowledged

---

[20] This point is developed in the complementary volume *Who is Truly Human?*.

dependency" (MacIntyre 1999). That is to say, they gave dependency its due.[21] Baltes speaks of this strategy as "managing dependency." It is reminiscent of the strategy Irving Zola adopted and which he chose to call "independence." But we avoid buying into the myth of independence when we think of it instead as "managed dependence."

If we manage dependence, we acknowledge its presence in our lives, select and optimize the opportunities that such acknowledgment makes possible, and thereby can better detect and protect against the fault lines that are part and parcel of our condition as dependent beings. What are these fault lines? Aside from the fully dependent period of our infancy, the dependency can emerge as a minor quake—a temporary illness—or a major one—a child with a congenital disability, an accident that leaves us with reduced functioning, a debilitating illness, the disability of old age. Most of us will experience the dependencies that come with frail old age. In the name of managing dependency, we can reorder our priorities and assert entitlements to care and support that are our due, not because in that way we can be independent and productive, but because our value derives from the chain of dependent relations that make all our lives possible.

Bringing this understanding of dependency into the lifeblood of society can be a precious contribution bestowed upon us from the community of disabled people. More broadly, it presents a saner view of human life, and particularly contemporary life in complex societies where we all are both inextricably interdependent and dependent on the actions of other individuals and social institutions.

Coda

The first chapter of part II has been a lesson on dependency. It is what I have learned from my daughter about what MacIntyre called "the virtue of acknowledging dependency" and about the extraordinary possibilities inherent in relationships created in caring for someone like her, someone who reciprocates but not in a like coin (say, by caring physically for another), but by bestowing her warmth and her love. It is Sesha's lesson. The remainder of part II comes from engaging in and observing how others perform the labor and love of giving care. It is the lesson of the caregiver. An ETHICS OF CARE derives from the best practices of the care for vulnerable dependent persons.

---

[21] One should acknowledge that it is possible to become manipulative in deploying the strategy of allowing oneself to be helped with tasks that one could with some effort carry out oneself. This is most likely to be a problem when the carer is not given due respect.

7

An Ethics of Care

> When women who are not mere students of other persons' philosophy
> set out to write it, we cannot conceive that it will be the same in viewpoint
> or tenor as that composed from the standpoint of the different masculine
> experience of things.
>
> —John Dewey (1993, 40)

> The philosopher who begins with a supremely free consciousness—an
> aloneness and emptiness at the heart of existence—identifies anguish as
> the basic human affect. But our view, rooted as it is in relation, identifies
> joy as a basic human affect.... It is the recognition of and longing for relat-
> edness that form the foundation of our ethic, and the joy that accompanies
> fulfillment of our caring enhances our commitment to the ethical ideal
> that sustains us as one-caring.
>
> —Nel Noddings (1984, 6)

7.1 Is Care an Important Concept for Philosophy?

All Western philosophy, said Alfred N. Whitehead, is a series of footnotes to
Plato. This frequently cited declaration is meant to express the idea that in Plato's
magnificent corpus, all the important ideas that philosophers have grappled with
are laid out, and all the rest is commentary. Truly, it is rare that any genuinely
new ideas enter into philosophy. Most philosophical treatments of ethics and
political theory have their roots in Plato. Seemingly new and too often ignored
philosophical issues, such as women's equality, love, and the education of children, were already present in his work.

Care too makes an appearance as *therapeia*, "care of the Gods," and as *melô*—
the notion of improvement, in the sense of self-care or care of the soul.[1] Just as

---

[1] Thanks to my colleague Alan Kim, who writes: "First, it seems that in Plato, the notion of
'care' is importantly connected with the Good and the dialectic between 'improvement' (motion
toward the Good) and 'corruption' (the opposite). Socrates appears as the improver and hence
the carer, whereas Meletus, in name the Carer, is in fact the corrupter. In Aristotle's *Nicomachean
Ethics* (chapter 1, section 2) too, we find the idea that the statesman's job boils down to tending

the midwifery of Socrates, bringing forth the ideas created in the minds of men, is a metaphoric appropriation of women's role as midwives of flesh-and-blood children from the bodies of women, so these references extend the metaphoric appropriation of women's carework, beyond childbirth and onto the rearing of the child. As women care for children past infancy, men are engaged in the care of the Gods or care of the soul.

The source of the metaphor, care of dependents and the ethical concerns that emerge from this enterprise, do not take center stage anywhere in the grand opus.[2] Nor are these present in the many "footnotes" to Plato. In contrast, in our quotidian lives, the care that we offer to an ailing friend, that a parent gives or fails to provide for her child, that we devote to an older parent or a stranger in need, or even how we care for our nonhuman fellow creatures and our earth,[3] are all matters that figure in our moral evaluation of ourselves and others. These constitute the heart of our moral selves. We think of a caring person as having lived a morally good life, and a deeply caring person as having lived even a saintly life. The deep divide between the philosophical conceptions of a good person and ones that ordinary people accept are at least as striking as the difference between what philosophers insist is needed for a good life and what many good and thoughtful people value in a life.

Although care as a moral value is not new, what is new is the claim that care requires articulation as an ethical perspective, as an ethical theory. In her studies of how women deliberated about moral dilemmas, Carol Gilligan (1982) claimed she heard "a different voice," the voice of an ethic of care. Gilligan's studies brought something fresh into philosophy: a new conception of ethics, and the beginnings of a new ethical theory.

---

to the citizens of the state in much the way Socrates describes the shepherd in the *Republic*. He is supposed to create or maintain the conditions for maximal thriving of his wards. But we clearly also see in Socrates, Plato, and Aristotle the idea that Foucault calls 'the care of the self.' The person who knows how to care for others in the first place cares for him or herself, and this self-caring is, it seems to me, the prime expression of Greek virtue. It means getting your soul in order, and thus into a healthy condition, which is the equivalent of happiness or 'living well' (*euzên*)" (personal communication, October 27, 2014).

[2] It seems like philosophy here can take place only where women step aside and men play their role in education, statesmanship, and philosophical improvement.

[3] The increasing moral importance of care of the earth and its creatures is beautifully highlighted in both the substance and the title of Pope Francis's Encyclical Letter, "On the Care of Our Common Home" (2015).

7.1.1 An Ethics of Care Emerges on the
Philosophical Horizon

Gilligan's empirical work led her to claim that the abortion debate, structured as a conflict of rights—those of the fetus versus those of the woman—fails to reflect the decision-making of women faced with an unexpected pregnancy. Rather than ask if the fetus was a rights-bearing person, the women in Gilligan's study asked questions such as: Is it responsible to give birth at this time of my life? Am I prepared to take care of a child? How will giving birth to a baby now affect my relationship to my lover, my spouse, my parents, my children? Will I be true to myself or cause harm by my decision? Rather than asking about rights, these women were asking about their responsibilities. Rather than framing the dilemma as a conflict between oneself and the unborn, they tended to think in terms of their relationships to a future child, current children, a spouse or lover, and other family. In particular, they were concerned how their decisions would affect those about and for whom they would be caring.[4] Other philosophical work by feminists soon took up the notion of care. Of particular importance were Nel Noddings's phenomenological treatment in *Caring* (1984) and Sarah Ruddick's *Maternal Thinking* (1989). These three works laid the groundwork for subsequent treatments of care.[5]

There is a plausible explanation for why there is little in the long history of moral thought that highlights care, whether as a virtue or as the basis for right action. Very few of those who have penned moral theories have been women or had access to the experiences of women when not in the company of men. Women, moreover, have been in a position neither to make decisions in the sphere that men have dominated, nor (as John Stuart Mill shrewdly observed) have they been sufficiently independent of a man's power to say what it is that they really think. The systematic moral scrutiny applied to promises, contracts, and conduct in battle and business was not applied to areas that men didn't occupy, like care for children and the ill.

---

[4] Gilligan's claim was that the dominant discourse in moral theory is what she called a justice perspective, while the ethical life of women traditionally has revolved about issues of care. Her theorizing and its subsequent development has set up an opposition between an ethic of justice and an ethic of care. The dichotomy has vexed theorists since, and I attack it in my own way (2015). Because I no longer hold the dichotomy to be valid, I refrain from opposing care to justice.

[5] If we grant that care has a role in Plato and the footnotes that follow, then perhaps we can say that rather than introducing the notion of a care ethics that is a break with the philosophical tradition, women have provided still another footnote to Plato, one that develops a different conception of care. Other predecessors who have come closer to the notion of care that contemporary feminist philosophers are developing include women philosophers such as Jane Addams, who are generally given short shrift or entirely excluded in the canon. I thank Richard Rubin for these insights.

Caring has been treated less as a moral virtue and more as the fulfillment of nature's plan. For example, a woman who failed to care for an ill spouse was doing something unnatural, something unfeminine—but not necessarily something to be accounted for within a conception of ethical behavior. And while a woman who leaves her child is viewed as monstrous, a man who abandons his child is viewed instead as doing something immoral. Women's position has changed, and we have discovered that men too are capable of caring for children and whomever is in need of care. Such a statement is not meant sarcastically. It hasn't been until the late twentieth century that feminists have even begun to demand that men share in childcare. Once care is no longer regarded as an instinctual and a natural disposition found mostly in women, we can de-naturalize and de-gender care and understand it as a mode of moral conduct. In this way feminism has, as Julia Driver (2005) puts it, added more data into the data bank that moral philosophers now need to consider.

Some aspects of care have entered the philosophical canonical literature. We have already alluded to Plato's work. *Love* is motivationally close to care, and it has had a small but important place in Western philosophy. Notions of *sympathy* (important to Sentimental philosophers), *benevolence* and *beneficence* (in utilitarianism and Kantianism), and *altruism* are important counters to *egoistic* theories of morality. These concepts share some of the attitudinal features of care. They all do some of the work of care: they all enlist other-directed motives, motives that arise out of a felt concern for or attachment to another. Often, however, the place of these attitudinal other-directed concerns lies not with right action but with supererogation. They cover those acts that are good (even saintly) but not required, and so are supererogatory. In contrast, the caring that is part of quotidian life includes not only a benevolent attitude and altruistic actions, but also actions that are *required* of a carer and so are not supererogatory, even when they demand significant sacrifice on the part of the carer. For instance, no one thinks to call the care a parent gives her child supererogatory.

Care has more recently become a concern in Western philosophy from a number of quarters. Within Continental philosophy "care" or *Sorge* entered into the philosophical lexicon via Heidegger.[6] But like Plato's conceptions of care, Heidegger's is far from the examination of care that has preoccupied more recent feminist thinkers. His is a feature of his metaphysical views of the nature of Being. The work of Levinas has been thought to have a close affiliation to a

---

[6] The Heideggerian notions of *Sorge, Fürsorge,* and *Besorgen* designate caring about, taking care of, and being concerned, and they are the ways in which *Dasein* is manifested in the world (Heidegger 1962). There is, however, a question as to whether the Heideggerian notion can be used for examining caring for another, since *Sorge* is a condition of *Dasein* rather than a relation to one in need of care (see Lavoie, De Koninck, and Blondeau 2006).

feminist ethic of care.[7] Harry Frankfurt (1988; 2004) and some of his followers have made a major contribution bringing care into the philosophical literature of Anglo-American philosophy. In their work, care is recognized as a central motivation in all human life. The most extensive contribution to the articulation of an ethic of care, however, has come from feminist moral philosophy.

Once we begin to think about it, it seems extraordinary that philosophers have taken this long to consider care as a central moral concept. A world without care would not only be a dismal world, it would be a world in which great harm would be done. A world in which nobody cared about anyone else would be a world in which needs of those who could not attend to their own needs (and that is all of us at some point in our lives) would be neglected. Although an implicit ethic of care has been indispensable to the survival and development of human society, its development into an articulated moral theory is still in its infancy. The idea, first put forward by a woman psychologist about the moral life of mostly women, has prompted a number of female philosophers (and some women-friendly male philosophers) to till new theoretical fields and come up with a set of notions that justify the claim that there is an ethics of care that governs the best practices of care and whose values spill out onto other moral domains. Furthermore, this ethic is different from the trio of ethical theories that have hitherto claimed the territory: a Kantian deontological ethics, utilitarianism, and virtue ethics.

7.1.2 An Ethic of Care: Descriptive or Normative?

A question that continues to haunt debates around an ethic of care is whether the concerns expressed in terms of care are fully normative ones. Calling something "an ethic" has always been ambiguous between an anthropology (that is, a descriptive account of the rules or codes that govern activity within a certain community—even a band of thieves can have an ethic in the descriptive sense), and a fully normative account (that is, whether the rules that are descriptively adequate are also rules that *ought* to be followed). Insofar as the idea of "an ethic of care" arose out of a set of psychological studies, it might be taken to be a description of what people think it is appropriate to do rather than an account of what in fact is the right thing to do.

---

[7] Levinas's conception of our responsibility to the other is close to the feminist concept, but it supposes an obligatory relation to the other that is not essential to a feminist conception of care. There is a literature that has developed regarding the applicability of Levinas's notions as they pertain to a feminist ethic of care. See Lavoie, De Koninck, and Blondeau (2006); Diedrich, Burggraeve, and Gastmans (2006); Bookman and Aboulafia (2000); Reynolds (2016); and Nortvedt (2003).

What makes the question especially confounding is that care is always embedded in a practice of care, for example: mothering, nursing, eldercare, or assistance for a disabled person. And practices are themselves a source of normativity. Practices provide the context by which we make claims of truth or falsity (Winch 1958) and within which we practice the virtues (MacIntyre 1981). A practice (that is, that set of activities with structures, rules, values, and virtues) has an aim (*telos*) by which we evaluate a behavior as good within that practice. Killing someone who is your enemy is generally commendable in the practice of war, but killing someone who is your enemy, even your mortal enemy, is generally not a good or right action.

Sarah Ruddick speaks of a gender-neutral *practice* of "mothering"—that is, a set of activities that have as their goals the preservation, nurturance, and socialization of children (whether done by women or men, and whether the parents be biological or adoptive). In respect to these aims of mothering, one can be either a good or a poor mother. We can speak similarly of nursing. The norms of nursing govern what counts as care from a nurse, allowing us to speak of good nurses who assist in comforting and healing their patients and poor nurses who are careless, neglectful, or incompetent. The *telos* is the regulative ideal by which we evaluate not only the behavior of individuals, but also the activities and structures, the rules and conventions that characterize the practice. When rules run counter to the *telos* of nursing, a good nurse should be willing to break those rules, weighing only if doing so will undermine her ability to continue to do good nursing.

Gilligan, however, in speaking of an ethic of care, was trying to get at something less descriptive and more fully normative. Women trying to decide whether to terminate their pregnancy were deliberating on what *the right thing* to do would be. They were assessing what a good person would do in her circumstance.[8] If care is a fully moral concept which tells us what is and is not right to do, what is good and what fails to be good, then the practice and its regulative ideals must themselves have moral validation. Thieving is a sort of practice. But honesty among thieves does not make a thief honest. The point of thievery is simply to enrich the thief. A moral practice is one which, when meeting its regulative ideal, is a morally good or morally right practice.

What gives a practice such moral validation? Consider mothering. It may seem that a good mother can be one that does everything for her child regardless

---

[8] More precisely, the women were trying to determine if their decision was *the right thing* to do (a moral judgment), and what would be right *for them* (a prudential judgment). Those committed to a religiously based belief that abortion was a moral wrong took a prudential decision to be merely selfish. For those not committed to an exterior moral authority, the deliberation was to come to a morally acceptable determination.

of the cost to others. But one of the aims of mothering is to socialize her child, to guide the child in becoming a member of her community. A mother who is ruthless in obtaining things for her own child may appear to be the good mother. But viewed from the perspective of the practice understood as a whole, she will actually be doing a poor job, for such a parent does not model behavior that is acceptable. Mothering does not set its own aims apart from the world in which the child must live, and we see our role as parents to equip the child with a grasp of what is morally acceptable in that world.[9] What caring practices share is an ideal that leaves no one's genuine needs and legitimate wants—needs and wants that can result in real harm—unattended. More positively, caring practices tend to people's CARES, to those things people care about, which figure in their flourishing, and which they cannot accomplish without the proper assistance. Avoiding harming another and allowing others to flourish are conceptions that are familiar to all moral theories.

A moral theory based on care gives special consideration to the avoidance of neglect, to the importance of attending to those who are inevitably dependent (and so cannot attend to what they require themselves), and to a motivational structure based on affective ties and empathetic capacities. If we are correct about the moral validation of practices of care, then we have a basis for thinking that there is a notion of care that is fully normative and not merely descriptive and can serve as the guiding virtue for a true ethics of care.

The way we normally speak of caring is the way we speak of mothering or nursing. You can do it well or poorly; you can be a good carer or an inadequate one. You can care "too much" ? (e.g., a parent constantly hovering over a child—the "helicopter parent"—or a nurse who, in her vigilance, causes more irritation than comfort to the sick patient) or "too little" (e.g., being callous, negligent, or even abusive in carrying out presumed acts of care). This is a perfectly service-able way to speak of care most of the time.

But if we want to speak of a fully normative conception of care, then can we really speak of "caring too much"? Consider that we never speak of a person as being "too just." We may speak of a person being too rigid in the application of laws or principles, or we may say that a person serves up too stern a form of justice. What we do not say is that someone offers up bad or poor justice. If it is bad, it is not just. For the outcome to be just, it must be something worthy of approval, even if we have reservations about the outcome that comes from

---

[9] Studies indicate, however, that parents are most likely to act dishonestly to benefit their children. However, when parents are in the presence of their children they are more likely to behave honestly, although they were more prone to act dishonestly in front of their sons than their daughters (Houser et al. 2016).

a different set of values or another practice—for example, that a particular just judgment was not sufficiently merciful.

Moral virtues such as justice are already defined normatively, and, as Aristotle tells us, they are generally a mean between two vices.[10] So, we cannot be *too* courageous, for then we are tending toward recklessness. As the guiding virtue for an ETHICS OF CARE, CARE too is a mean between too extremes. On one extreme is over-solicitude, that is, the unwanted attention to another person and their needs. Alternatively, there is the paternalistic imposition of someone's idea of what good is for the cared-for, without consideration of what the cared-for regards as their own good. On the other extreme is a neglect borne either of indifference or a misplaced "respect for another's autonomy" that involves a failure (or unwillingness) to perceive another's need, an insufficient concern for the other's well-being, or a failure to seize the opportunity to act upon the perception of another's need. The point of caring is to benefit the cared for, but when the person who is presumably being cared for says that the carer cares too much, they are complaining that the benefit the carer assumes she is bestowing is not a benefit at all. In chapter 8, we will speak of the need of the cared-for to take up the actions of the carer as care. This last requirement is essential if we are to have a way of identifying whether what we do for another's benefit is indeed a benefit for that person.

7.2 Features of an ETHICS OF CARE

The concept of an ethics of care has now been around for approximately thirty years, and some of its core features have been identified. I incorporate these into the particular conception I am offering here. An ETHICS OF CARE needs to hold together a tripartite conception of CARE as labor, an attitude (or disposition), and a virtue. As a labor, caregiving requires attending to the needs of another, putting aside one's own needs for someone more vulnerable, and often becoming intimate with the body and the bodily functions of the cared-for.[11] The labor of care is, for the most part, carried out on the body of an individual. An ETHICS OF CARE is one in which the embodied existence of each, in both our unique individuality *and* in our material connectedness to one another, is never eclipsed. As such, it must be able to dignify each morally significant individual in his or her embodied existence.

---

[10] When we are courageous or virtuous in any regard, we act according to the mean between these extremes: we do the right thing "at the right times, with reference to the right objects, towards the right people, with the right motive, and in the right way" (Aristotle 1908, Book 2 Sec 6).

[11] See MacIntyre (1999); Gastmans, Dierckx de Casterlé, and Schotsmans (1998).

The custodial maintenance of the body is not yet CARE. The attitude of CARE, the open responsiveness to another—so essential to understanding what another person requires—is needed if the work is to constitute caring labor. Sarah Clark Miller captures the nature of caring labor when she defines care as "the process of responding to another's need by understanding their self-determined ends, adopting those ends as one's own, and advancing them in an effort to cultivate, maintain, or restore their agency" (2005).[12] For this to take place CARE requires a "shift . . . from the interest in our life situation to the situation of the other, the one in need of care" (Gastmans, Dierckx de Casterlé, and Schotsmans 1998) and what Nel Noddings (1984) calls "engrossment" in the other. That is, attitude must accompany the labor.

CARE, as we said, is also a virtue to be cultivated, a disposition to make the attitudinal shift as it is called for. Those in whom this virtue is present are able to respond to people in need of care even when the parties are not bound by intimacy. Carers not only care about and for those whom they encounter, they also care about CARE (Dalmiya 2002).

The skills and virtues of caregiving are many, and the degree to which the caregiver must become enmeshed (in Nodding's words) in another's needs in order to adequately meet those needs varies with both the urgency and extent of the other's dependency and with the degree to which one has cultivated the virtue of CARE. Because it involves a shift from one's own interests to those of the person in need of care, it often requires the caregiver to defer the fulfillment of his or her own needs. When caring for someone who is extremely (and inevitably) dependent, the deferral can take too long to ever be fully compensated, and it is effectively a loss for the caregiver. Another must come to the aid of the caregiver. The caregiver herself becomes dependent on someone who will look after *her* interests and attend her *own* (first-person) CARES, as well as allow her to care for the dependent. The self of the caregiver and her relation to the dependent have a moral value no less than the person for whom she cares, even if attention to the caregiver's concerns must be deferred given the urgency of the needs of the cared-for.

In addition, an ETHICS OF CARE can be characterized by concepts that one can find in other moral theories. One way to sketch out an ethics of care is to consider how it differs from other moral theories in treating the concepts of

[12] Because I want to speak not only of needs, I use a more inclusive term, CARES, to cover both needs and wants. Doing so also has the virtue of avoiding the difficulties of delineating what constitutes a need. However, since the term "needs" is so naturally employed when speaking of care, it is often too stilted to speak always of CARES, and I will slip into speaking of needs, unless the context requires a careful demarcation of terms.

moral selves, moral relations, moral deliberation, the scope of moral judgments, the aim of morality, and moral harm.

7.2.1 Moral Selves and Moral Agency

Most ethical theories begin with an explicit or implicit understanding of the self, or the moral agent. Modern theories of ethics generally begin with independent autonomous individuals as moral agents in rational pursuit of their own good, as they see it. An ETHICS OF CARE begins with embodied selves who are regarded as inextricably connected to other embodied selves. Such a self is vulnerable and embodied in a particular way: that is, this self, unlike the idealized self of many other theories, has a gender, a race or ethnicity, a social position, and a set of abilities and disabilities as these are, or should be, realizable within the context of their lives. Their relationships play a constitutive role in the formation of their desires and in their identity.[13] Moral deliberation must contend with the way in which differences among selves make a difference in the outcome of our practical actions.

While (in dominant ethical theories) the self is a self-determining adult who is an independent agent and party to an ethical determination, an ETHICS OF CARE does not presume that all parties in an ethical exchange are adults capable of self-determination and independence. Some are deeply dependent on others for care. The fact of our dependency does not take us out of moral consideration, but rather constitutes a ground of our moral world. We cannot extricate ourselves from our vulnerability to dependency and our interconnectedness.

The self who is engaged in a caring relationship is a *relational self* that is capable of being motivated by the CARES of the other. The CARING self needs to be able to make itself transparent to the needs of the other, that is, it needs to bracket its own CARES so that these do not cloud its ability to apprehend the CARES of another. Yet such *transparent selves* do not become mere ciphers—they must be capable of self-direction, self-rule, and self-reflection (Meyers 1989;

---

[13] That our relationships are a constitutive part of what it is to be a self does not mean that there is no self apart from the relationships we have with others. But from the first breath we take we are already in relationships: with the birth mother, with those who care for us so that a fully dependent being can survive, and with all who have helped in our birth. We also occupy certain relational roles. For example, we are a child of some human being. But it is not the case that anything can be a child of someone. All relations already specify something about the nature of the relata. Gravity is a relation. But it doesn't relate entities that lack mass. The relationship arises out of the properties of the relata, but the relationships also constitute the relata. For an account of the importance of these relations in the recovery of a shattered self, see Brison (1997; 2002). For a discussion of the relation of autonomy and relationality see the essays in Mackenzie and Stoljar (2000), and see Friedman (2003). For a discussion of the relational self and identity see Brison (2017).

1994). Self-reflection allows them to consider how their own desires might continue to obstruct their ability to be attentive and responsive to the other; self-rule and self-direction allow them to evaluate and determine the extent to which the other's CARES should direct their own actions. An ETHICS OF CARE ought to preserve the caregiver's ability not to stray from her own moral compass in her willingness to become "engrossed" in the other.[14] Similarly, a fully normative theory ought to encourage caregivers to be alert to the exploitation or abuse that caregivers can be subject to. They also need to be sufficiently self-reflective so they do not subject the cared-for to some abuse that they themselves might unwittingly or carelessly inflict.

7.2.2 Moral Relations

In contrast to the presumptions we find in many other ethical theories, the relationships in which such relational selves stand may not be self-chosen and are not always among equals—and so there is no presumption that reciprocity is possible, much less that it is obligatory. Care ethics then deals with our obligations and responsibilities in relationships of asymmetry in situation and power.[15] In such asymmetrical relationships, the carer needs to be attentive, mindful, and responsive to the genuine needs and legitimate wants of the other, and respond in a way that addresses the other's particularity. Although all moral relationships require a level of trust and trustworthiness, those qualities have a heightened importance in care relationships, given the special vulnerability of one party to the actions of the other. Nonetheless, as I will argue in the following chapter, there is a legitimate expectation that the ones cared for (when and to the extent that they are able) do their part by taking up care offered in good faith and with the requisite competence.

7.2.3 Moral Deliberation

Love, empathetic concern, commitment, loyalty, compassion, and other attachments and emotions are important motivations to act on behalf of another. Within an ETHICS OF CARE they play a part in moral deliberation both because they direct our motivations, and because they are a rich epistemic resource.[16]

---

[14] Noddings (1984) uses the apt term "engrossment," but it is a term that can be taken to mean that in this sort of involvement one loses oneself and one's own good judgment.

[15] While the caregiver may be more powerful along some dimensions, the cared-for may have more socioeconomic power. Each party who has an advantage over the other party has the obligation not to abuse that power, turning the advantage into dominating the other. I discuss issues of power and domination in Kittay (1999, chapter 2).

[16] See Gallegos (2016) for a fine discussion of this point.

However, as emotions and attachments have been thought to be unreliable moral guides that give rise to skewed and arbitrary decisions, most moral theories, especially Kantian and Utilitarian ones, prefer generalized principles that rely on reason alone and result in conclusions that are impartial. But care ethicists point out that caring for a sick child is motivated more by empathy and concern than by algorithms utilizing a calculus of maximizing pleasure and minimizing pain; kindness to an elderly person is more reliably evoked by a feeling of sympathy than by a sense of duty; and (as the moral sentimentalists have already told us) even keeping a promise is more readily motivated by moral sentiments such as honor, shame, or loyalty than an application of the categorical imperative. To counter the charge that emotions are unreliable, the care ethicist (in common with other virtue theorists) would reply by calling for the active cultivation of moral emotions and for the modeling of their appropriate use.

What a care perspective adds to virtue theory and sentimentalist ethics is the understanding that these motivational forces also make us more alert to what is required in this particular circumstance. The attentive responsiveness critical to successful caring is made possible—often, at least—by an empathetic connection to and understanding of the other. These enable us to "read" the mind of another, especially in cases where the other is either temporarily or permanently incapable of communicating through speech. As such, these affective connections are a needed moral epistemic resource. They have this epistemic reach because moral emotions draw us into the subjectivity of the other, allowing us to respond to this particular concrete other, not a generalized other (Benhabib 1987).

Our relationships to others come with additional (although not always privileged) epistemic access to the other—and with such knowledge come special responsibilities to respond to that individual's CARES. Giving priority to one's spouse or children in situations of crisis is not immoral. Rather, as Bernard Williams memorably pointed out, hesitating to do so is to have "one thought too many" (1976). Surely not all of our ethical life is circumscribed by such relations, but having them allows us to understand the importance care has as a moral conception. Further, if we care about care, we come to understand how we enlarge the circle of those whom we care about and why we must see to it that all can be cared for through meaningful relationships.

7.2.4 The Scope of Moral Judgments

Most dominant moral theories are supposed to give us judgments that are universal in scope. That is to say, if it is morally right to treat a person in such and such a manner, this is true of whosoever that person may be. For example, it is no more permissible to lie to a stranger than it is to lie to someone near and dear. Such universality works well when the injunction is a negative one, such as "one must not lie" or "one must not trample on another's basic rights." But such universality is not always appropriate when we are thinking about CARE. An injunction as presumably universal as not lying gets complicated when we try to apply the best standard of care for a person with Alzheimer's disease. A fellow philosopher and caregiver of a spouse with Alzheimer's disease remarks:

> Lying becomes especially problematic with dementia. One woman in my support group used to say, "You have to learn *how* to lie." I don't regard it as lying per se, but simplifying communication to take care of the cognitively impaired person. Indeed, it's better to deflect than to lie. If a woman in a nursing home thinks you are her sister, you don't want to tell her that her sister is dead, but you also don't want to pretend to be her sister. It's better to get her to talk about her sister and to inquire indirectly why she is thinking of her.[17]

Another injunction that is generally seen to have universal scope is a principle of noninterference. Except when we act in ways that are harmful to others, we should not be interfered with in our pursuits.[18] But when we are dealing with those who require care, "noninterference" is often neglect and the source of great harm. More generally, however, the idea that noninterference is of upmost importance arises from an understanding of moral life as occurring amongst nonrelational, self-sufficient selves. If we begin with our interconnectedness, we want to look instead at the inevitable impact each of our actions has on others. We also recognize that the impact of our actions is often (though not always) proportionate to the closeness of our relations to others.

Within an ETHIC OF CARE, impartiality, along with noninterference, loses its moral supremacy. Helping another to flourish (according to the cared-for's conception of her own flourishing) takes precedence over a principle of non-interference. But as such intervention is demanding on the caregiver, it is quite unreasonable to expect everyone to be fully engaged in caring for everyone else—or even to be equally caring toward all. The limitations of our ability to

---

[17] Richard Rubin, personal communication, June 21, 2015.

[18] A classic statement is John Stuart Mill's harm principle: "The only purpose for which power can be rightfully exercised over any member of a civilized community, against his will, is to prevent harm to others" (1860 [1978], 9). Similarly, John Rawls's conception of the basic liberties is to guarantee that each one has the freedom to pursue their own conception of the good, without interference, as long as doing so is compatible with others having the same freedom. The priority of the right over the good is another form of the idea that noninterference is more important than fostering another's good—at least in the realm of justice.

form significant emotional engagements beyond a rather narrow sphere, as well as the demanding nature of care, means that a CARE-based ethics is inevitably sensitive to proximity, whether it be the relational proximity of family or friends or the geographical contiguity of neighbors and fellow citizens. The scope of care is therefore partial and contextual, and not universal.[19]

An ETHICS OF CARE, which is anchored in our relationships with and connections to others that are at least partially constitutive of who we are, nonetheless requires a cultivation of care for those who are distant. If CARE itself is a fundamental value, as we averred in section 7.1.2, then it should be a value that is not confined to our relations to intimate others, but needs to characterize a certain moral stance we take in the world, one we can call caring about CARE (Dalmiya 2002). If we understand that we are all connected, we see that noninterference can too easily morph into neglect globally as well as locally. How to properly adjudicate and execute such obligations and responsibilities is something for which an ETHICS OF CARE needs to provide guidance, guidance that may be based on degrees of intimacy, proximity, urgency of need, or a general concern that adequate care be available when needed. Acknowledging our relationships is a first step toward understanding the many ways these connections risk becoming forms of domination or occasions for neglect, and thus an ETHICS OF CARE must guard against both an indifference to those who are distant and a temptation to dominate those to whom we are connected.[20]

7.2.5 The Aims of Moral Relations

Perhaps the most fundamental difference between moral theories resides in how they conceive of the point and purpose of moral interactions. Ethical theories within a liberal tradition stress the importance of people being able to live their lives according to their own lights, free of unnecessary interference from others. Utilitarian theories understand moral theory to provide the greatest good for the greatest number. Communitarian theories understand the point of moral relations to serve a communal good.

An ETHICS OF CARE stresses, first of all, the concern for the well-being (or flourishing) of a person *for their own sake* and the moral importance of enabling each one to flourish. Like other moral theories, an ETHICS OF CARE is primarily one that is concerned with the interactions among selves, each of whom have a subjective life. Such selves have a well-being to which a carer is responsive. I will

---

[19] Universality, however, makes an appearance in the notion that a care ethics is one in which care is a universal value. I may not have a duty or responsibility to care equally for all, but I do need to acknowledge the equal right all have to receive care.

[20] For a good discussion of domination see both Young (1990) and Pettit (1997).

not here engage in the disputes that surround the nature of well-being. The view to which I subscribe, and which I believe inheres in an ETHICS OF CARE, is that the well-being of an individual (who is also a subject) is a form of *flourishing*. In the context of an ETHICS OF CARE an understanding of flourishing requires the following:

1. A person flourishes when the person has (or has access to or can strive to attain, either on her own or assisted by another) the things an individual truly cares about (in the sense that these are the things that make it worthwhile for a person to get up every morning).
2. The things the individual truly cares about that are genuine needs are met (that is, needs which if they fail to be met will result in a genuine harm to the individual), and legitimate wants are satisfied (that is, wants that can be met without sacrificing the equally legitimate wants of another).

That is, when we CARE for another, we are concerned with that person's welfare as it contributes to that individual's flourishing. Furthermore, this caring is not for the sake of the larger community or some abstract conception of goodness, but for the sake of that individual. It is this concern with the other's well-being for his own sake that places *responsibilities* on us for the other's care. Because relationships of affiliation and affinity are themselves constitutive of how selves-in-relationship understand themselves, the other's care and the other's CARES are not external to our own well-being.

7.2.6 The Nature of Moral Harm

Ultimately, the point of moral theories is to help us prevent harm: harm to ourselves and harm to another. Within dominant moral theories, moral harm is identified as the violation of rights or the unwarranted intrusion in the form of paternalism, domination, or violence. In an ETHICS OF CARE, moral harm results when important genuine needs and legitimate wants (especially of vulnerable persons) go unmet; when our concerns elicit only indifference, when vulnerability arouses disdain and abuse rather than care, and most especially, when human connections are broken through exploitation, domination, hurt, neglect, detachment, or abandonment.

7.3 Temptations and Critiques of an Ethic of Care

A moral theory that stresses the importance of relationships and moral emotions comes with a host of "temptations" (Ruddick 1989, 30). Temptations are vices that result when otherwise beneficial tendencies are overindulged. We encounter the lure of temptations when we consider critiques of care ethics that question whether women and people with disabilities should embrace an ETHICS OF CARE. As a feminist and an advocate in solidarity with people with disabilities, I have sympathy for both critiques, and some of these were addressed in chapter 6.

An ETHICS OF CARE should acknowledge the temptations pointed to by feminist theorists and people with disabilities and address them. Once we have an ETHICS OF CARE properly articulated, we will come to see that it is the moral theory that best serves the interests of both, and it may well be the ethical view best able to provide a vision for a fully realized human existence.

7.3.1 Indifference to Distant Others

Although our connections to those who are close have special moral importance, we also need to guard against indifference to those who are distant (whether through geographic proximity or social position) from us. Ignoring the plight of others is a temptation of an ethic for which partiality and the restricted scope of moral obligations are a feature. Nonetheless, we are inextricably connected to others through vast and often unfathomable networks, making others susceptible to our actions regardless of our distance and our intentions.

Within an ETHICS OF CARE, connections generate responsibilities, and while such responsibilities to distant others are weaker than to those close at hand, they are nonetheless morally significant. We do, of course, have laws and principles to govern our relationships to distant others, but these cannot do all the moral work required to ensure that we act well and responsibly toward distant others. As Alasdair MacIntyre writes:

> The networks of giving and receiving in which we participate can only be sustained by a shared recognition of each other's needs and a shared allegiance to a standard of care . . . [without which] laws will often be observed from fear of the consequences of doing otherwise, sometimes grudgingly and always in a way that has regard to the letter rather than to the spirit of the laws. (1997, 84–5)

7.3.2 Undesired Benevolence—Especially as Care is Directed at People with Disabilities

A feature of an ethic of care, which we cannot really term "a temptation," is that we should be attentive to people who may need care and anticipate the need even before help is requested. We should not wait until a person has already struggled getting a suitcase up three flights of stairs before asking if that person needs help with the fourth flight. Yet many people with disabilities regard unsolicited help as intrusive, paternalistic, and sometimes outright insulting. Adam Cureton, a philosopher of disability, has zoomed in on this conundrum. He writes, "Simple acts of kindness that are performed sincerely and with evident good will can also, paradoxically, be received as deeply insulting by the people we succeed in benefiting" (2016, 74). Yet for people without speech or another form of expressive communication, such careful attention to their needs is necessary precisely because they cannot ask for help.

But is this anticipation of need always appropriate? Imagine that you see someone who is blind and using a cane, who is about to head for a store window rather than a street crossing. You take his arm and start walking with him to the crosswalk and escorting him to the other side. The man needed help but does not display much gratitude. Have you acted wrongly, or has he not been gracious in accepting needed help? Imagine that you are vision impaired and moving through an airport you have traversed many times before. Your journey is interrupted several times by some kindly airport attendant who suggests that you request wheelchair assistance. The first time you answer matter-of-factly that you are very familiar with this route and when you need help you will ask for it; by the third time you are stopped you repeat the same words brusquely, almost rudely. At the end of chapter 8 I will argue that we have an obligation to accept care graciously when offered with good faith and with competence, and when there is a need. Has the disabled person in these instances failed to meet this obligation, or is the fault in those who have intervened? Why do we encounter the hostility to our efforts to assist? How and when should we make offers of assistance?

Cureton alerts us to one difficulty that the instrusive benevolence generates. Generally we feel the need to reciprocate when another does us a kindness. Without the opportunity to reciprocate we feel indebted, and we can even feel inferior if we are unable to reciprocate. Therefore unsolicited acts of kindness, when directed at people who are frequently stigmatized and regarded as inferior in ability, need careful consideration. The temptation to assist may be just that: a temptation. Unless we have checked in with the person in question or accurately observed that the person desires our help, we may be gratifying our sense of our goodness rather than the need of another. Cureton's caveat suggests that attention needs to be directed not only at what we perceive as another's need, but also at whether or not the person we are tempted to assist desires this assistance. If they do not, then the caring thing to do is to leave them be.

7.3.3 The Cult of Self-Sacrifice and the Collapse of Relationality

Another temptation of an ethic of care arises directly from the need for the caregiver to set aside her own needs when the needs of the cared-for are pressing. This can lead to a cult of self-sacrifice that, as Carol Gilligan so astutely remarks, undermines the very connectedness that sits at the heart of care. A relationship involves more than a single self, but when one self sacrifices for another, there is no longer a relationship between two integral selves—one self is lost in the process. Gilligan writes that in an ethic of care, the transition from a conventional to a postconventional morality "begins with reconsideration of the relationship between self and other, as the woman starts to scrutinize the logic of self-sacrifice in the service of a morality of care. . . .The woman asks if it is possible to be responsible to herself as well as to others and thus to reconcile the disparity between hurt and care" (1982, 82).

A contrary but related temptation, one that people with disabilities who need care are especially wary of, is the potential for the carer to lose sight of the separateness of the person for whom she cares. The danger is that she will impose her own conception of the good (or alternatively an abstract notion of what is good) upon the cared-for without sufficient attention to the subjectivity of the one for whom she cares. Once again, to affirm the relationality of the self, it is also imperative to affirm the distinctness of each self in the relation. Another way to put this is to say that an ETHICS OF CARE needs to be sensitive to the rights and individuality of both caregiver and cared-for, even as it stresses the responsibilities that arise out of the relationship of care and the intermingling of desires and interests to which such a relationship gives rise. The self, in an ETHICS OF CARE, is at once deeply enmeshed with others and yet always also a distinct self.

7.3.4 Care Ethics as a "Slave Morality"

A frequent criticism lodged at an ethics of care comes from feminists who have argued that care is, as Nietzsche would have it, a "slave morality." Feminist critics of an ethics of care claim that if it is empirically true that women exhibit an ethic of care, it is an ethic borne of their subjection, arising as it does from women's traditional labor, labor that women have been compelled to perform by custom and law. They argue that if women are to emerge from this subjugated condition, they need to adopt an ethic more suited to liberation from traditional roles. These criticisms have a bearing for disabled people as well: If disabled people are to demand their place in the world as equal citizens, then why subscribe to a "slave morality," a morality of the powerless?

In response to such criticisms, proponents of an ETHICS OF CARE can argue that an ethics arising from a subjugated position reveals that the subordinated in fact do have a voice. This different voice can inject new values into an oppressive society. To aspire to dominant values is often to collude with the very values that serve to oppress. The discussion in the previous chapter concerning the relationship between disabled people's embrace of "independence" and the invisibility of the personal attendant exemplifies this conundrum. I don't believe that people with disabilities want to perpetuate what Annette Baier called the "moral proletariat," the position of domestics and care workers within a theory focused on rights and independence (1995, 55).

7.3.5 Unequal Relationships

One still may want to ask whether people with disabilities should embrace an ethics based on the inequality of parties in a moral relationship, rather than one that presumes and works toward equality. An ethic of care has often used the care of an infant as a paradigm of care, which can then lead to the same error we identified in chapter 6: assuming that all dependency is infantile. Treating an infant as an incapacitated adult or an incapacitated adult as an infant will not be providing good care for either, but neither will the pretense of equality serve either in the relationship well.

Addressing the limitations of a rights approach to morality, Annette Baier speaks of the sham in the "'promotion' of the weaker so that an appearance of virtual equality is achieved . . . children are treated as adults-to-be, the ill and dying are treated as continuers of their earlier more potent selves." She continues:

> This pretense of an equality that is in fact absent may often lead to a desirable protection of the weaker or more dependent. But it somewhat masks the question of what our moral relationships *are* to those who are our superiors or our inferiors in power. (1995, 55)

She goes on to suggest that a morality that invokes a mock equality and independence, if not supplemented, may well "unfit people to be anything other than what its justifying theories suppose them to be, ones who have no interest in each others' interests" (1995). That is, it may leave us without adequate moral resources to deal with the genuine inequalities of power and situation that we face daily, and which not infrequently are conditions that certain impairments (apart from social arrangements) impose on us.

Instead we need an ethic that can guide relationships between different sorts of care providers (nonpaid family members, hands-on paid care assistants, professional medical personnel) and people with different sorts of care needs. The urgencies of need, whether they arise from medical emergencies, a break-down in critical medical equipment, or disabling conditions not addressable by accommodation, are ones that render disabled persons (and often those who care for them) vulnerable. Many able people are also subject to such circumstances, and when they are, they do not want to be "abandoned to their autonomy" (Pellegrino and Thomasma 1987, 31).[21] An ETHICS OF CARE walks the line between the Scylla of paternalism or domination and the Charybdis of neglect.[22]

---

[21] See also O'Neill (1984).

[22] The inequalities extend beyond the relation of carer and cared-for. Where a child needs professional care from a physician, for instance, the parent and the child are both vulnerable and dependent on the physician. The same is true for a disabled adult and her carer when the disabled adult is in need of specialized care. For an excellent discussion of this sort of vulnerability see Feder (2002).

8

The Completion of Care—The Normativity of Care

8.1 Starting with the Completion of Care

Descriptions of care usually begin with the obligations and responsibilities of the carer: at the front end—so to speak—of the caring relationship.[1] If, however, we look at an ethic of care from its endpoint, that is, from its reception, certain important features of the caring relationship and of a care ethics become newly and especially salient. In particular, care as a fully normative conception comes into relief. That is, we can identify in the concept of care the particular conception of CARE that functions in an ETHICS OF CARE.

The way into the question I pursue in this chapter comes from an aspect of care first remarked upon by Nel Noddings and later by Joan Tronto. Noddings writes: "My caring has somehow to be completed in the other if the relation is to be described as caring" (1984, 4). Fischer and Tronto write that care-receiving, the final phase of caregiving, "involves the responses to the caring process of those toward whom caring is directed" (1990, 40).

Most moral concepts that we call "virtues" do not behave in this fashion. I can be prudent, gracious, honest, charitable, and temperate even if no one responds to my efforts as instances of such virtuous action. If I succeed in rescuing an unconscious person from a burning building, my courage is already demonstrated, and it does not depend on the person recognizing my actions as courageous, nor does it depend on that person having wanted to be rescued. For the most part, virtues are virtuous insofar as the person acts with a right intent and in the right manner. Whether an action is taken up by another as an instance of such a virtue is not an issue.

---

[1] Portions of this chapter have appeared in the following (Kittay 2014; 2018; 2011b).

There are, however, other moral theories where the endpoint matters. Classic utilitarianism holds that right action is the maximization of pleasure (or happiness) and the minimization of pain (or unhappiness). An action is right, then, only if utility is thereby maximized. "Mercy" and "respect" work the same way. We act mercifully toward someone insofar as we want her to be relieved of a burden. If a governor with the ability to commute the sentence of an inmate on death row decides to be merciful and spare the prisoner's life, but the inmate sees the commutation of his sentence as a form of torture, not mercy, then commuting the sentence may not, in fact, be merciful.[2] If I think it is disrespectful to ask about another's mortal illness because I believe such a question would be too personal and so presumptuous, but the afflicted person regards my silence as coldness and aloofness, then my attempt to be respectful has misfired. CARE, I believe, is this sort of moral concept.[3]

That is to say, "care" is CARE only when it is completed through its reception. To put the point still more strongly, the normative content of CARE—that is to say, what distinguishes CARE from care—is that it is taken up by the other as CARING. As I begin here to consider its uptake as critical to CARE, we can see a number of things about CARE that otherwise might not be apparent. In particular, we can see why a CARE ETHICS requires action and is not based only on intention; how realizing the moral worth of an action requires some sort of relationship between the carer and cared for; why CARE should be distinguished from paternalism; and why moral luck plays a big role in caring successfully. I will end with a surprising implication that I have already hinted at earlier: That not only do we sometimes have a *duty to care*, we also have a *duty to receive care graciously* if it is offered with a good will and with the requisite attention and competence, insofar as we have the capacity to discharge such a duty.

8.2 The Taking-Up of Care—The Logic of Care

Why has the reception of care received so little attention? I do not know why others have missed its importance. But I do know why I failed to do so. The model that informed my thinking about care also shaped my views about its reception. That model was care for my daughter. My criterion for the adequacy

---

[2] I say "may" rather than "will" because it can happen that the prisoner whose life is spared eventually finds happiness or meaning even though he did not think it was possible prior to the intended act of mercy.

[3] I hope I will be forgiven for repeating some of the thinking of Tronto and Noddings as I integrate this notion into my own way of working through the idea of an ethic of care. A good idea is well worth repeating and worthy of new framings.

of any ethics—including care ethics—was whether it would be true to the care of Sesha and people with similar disabilities. Although now an adult woman of forty-eight, she remains incapable of doing anything that falls within the conventional understanding of acknowledging or refusing another's care: she can neither say thank you, nor flee or otherwise refuse the care she receives. It was absurd to say that because of her incapacities, what we do for her is not care because there is no way she can "complete our care."[4]

It was only when I found myself having to care for my ninety-two-year-old mother that I came to appreciate the idea that care needs to be completed in the other. Unlike my daughter, my mother would sometimes acknowledge my care with words of praise and thanks, but more often, she would fiercely resist my attempts to help her. Sesha's response to our caring presented a stark contrast to my mother's bitterness at her powerlessness and lost capacities. Faced with the intransigence of someone in need of care but who refuses it, I came to recognize that Sesha did in fact receive our care. I realized that she could in fact turn away; could, even with her limited means, resist; and get angry at her impotence, as do some folks with whom she rooms. It suddenly became apparent that Sesha is much less passive than I had acknowledged. There are times when she makes it difficult for us to give her medication, when she turns away at something unpleasant we have to do, and there are other times when she clearly helps us to help her. I have come to see that Sesha's thriving is itself a responsiveness to our care; that the hugs, smiles, and her own distinctive "kisses" are still other forms of receiving our care.[5] All this she does with a beautiful graciousness. It is precisely because Sesha receives her care with such grace that I was able to miss the fact that she does indeed complete our care.

The general assumption is that to be a recipient is to be passive. To resist is instead a mark of agency. But this is false. To be receptive to care can itself be an active affirmation of a willingness to be helped and to embrace the relationship that care establishes. To refuse care may be a form of passivity in the face of suffering, and a refusal of care can be found in a passive resistance to actively engage with another. Care is not something we do *to* something or someone. It is something we do *for* another's benefit. There has to be an uptake on the other's part if our action is to count as a benefit for the other. If the other is not benefitted—has not taken up our actions as a good—we have failed to confer a benefit. To underscore the active element in the reception of care, I will speak of the completion of care as the "taking-up of care."

---

[4] Although Tronto speaks of caring for things as well as people, there is no discussion of the reception phase that could clarify how those persons or things that could not acknowledge or refuse care could be involved in care's reception.

[5] For a description of Sesha's kisses, see my depiction in Kittay (2000).

How important is the taking-up of care to the act of care?[6] Let us begin by considering a very simple example: caring for a plant by watering it. Now suppose that unbeknownst to me, I pick up a glass of *vinegar* instead of a glass of water to pour into a dry wilting plant. Predictably, the plant begins to wither instead of perk up. Have I cared for the plant? Most of us would answer, "No."[7]

Of course, pouring vinegar rather than water was an error on my part. Some errors result from incompetence or carelessness. But if I had no reason to suspect that someone would leave a glass of vinegar in my vicinity, the error was not due to my carelessness, thoughtlessness, or lack of competence. My action was not perfunctory. Yet even if my act was motivated by my love or concern for the welfare of the plant and my desire to see it thrive, I could not be said to be caring for the plant. Although I may not be blameworthy, I failed to carry out a responsibility I took upon myself, namely to care for the plant. If, as it appears, pouring vinegar when I intended to water the plant was not care, then this simple case illustrates that: *We have a strong intuitive sense that a thing's or person's well-being must be positively affected by our actions if our actions are to be counted as care—at the very least, it ought not to be negatively affected.*[8] This intuition helps to ground what I have called the normative sense of care. Of particular importance to the development of a fully normative account of care—CARE —are the following three claims:

Proposition 1. Caring requires action, or it is not yet CARING. This is because nothing can have the effect of CARE, if it is not put into action.

Proposition 2. CARE is an achievement and *"to CARE"* is a success verb.

Proposition 3. CARE requires that the object of the care *respond* in some way that results in the achievement of the act—that is, CARING requires that the cared-for *"take up the action as care."*

These are first, and not final, formulations of the propositions. Each of these propositions are contentious claims, and there are important nuances and qualifications that are needed to make them cover all—and only—those cases that should be included in the notion of CARE. Let me take these considerations in turn.

---

[6] For the moment I drop the distinction between care and CARE. There is a deep logic to the general concept of care that concerns us here. That logic will figure into the more precise sense I mean to capture in the use of the locution CARE.

[7] Since I first presented this thought experiment, the response of many and diverse audiences is overwhelmingly "No, I have not cared for the plant."

[8] I use the term "well-being" here as a neutral term covering different conceptions of well-being such as welfare and flourishing.

8.2.1 CARING Is an Action or a Disposition to Act

The claim I wish to defend is that while the term "care" is used in many different ways, when it is used with normative content, then "to CARE" is to *act* in a certain way, or to have the *disposition to act* in this manner. That is to say, care or caring is *not only* a frame of mind (though it is that as well), nor is it simply an intention. To be in a caring frame of mind or to have caring intentions would mean nothing at all if these were not tethered to a willingness to act in certain caring ways when the appropriate circumstance pertains.

Let us take a moment to consider Tronto's phases of care and see if this claim is defensible.[9] "Caregiving" is the phase of care that clearly involves action. "Taking responsibility" similarly implies that we will act in such a way that the other's needs get met, whether we ourselves meet these needs or ensure that a third party does. We can't claim, for instance, that we are taking care of someone's financial matters, and do nothing to assure that their financial matters are taken care of.

"Caring about" less obviously involves action, since that term is first of all attitudinal. We can care about many things without actually *doing something*. We believe we care about the hungry children in the world even if we do not travel the world feeding hungry children. But if we never give a dime to organizations who try to feed the hungry, nor vote for the candidate who is most likely to pay attention to world hunger, nor engage in any action whereby we can say this is our small part in doing something to alleviate world hunger, then we vacate the claim that we care about world hunger.

Two senses of "care for" seem to require no action at all and seem to offer counterexamples to the claim I am pressing. One is used to convey a preference (as in "I care for some ice cream"), and the second is to express warm feelings (as in "I care for Sally, but Sally doesn't care for me"). These carry no requirements for correlative action. I can care for ice cream—really love it!—but refuse to eat it because I want to reduce my caloric intake. Because Sally doesn't care for me,

---

[9] Theorists of care have made important distinctions between the many ways in which the term "care" is used. Bernice Fischer and Joan Tronto sequence some of these senses when they speak of the phases of care. According to their model, we first care about something, then we take responsibility to take care of it, and then we do the caregiving required. The care is completed when the cared-for receives the care. Fischer and Tronto distinguish taking care of and caregiving, but frequently both are thought of as aspects of caring for another rather than caring about them. Even though it is useful to make the lexical distinctions that Fischer and Tronto make, I do not follow them in their sequencing of the "phases" of care. The sequencing is neither conceptually nor temporally necessary. For example, sometimes one is thrown into a situation where we must care for another without actually caring about that individual. What frequently will happen is that the relationship that forms gives rise to a "caring about," which becomes a motivational attitude. Once such a bond is formed, we want to care for a person because we care about her.

I may do nothing to express my feelings toward her, nor act in any way that betrays my feelings for her. In itself having a preference or "having tender feelings" toward someone or something is not a moral attitude or a moral disposition, and so neither operates in the sense relevant to CARE. Feelings toward something or someone will often serve as important moral motivations propelling us to act. Except when they are motivations for caring actions, these uses of "care" and "caring" are not relevant to an ETHICS OF CARE.

What are we to say of the use of the term "cares" in the sense of a set of worries, burdens, or needs? I use the term CARES in the previous chapters to speak of those things we attend to when we attend to an individual's legitimate wants and genuine needs.[10] When we give CARE, we are taking care of another's CARES: we are assuming responsibility, and then doing what needs to be done about the CARES another has. Thus CARES are what people acting in accordance with an ETHICS OF CARE respond to by some action.

With respect to my own CARES, I can worry myself to death without doing anything to take care of the matters that I am concerned about. Here again, the failure to act—when action is warranted and when I am capable of it—raises the question of how much importance to place on these concerns, or even whether or not they, in fact, are cares or concerns of mine. While it may not be infelicitous to speak of CARES about which I do nothing (when I can and should do something), it does somehow impugn my character. We soon lose sympathy with someone whose only response to his CARES is to fret over them. One more use of caring is worth remarking upon, namely to describe someone's character. We speak of someone as a caring person, a person with a warm heart. What is implied is that this person is emotionally attuned to the concerns of another. Once more, if these attitudes do not impel a putatively "caring" person to perform *acts* of care when the opportunities present themselves, we revise our conception of them. A caring person is just a person with a disposition to act in a CARING manner.

To conclude, we can say that, in all its senses, action has a bearing on anything we want to call CARE: To care (for or about) or to be a caring person is to engage in caring activities or to be prepared to engage in actions that such care demands. To have cares is to have concerns about matters we believe are important to act upon, if such action is doable and advisable. To care for a person in the sense of having affection for that person is to be motivated to act to benefit the person when we are able to do so. And to be a caring person is to act in a caring manner when the occasion demands it.

---

[10] See chapter 6 for a discussion of this formulation.

8.2.2 CARE as an Achievement Term

Our withered plant thought experiment carried the implication that CARE is a particular kind of action, namely one that is an achievement. The British ordinary language philosopher Gilbert Ryle drew a distinction between verbs that named tasks (e.g., "running"), those that signaled failures (e.g., "losing"), and those that marked achievements (e.g., "winning"). The meaning of an achievement verb includes the idea that the action aimed for was successful. If we say of someone that they can spell a word, it means that they provide the correct letters in the right order. It also implies that the actor was competent to do this and that this was not a random action. If you can spell the word, you know *how* to spell it—a typewriter mechanically spewing out letters will at times come out with recognizable words, but we don't presume that the typewriter spelled any of these words. Most importantly, achievement terms include the end result, and not merely the tasks or conditions needed to achieve the end.[11] Ryle writes:

> For the runner to win, not only must he run but also his rivals must also arrive at the tape later than he; for a doctor to effect a cure, his patient must both be treated and be well again; for the searcher to find the thimble, there must be a thimble in the place he indicates at the moment when he indicates it. (1984, 150)

Just as there must be a thimble in the place that a person indicates if we say that the person found the thimble, so the person caring must have something or someone in need of her care. Just as the doctor must not only treat a patient but the patient must be well again if we are to say that the doctor cured the patient, so must the carer not only attend to the cared-for, but the cared-for also has to receive these attentions as caring (something which is not always as clear cut as a cure, but is nonetheless something which we can articulate sufficiently well for it to count as an achievement). Activities that are intended as caring must involve the achievement of caring or they are not yet CARE. For CARE there must be:

1. Needs or wants of those cared for that require attention.
2. A carer who has the requisite competencies called for in *this* situation.
3. The individual (person or thing) cared for should be better off than before by some specifiable criteria.

---

[11] Ryle tells us "some state of affairs obtains over and above that which consists in the performance, if any, of the subservient task activity" (Ryle 1984, 150).

A thing may need to be properly maintained or repaired. The plant needs to be replenished with the right sort of liquid. An animal that needs care may need to be restored to its previous condition or have its habitat restored.

What counts as uptake depends on the nature of the cared-for. The cared-for may be a living thing, but one that has no subjectivity. In that case, uptake is a physical process, such as the revival of a withering plant if it is watered (with water, not vinegar). But when the cared-for individuals are subjects, which is to say that they are capable of a subjective life, caring aims to do more; it aims to contribute to their flourishing.[12] In sum, *an action will count as* CARE *if it contributes to the well-being, restoration, or flourishing of a being or a subject.*[13] In the previous chapter I proposed the following aim of CARE, as an ETHICS OF CARE conceives it: *a concern for the flourishing (or minimally the well-being) of a person for his or her own sake, that is, not for the sake of the larger community or some abstract conception of goodness.* The concern takes the form of actions directed at the genuine needs and legitimate wants of the individual requiring care.

A care ethics also specifies a constraint on how the aim is legitimately achieved. Just as one does not win a race by knocking down opponents to ensure that one gets to the finish line first, so CARE is constrained by what care ethics recognizes as moral harm, most importantly exploitation, domination, and the neglect of others' needs. To insist that an action that fails to achieve its end (even when it is carried out with the intention to care or with the attitude of care) is insufficient to make it an act of care is not to propose a stipulative definition. As our plant example shows us, insisting that care is an achievement verb is based on a strong intuition that is very widely shared. It is this intuition I am isolating in the use of CARE (that is, care in the fully normative sense) when I insist that the achievement of CARE requires uptake on the part of the cared-for.

---

[12] I will be using the term "flourishing" to mean having a flourishing life across one's lifespan. At times this may mean no more than making a person comfortable and to the extent possible, feeling cared for, because that is all the person is capable of experiencing at that point. At life's end, it may mean having what we may call a good death, and by this I mean a death without much pain, in the company of people we care about and who care about us, that is, in circumstances that provide us with comfort and love.

[13] Some care theorists, such as Fiona Robinson, "the ability to care with commitment about another can emerge only through sustained connections among persons and groups of persons" (Robinson 1999, 157). I think the plant example makes it clear that we can and we do care for and care about nonhuman beings. Our care for pets is still more evidence. But we can also care for a painting, by ensuring that it remains well preserved, or fail to care for it by subjecting it to conditions under which it will deteriorate. Some would deny that we care for the thing itself and not for the humans who care about the picture. Its an interesting question but it takes us too far afield. Tronto's most expansive concept of care (which is too expansive for CARE)—that caring is any activity that maintains or repairs the world we live in—allows that we can care more broadly than for persons (1994, 103).

This may nonetheless sound too demanding. If we say "Sue intended to care for her sister, Ann, but didn't succeed—because Sue did more harm than good," we can admit that Sue cares about Ann and tried to do what she thought would be best for her (and so went beyond mere feeling into action). The intent and the effort may have been admirable (even commendable),[14] but Ann did not get the care that she needed, and Sue did not provide it. Sue might also have tried to take care of what she *assumed* Ann needed, when that was not what Ann felt she herself needed. When help is not needed, but a would-be carer insists on helping, her action may not even be commendable. As we pointed out in previous chapters, disabled people resent help that is unasked for, and when combined with incompetence, such attempts at care can easily turn into harm.

If care in the normative sense is an achievement term, then Sue fails to CARE for Ann just as we would say that I failed to care for my plant when I poured vinegar onto it. Can we then conclude that nothing is CARING unless it hits the mark—that is, unless it in some way contributes to the recipient's flourishing? Before we can adopt this position, there are important questions and one important qualification.

The qualification first: The one who is cared for may at once recognize her carer's sincere effort to care, while knowing that these efforts will fail to meet her actual needs. Sometimes merely experiencing the other's *desire to care* for oneself can be a contribution to one's flourishing. As clumsy or inadequate as these efforts may be, we can be moved by the evident tenderness and concern, and these efforts can make us *feel better*. It is important, however, that inducing in another the sense that they are being cared for requires sincerity and good faith. A carer who feigns the intention to care, for manipulative or exploitive reasons, morally fails on several grounds: she has not met the cared-for's needs, she lacks the appropriate attitude for caring, and she may even envision using the deception for harm. Should her genuine motives ever come to light, the *feeling* of being cared for will quickly dissipate.

It is plausible to consider whether or not we are wrong to insist that the *achievement* of care is part of the *moral* content of care. There are many reasons why care may not be, or could not have been, completed in the other, and the fault may not lie with the attitudes, intentions, or sincere efforts of the carer. It seems problematic to claim that the carer is not to be morally commended for her attempts to care, and that she should not be given moral praise for being caring.

To respond to this objection, we need once again to consider the point of caring. I have maintained that the act of care is meant to meet the genuine

---

[14] I thank Michael Slote for this observation.

needs and legitimate wants of another, especially when the one who has them cannot meet them him- or herself. Harm that results from a failure of care occurs not merely if we fail to act, but if we fail to succeed. This is because the harm we aim to avoid within an ethics of care is not only the unwarranted interference into another's life and affairs prominent in most modern ethical theories. Rather, within an ethics of care, what is often required is the active intervention on another's behalf.[15] If we fail to succeed in caring, we are willy-nilly causally implicated in an ethically important harm. A Kantian good will, which Kant maintained was the only unqualified good in the world, without the *successful* action, does not feed a hungry infant. And unless the infant is fed, it dies. The well-intentioned person may not be morally culpable for the death, but neither can she be praised for bringing about a moral good or preventing a moral harm.

Just as importantly, the way in which a carer goes about meeting these concerns is also a factor in whether the care is taken up as care. A patient with advanced Alzheimer's disease who is incontinent and needs to be refreshed by an attendant might resist the action and have enough awareness of personal shame to be humiliated by the carer's efforts. The attendant who proceeds without regard for the shame felt by the patient *does* meet the bodily need for being cleaned, and in this limited sense provides care—the body is cleansed as a consequence of his actions. But at the same time, the attendant has failed to contribute to the patient's flourishing if his actions result in making the patient feel demeaned, and in this sense the attendant has failed to care. If there is no gentle and dignifying way to accomplish the task, then the attendant is in a quandary.[16] When the caring is taken up as caring, the carer contributes to the others' flourishing and to the avoidance of harm (especially as an ethics of care defines harm).[17]

That we missed our mark may simply be an instance of bad moral luck:[18] the carer has a patient with Alzheimer's disease who is unrelenting in fighting her as she attempts to clean up her incontinent patient. Or some unjust circumstance has made our attempt to care impossible to carry out: the parent, herself starved, has nothing to feed her infant and so cannot care for her child.

We can mitigate the harshness of the moral position that only care that is taken up as care is CARE, if we follow G. E. Moore: "That we didn't act other than

---

[15] In Kantian terms, these are not the perfect duties but the imperfect ones. While the imperfect duties of benevolence are not required of anyone in particular, unlike perfect duties which are required of all, the duties within a care ethics are more properly *responsibilities* that fall on whoever is in the appropriate role or the contingent situation of one in a position to assist.

[16] Sarah Clark Miller (2012) refers to care that attends to the person's dignity as "dignifying care." I am making the claim that all care that is CARE needs to be dignified care.

[17] I use the plural form here to acknowledge that one carer may be caring for several people at a time.

[18] See the section below, "Moral Luck," for a fuller discussion.

how we acted, even though our actions did not result in right action, does not necessarily mean that we acted *wrongly*" (2005, 14, emphasis mine). Similarly, Julia Driver (2005, 192) who, in developing a "sophisticated consequentialism," uses Derek Parfit's term "blameless wrongdoing" (Parfit 1984).[19] It is interesting to note that many carers, in fact, do feel this way when their caring efforts fail: "I did the best I could, but sadly I failed and she is just as bad off as (or worse off than) before." Moreover, carers at times are irked when people attempt to console them with praise, and that is precisely because they recognize that their actions did not warrant the praise, even if their intentions might.

But what about those intentions? Are they of no moral value in and of themselves within an ETHICS OF CARE? If they are not of any moral significance, then an ETHICS OF CARE is simply another form of consequentialism.[20] But they clearly have moral significance in an ethic of care. That someone's needs are met without anyone's intent to give care signifies only that a need has been met, not that CARE was given. Consider a man who has lost all interest in the world, throws his money out the window, and says to himself (as he watches the bedlam below): "Look at the fools below picking up the useless paper!" This misanthrope has doubtless met the needs of many, but he will have cared for none, and no one who has benefitted from his actions will feel cared for by him. What remains crucial to CARE is that the action is executed *out of concern for the other's welfare or the other's ability to flourish*.[21] This is a motivational or, better still, an intentional constraint on the part of the carer. [22] Such intentionality is essential to our evaluation of the outcome as CARE. Even actions one might have experienced as caring at the time they were carried out might be revalued as uncaring

[19] Consequentialists use the notion somewhat differently from the way I do as I adopt the notion. They are generally concerned about two conflicting motives, one which would lead us to do the right thing because it is the better thing to do, while the motive we acted upon displays a good disposition but would not be the better thing to do. In my case I am not speaking of two sets of motives. But if the attempt to care arises from a caring disposition, then one can say that the act is blameless, even if the desired result did not occur and so is not praiseworthy.

[20] Although John Stuart Mill insisted that intention is everything in utilitarianism as well: "the morality of the action depends entirely on the intention of the action, that is on what the agent wills to do."(2001, 18-9)

[21] Here again I am not drawing a sharp distinction between welfare and flourishing.

[22] We can appeal to Mill's (2001, 18-9) distinction between a motivation and an intention. Intention is part of what makes an act what it is and hence the morality of the act depends on the intention. We can have a motive to act out of empathetic concern, where the action is one that intends that we express our empathetic concern for the other's well-being. Alternatively, we may provide care out of a sense of duty, where the intention to act caringly is just the intention to act out of a sense of duty. While I may not be acting out of an empathetic concern for the other, I could nonetheless be acting caringly if I act with the intention to benefit the other when I meet their genuine needs and attain their legitimate wants.

if it turns out that the intentions were not appropriate. The point is nicely illustrated in a segment of the movie *The Blind Side*. Big Mike is an African-American teenager who is adopted by a white family when he is already in his teens. With their help, Mike becomes a successful high school athlete with an academic record strong enough to make him an attractive recruit to many colleges. When someone suggests to him that all the efforts on the part of the family were to groom him to become a player for the mother's alma mater's team, he confronts his adopted mother and asks her accusingly, "What was this all for? Was it for me or was it to acquire a winning football player for your school?" As implausible as that accusation is, the mere suspicion of such an intention was sufficient to throw into doubt all the manifestations of care: the sacrifices, efforts, apparent trust, and affection.

Although the nature of the inner state typical of CARE may generally be characterized as empathy, and empathy may be critical to successfully caring, it may not be critical to having the intention to care.[23] The empathy may arise from a history with the cared-for or out of an empathetic disposition that can be extended to strangers no less than to intimates. Yet I think one cannot rule out an inner state that is equally well characterized as a Kantian good will.[24] Duty seems inimical to care, and in many circumstances it is. Still, a hired caregiver who has to attend to a cantankerous but very ill older person may still take it to be her duty to attend to this person's needs (and do as well or better than a relative who lacks the requisite skills but would be caring out of a more affective tie). Care can be so costly to the caregiver that it may even require some element of duty to sustain it through periods of difficulty. Although an ETHICS OF CARE is not a deontological ethics that *demands* duty, duty may be able to compensate for the absence of feelings of affection if it is sufficiently responsive to the other's needs and wants and is administered so that it can be taken up as care by the cared-for.[25]

It is, however, difficult to carry off care over the long term without some inner state that conforms to what we normally take to be a caring attitude arising from an emotional connection we have to another. Parental care requires such an emotional connection, specifically love, if we are to provide the benefit children require. The absence of such love in a parental relationship may not only diminish the quality of care. The lack of love may itself be harmful. Like empathy, love and an emotional connection, however, are not always required. Those who

---

[23] See Michael Slote (2007) for an alternative but not inimical understanding of the relationship between duty and care, understood in terms of empathy.

[24] Also see Sarah Clark Miller (2012), who develops a Kantian account of a "duty to care."

[25] This is an interesting twist on Kant, since for Kant only acting out of duty (and not merely in accordance with duty) makes the action a moral one.

acquire a caring disposition are capable of acting in a caring manner to a total stranger. If the relationship is sustained past the initial contact, the emotional bond usually *arises from*, rather than gives rise to, the caring relationship.

A caring disposition is a virtue and, insofar as the intention exhibits that disposition, it is worthy of praise. Acting caringly out of love or a strong affective bond short of love, or even out of a sense of duty, is also praiseworthy. Still, the value that we attach to a caring attitude (whatever its source) tells us primarily that a caring attitude is necessary, not that it is sufficient. If the action fails to provide the benefit or offers a benefit but causes more harm than good, then the action isn't praiseworthy as a caring action, no matter if it reveals a praiseworthy character and a praiseworthy intention. To return to the analogy with other achievement terms, someone can be praised for entering a race and trying their best to win. If they failed but exhibited good sportsmanship in the face of their loss, they are rightly praised for good sportsmanship. If they prepared well for the race and gave it their best effort, these efforts deserve praise irrespective of the outcome. But if they fail to get to the finish line first, they still have not won the race and do not get the credit that is due to the winner.

If the field of ethics is parsed into deontology, consequentialism, and virtue theory, it appears an ethic based on care fails to neatly fit any of these.[26] It is sui generis. What will count for an ETHICS OF CARE, then, is whether the person in need of care is attended to in such a way that they receive the care they require (and the tenderness or concern of another may be part of the care a person requires), and that the care is being received as care.

That care is an achievement term both determines the normative condition of an ETHICS OF CARE and helps mark an ETHICS OF CARE as a distinctive ethics, if not a self-standing theory.

Thus far we have argued that an ETHICS OF CARE is a sui generis ethics that requires:

1. An intentional agent, that is, a moral agent who intends to and succeeds in benefitting the subject (or object) of care.
2. Intention based on an affective relationship to the cared-for, or in the absence of a prior relationship or the affective sentiment, on a sense of duty or of concern born of a caring disposition.
3. A benefit for the cared-for, for the cared-for's own sake, which comes about through the successful actions of the carer.

[26] Whether it can handle all the problems that other ethical theories can is still an unsettled matter, just as is the question of whether an ethics of care is a stand-alone theory or a supplement to another moral theory. These are not questions that can be resolved at this point of the development of an ethics of care.

An ETHICS OF CARE also requires the following, which we will discuss in the next section: If the cared-for is herself a subject who is at all capable of endorsing the intended benefit, then the action needs to be taken up as care by the cared-for, if not at the time it is performed, then in hindsight.

8.2.3 Our CARING Must be "Taken Up as Care"

What does the taking-up of care on the part of the cared-for look like? In the case of the plant, that participation is akin to a heliotropic response: that is, it is without intention, will, or agency of any sort, but it is a responsiveness that is inherent in that sort of being. As there is no subjectivity on the part of the plant, whether or not care has been given can be determined entirely from a third-person standpoint. Either the plant survives or it dies. I contend that such purely objective measures of the success of caring are insufficient when the cared-for is a subject, and I will consider the many different ways we might consider how beings, in different states of awareness and stages of development, take up care as beings with a subjective self.

But first, I want to point out how the claims made here about the taking-up of care exhibit the intimate connection between this conception of care and the normativity of care. I suggested earlier that one test of whether we can say we are using care in a fully normative sense is whether the claim that someone "cares too much" is incoherent, in a way similar to the claim that someone is "being too just" is incoherent.[27] The two propositions—that CARE has to be taken up by the other *as* care, along with the added one that the subjective endorsement of the carer's actions as care is necessary when the cared-for is a subject (and an ethic of care applies primarily to care directed at subjects)—do in fact lead us to conclude that caring too much is as incoherent as being too just.[28] The carer who "cares too much" is providing something that the person who is cared for doesn't care about. A caregiver whose ministrations are rejected (or criticized as "caring too much") may tell herself that her charge in time will come to see that her actions were caring. Her longings to be seen as caring may be so powerful, or

[27] When I speak of "caring too much," I am not speaking about a distributional matter. One can tend to "care too much" about people of one's own race and ignore the well-being of those of other races. This is like saying wealthy whites are given "too much justice" compared to poor whites or people of color, when we mean to say that the legal system gives too much deference to wealthy persons who are accused of white collar crimes compared to other groups who are given "too little justice," that is, too little fair consideration by the justice system.

[28] One could coherently "care too much" for an inanimate object, a car for example. One could spend hours on end polishing it, cleaning it, gazing affectionately at it, and ignoring other things one ought to be doing. If we do the equivalent to another subject, we may well get responses telling us that this is unwelcome attention.

her concern or love is so strong, that she cannot imagine that her actions may be anything but caring. Yet if we think of care in its normative sense, she may well be *wrong* in thinking that she is CARING at all.

8.3 The Requirement of Subjectivity

I have claimed that the conception of care I am proposing is one in which a carer assists another in flourishing, especially when the other is inevitably dependent on another to meet genuine needs and legitimate wants. The claim we want to look at more carefully now is whether, in caring for a subject, there has to be a subjective taking-up of care as care. Although there are objective measures by which we can determine that a person is not flourishing, these cannot definitively tell us that a person *is* flourishing, at least in the sense that I want to speak of it, because flourishing means that the needs and wants we try to satisfy are ones we truly care about.[29] At best, an objective list, such as Martha Nussbaum's capabilities list (2000), can provide the conditions that many or most people need to flourish (although Nussbaum's claim is that the list includes what *all* people require). To flourish as a conscious sentient being includes having the sense that we are flourishing, sensing that we are living the life we want to live, having a sense of well-being—as we ourselves conceive of well-being. To live a life that others might think is a flourishing life, and yet to feel no sense of well-being, is not yet to flourish. Let me clarify further how I am talking about flourishing in the context of an ethic of care.

8.3.1 Flourishing and Subjective Endorsement

I have said earlier that to care about someone and to take care of or give care to another is to take up the cares of the other as one's own. One can care not only about oneself, but also about others, about causes, about things. One may fail to care about oneself for legitimate reasons or for illegitimate ones. If one lacks any sense of self-regard or self-respect, because—say—these have been taken away through oppressive and unjust social arrangements, then a lack of caring about oneself is morally problematic. But it is not problematic for a mother to care more about her dependent child's life than her own and to take food out of her own mouth to feed her needy child. The same can be said of caring more about the poor and needy than about oneself and even (though perhaps more controversially) to deny oneself to the point of death for the sake of those who have

---

[29] See the discussion in the section of chapter 7, "The Aims of Moral Relations."

been oppressed. Martyrs, such as those who took in Jews during the Nazi regime, and people motivated by deep religious conviction or by a profound commitment to social justice, such as Simone Weil, come to mind.[30] Although it may seem paradoxical to characterize as "flourishing" the lives of people who willingly suffer for others, we could say that given the conditions under which some are deprived of flourishing because of cruel circumstances, those who willingly suffer for others live lives that are intensely attuned to the CARES of others; they regard the flourishing of these others as essential to their own flourishing, and (to the degree that they engage these projects) theirs are flourishing lives. They are living the lives they want to live; they are doing what they care about; they are attending to their most urgent CARES, to what makes their lives meaningful.[31] To flourish, on this account, is to be able to attend to the things one cares about. A carer serves as an affordance for another who cannot tend to the things they care about without another's help.

The claim that a subjective element is *necessary* for flourishing, however, does not endorse the view that subjective criteria are *sufficient*. We can care about things that are genuinely harmful and either be aware or unaware of how harmful they are, either to others or to ourselves. For example, malnourished poor Indian women will report being adequately fed, even though their diets are worse than their husbands, who themselves report that their own diets are inadequate. Yet these women are in fact starving (Sen 1990). The starved woman who reports being adequately fed is as likely to face a premature death due to malnutrition as the one who acknowledges her deprivation.[32] We also can be pretty sure that if conditions were improved and more food were made available to them, they would experience their lives as better, at least as far as their nutrition goes (Khader 2011b).[33]

[30] These are the cares that Katharine Wolfe speaks of as second-person needs.

[31] I conceive of one's flourishing as delineated by the things one cares about. See Frankfurt (1988; 2004), and see chapter 7 in this volume. This conception of one's good takes us out of the confines of our own skin since much that we care about concerns the good of others and the things in the world that provide meaning in our lives. It is, of course, possible to care about things that are harmful to others, to care about harming others. Such objects of a person's care—cares that interfere with the cares of others—are ruled out by moral considerations and are incompatible with an ETHICS OF CARE. Flourishing *at the expense of* others' flourishing must be disqualified as a morally acceptable ideal in any ethical view—more so still in an ethical view that takes CARE as a fundamental value.

[32] It's possible that they don't care about a premature death, but dying prematurely is a clear failure to flourish, except perhaps in the case of the sort of martyrdom I discussed above.

[33] Serene Khader, in her philosophical study of adaptive preference formation, makes the claim: "More generally, we may say that if people have a tendency toward their basic flourishing, preferences that are inconsistent with their flourishing . . . are not deep preferences. That is, nonflourishing preferences formed under bad conditions are not only amenable to being changed; it is likely that people with adaptive preferences can come to endorse changes that will increase their capacities to flourish" (2011b, 53). Khader, however, urges that what counts as flourishing can be

That it is necessary (though not sufficient) for subjects to have the subjective sense of living a flourishing life may be taken as an expression of the importance of autonomy. For example, in setting forth her list of capabilities, Nussbaum isn't mandating that any one person realize all the capabilities, but only that persons have the opportunity to do so—that is, that no government action or lack of resources prevent them from doing so. Someone can freely choose to fast, as long as they have the capability to eat. Otherwise they are merely being starved.

To say, however, that such endorsement must be a matter of autonomous choice is too strong. A conscious volitional being may be incapable of autonomy and still have a sense of its own well-being. It is difficult to insist that my dog has any autonomy, yet I can discern when he is no longer hungry or has had his fill of affection. When we are dealing with human beings who are nonverbal or who are cognitively or psychologically impaired, endorsement can be difficult to discern, or it may be questionable whether the endorsement is something that we ought to respect when it appears to go contrary to the person's best interests. A resistance to an action intended as care may be due to a failure to comprehend the nature of the care; similarly, the lack of resistance may not be an endorsement but only a mere acquiescence. But just because we cannot be certain of rational reflection, it is not to be assumed that endorsement need not be sought. A person impaired or disabled in these cases can nonetheless be assumed to have a sense of what fulfills her and what runs contrary to her well-being, as she lives it.[34]

8.3.2 The Subject Who Is Unconscious

The requirement that there is a subjective uptake of another's actions as caring is readily susceptible to objections. Most important are those objections that presume that care can be, and often is, paternalistic. Stephen Darwall's account of care builds paternalism into the concept. He writes:

> Consider the difference between the perspective we take when in caring for someone, we attempt to work out what is good for her, on

identified only in vague and general terms. A more specific understanding of flourishing requires the endorsement of the subject under relatively good conditions.

[34] One could claim that a good carer intuits what the other really cares about, and as long as what she cares about involves no harm to others and appears to be a genuine want or need—that is, not one that is coerced or adopted out of fear or undue influence—the carer constructs an understanding of what would be a rational autonomous choice given such a care or set of cares. In this way, the choices that the carer helps to support are not merely "wanton," as Harry Frankfurt calls a life or a set of choices that are arbitrary and without reflection. But this takes us too far afield for the project at hand.

the one hand, and the perspective that is implicit in her own values, interests, and preferences, on the other. . . . The former is a perspective we attempt to take on the person, whereas the person's own values are what seems good to her from her point of view. (Darwall 2002, 14)

A person's welfare, he avers, is what a rational carer should want for that person. Wishing to attend to another's welfare, he maintains, arises from what he calls a "natural disposition" to care. The rationality in "rational care" comes from adhering to an objective conception of a person's good, which the carer *should* want for the cared-for, for the cared-for's own sake. While care arises from a "natural disposition," there is another moral disposition which considers the person's own view on his good. This is "respect." It requires that we view the other as autonomous and an end in herself with her own perspective of what is of value.

Because, on Darwall's account, a carer has an objective standard for the other's good, the carer is justified in acting paternalistically and overriding the cared-for's own idiosyncratic view of what is good and right for herself. In doing so, we will be caring for her, but we will not necessarily be respecting her. Darwall's approach reflects, I believe, a rather standard view of care as sanctioning paternalistic interference with another.[35]

Such a conception of care, I suspect, underlies the distaste many disability advocates have for care, and it is a view that identifies care as infantilizing the cared-for, making the cared-for an object of paternalistic concern rather than a subject whose subjectivity demands respect.

Against this conception of care is the view that care has to be a moral concept and not merely a natural disposition, and that care is fundamentally opposed to a paternalistic imposition of a putative objective conception of a person's good. The carer who acts in accordance with the moral concept CARE takes CARE as her regulative ideal. She disciplines herself to have what I have called a "transparent self," a self that is respectful of the perspective of the other and the other's own conception of her needs and wants.

---

[35] Injected in the moral codes of certain caring professions is the idea that we act "in the best interests" of a person who cannot make an autonomous decision. A paternalistic conception of medicine would hold that a physician can and should override the wishes of a patient, if the patient's view of their own good is, in the judgment of the physician, not in the patient's best interest. This is a view that is now generally held to be permissible only in the case of the "incompetent" patient, that is, the nonautonomous patient. According to the newer understanding of the physician's role, the healthcare provider respects the autonomy of the patient. I reject not only a paternalistic conception of care, but also a stark contrast between the autonomous patient and the incompetent patient. All patients are better served by a nonpaternalistic conception of care based on the idea that the carer needs to make him or herself transparent to the needs of the other. See Kittay (2007).

Let us look at a number of possible counterexamples that favor a view like Darwall's, and see how the intuitions about care, paternalism, and respect are sorted out.

8.3.2.1 Case 1: The Permanently Unconscious Subject

A permanently comatose patient, who would otherwise be considered a subject, appears unable to take up the care of her caregiver either at the time the care is given or at a later time. Here I would submit that this patient can complete the CARE, but, while in a comatose state, the patient's response is closer to the heliotropic-like response of the plant. A nurse tending to a comatose patient has to content herself with a body that stays clean and, for example, free of bed sores. *It is the body—not the subject—that takes up the care.* It may be possible that persons at very advanced stages of a life-terminating brain injury or disease have nearly as little subjectivity as a person who is permanently comatose. Here too, it may be the body rather than the subject that takes up the care. But to the extent that traces of subjectivity remain, these people cannot be viewed as merely bodies to be taken care of.

8.3.2.2 Case 2: The Temporarily Unconscious Patient

Next, consider a less extreme case: an individual who is temporarily unconscious—say, a person undergoing a surgical procedure. A surgeon who cuts into flesh, something that on the surface looks very uncaring, has to have the confidence that she has the skill to turn this action into an act of care. The action will be completed as such when the patient recovers and the condition that required the surgery is improved. But the patient, once awake and aware, is no longer merely a reactive body. Therefore, successful surgery may not count as CARE if this cure is enacted on a patient who never wanted the procedure, who perhaps feels ready to die, or who would prefer to live with the impairment than be "cured" by the surgery. What such a patient received, we might argue, was not, in fact, CARE, since the surgeon cared not at all about what the patient wanted. It is a form of care that he would rather have lived without, and that fact alone can vitiate the good accomplished by a successful surgery.

8.3.3 The Conscious Subject with an Underdeveloped
Ability to Make Judgments

As we have already seen in the first two cases, there can be (and often is) a time lapse between the administration of actions intended as care and their uptake by the cared-for. In this way, care may seem different than many other achievement terms. There is no time lapse between the moment we reach the ribbon marking the end of a race and our winning the race. And yet, as we see in most compelling races, there are moments when the winner will be ahead and other times when she falls behind—only to emerge triumphant at the end. Winning may appear to be a momentary event, but between the start of race and its completion, time passes. What goes into winning a race also takes time. Most achievement terms have a temporal lag between the time the activity is undertaken and its moment of completion. Care too might not look like it is being carried out at every moment. Unlike the paradigm case of a race, however, there is a time lag, and often an indeterminancy, between the time the activity *ends* and the achievement is *ascertained*.

Again, unlike the race, the criteria of success are not always well marked out even after time passes. These factors often become justifications for care that is paternalistic. The following cases illustrate these indeterminacies and temporal dimensions that appear to challenge the claims I have made about care as an achievement.

8.3.3.1 Case 3: The Conscious Being with Underdeveloped Judgment of His or Her Own Good

There are cases where we cannot penetrate the other's mind, or we have good reason to believe that the other doesn't know their own mind or that their judgment is impaired, although subjectivity is still very much alive. Then it seems that paternalism is both called for and is benign.

The proper response to this objection is that when one's mind is underdeveloped, or temporarily impaired, the actions of the carer may only later be acknowledged as caring by the cared-for, that is, when the cared-for matures or regains function. Good (enough) parenting often depends on such deferred reception: "One day," we say, "the child will appreciate what we did for her." Sometimes we get it right; sometimes we get it wrong. We can only hope that on balance we succeed in our efforts to care. A telling case is the response to parents and physicians by adults born with ambiguous genitalia who underwent surgery to "normalize" them while they were infants and children. As adults, many who have undergone these interventions have revealed that the procedures have been detrimental to their flourishing. In light of these results, it is appropriate to say that these surgeries failed to be CARE, despite the good intentions of parents and physicians (Feder 2014), and their beliefs that they were doing the procedures for the sake of the children, that is, for the children's welfare.

The fact that we cannot tell *at the time* that we actually have succeeded in caring for a person can have a still more troubling correlate—namely, that we never find out. The problem of indeterminacy arises in both profound cases of life and death and in mundane cases, for example, getting one's child to eat the spinach. At the time, we cannot assess whether or not the child who rebels (and will not eat her spinach) will come to see that pressuring her to eat the greens was the right—that is, the CARING—thing to do. But as the child matures, if in retrospect she endorses the parent's choice, we can say that she has taken it up as CARE. Sometimes tragedy strikes. The child who resisted parental efforts to care will die prematurely from causes unrelated to the conflict and can never say, "Mom, you were right." We are left with an indeterminacy of whether to call our actions CARE. The case is similar to other situations in which an activity aimed at some achievement has been prematurely terminated. If a race were to be interrupted by a sudden violent storm, should we count the frontrunner as the winner, or declare that there is no winner, no matter how close the racers were to the finish line? When achievement determines the correct application of a term, indeterminacy is always a possible outcome.

What about the case of an ungrateful child who has been clothed, fed, educated, and even loved? Although the child has flourished, he exhibits no gratitude and grows into an adult resentful of his parents. Should we not say that the parents nonetheless cared for the child, and the only failure here is the child's unwillingness to acknowledge the care? The answer is yes and no. To the extent that the child truly has flourished, where the flourishing is attributed in part to the parent's efforts, the parent has succeeded. If the child is so resentful of his parents, it is possible that in certain ways their efforts at care did fail. But it is also possible that the fault may lie with the adult child who never learned to accept the care of the parents with graciousness.[36] I will discuss this sort of failure in the reception of care in the last section of this chapter.

8.3.3.2 Case 4: The Child or Adult with a Disability Affecting Judgment

My own experiences of caring for my daughter seem to condemn my theory. When I give my daughter her anti-seizure medication—which is bitter and difficult to swallow—I do believe that I am CARING for her even if she tries to spit it out, and even if she hardly feels cared for at such times. In fact, not to give her

---

[36] There is also the possibility that the child who walks away from the parental home without a willingness to acknowledge care has not been cared for well in one respect: he may not have been taught to acknowledge care and understand the gift of gratitude that the cared-for can bestow for care well done. This fine point was made by an audience member in a presentation at Boston College.

this medicine would be negligent and morally culpable. If the medication works, and she doesn't have seizures, I am CARING for her by any objective measure.[37]

In that case, either the subjective uptake is unnecessary or (counterintuitively) I am not being CARING. My response is that in such instances, when one is dealing with someone whose judgment or communicative capability is impaired in ways that preclude their endorsement of a vitally important issue of care, the carer must effectively construct a counterfactual: If the cared-for could understand, then she would endorse my actions as CARE. So I say, were Sesha to understand the purpose of the medication, she would take it willingly. This is sometimes referred to as "hypothetical consent" in the bioethics literature. One has to be careful with such counterfactuals. In principle, they can be used to justify all sorts of coercion. In my daughter's case, she has two sorts of seizures. There are the small quick jerks often ending in her giggling—hedonic seizures she might well have no interest in preventing. The other are grand mal seizures, which are frightening, leave her drained, and—were they to get out of hand— could be life-threatening. These are not events that she herself would want.

If Sesha and I could communicate better, not only would I be able to explain the importance of her taking the pills, but she would be able to explain her resistance to them. As it is, I must grope about and consider if the pills are too large, too distasteful, or perhaps have an unpleasant side effect. The closer I come to discerning the reason for the resistance and avoiding coercion, the more fully do I fulfill my obligation to CARE for her.

8.3.3.3 *Case 5: The Adult with a Degenerative Condition Affecting Judgment*

This case strides between case 3 and case 4. The person starts out needing care because of a degenerative condition. As the condition grows worse, judgment is affected and the individual grows increasingly unable to respond to our care or guide us in our caregiving by their responsiveness or lack of responsiveness. This is the situation of those caring for adults with Alzheimer's disease, for example. The person may at first not welcome care because they are used to doing things for themselves, and the need for care is a reminder of the condition that will increasingly limit their ability to function. The caregiver nonetheless has to provide the assistance because the person may well be harmed without it. A hindsight judgment that our carer acted in a caring fashion never comes, because in time the person loses the ability to make such a judgment. Here the caregiver is stuck in murky territory, not knowing if what she has done has been

---

[37] Note, I am assuming that the reason she would try to spit it out would be because of the unpleasantness of the pill itself and not whatever effects it has on her other than subduing her seizures (Fadiman 1998).

the right thing—the CARING thing. As the judgment of the one who is cared for is increasingly impaired, the case needs to be treated as case 4. This often requires a continuing readjustment on the part of the caregiver. Signals that were clear become increasingly unclear, and the question of where and when it is appropriate to use a notion of hypothetical consent or switch how we take care become difficult questions of judgment. The more we learn about the best way to care for people with conditions such as Alzheimer's disease, the more likely we will be in the position to make the right judgment call. This requires a personal and social commitment to make the necessary inquiry and refuse the assumption that there is no right or best way to care, that is, that uptake is unnecessary. But in a degenerative and terminal condition such as Alzheimer's disease, where the end stages can result in such diminished subjectivity that any sort of endorsement is beyond what is possible, we may face a situation that is best described as a modification of case 1. The person is still conscious, but has lost most all of the awareness needed for subjectivity. For the very end stage of such degenerative conditions, the best we can hope for is the uptake of the body.[38]

8.3.4   The Conscious Adult Subject

8.3.4.1   *Case 6: The Adult in Need of Care Refusing Medication*

What if a person did understand the connection between the seizure medication and the reduction in seizures, but still refused to take the pill? Then we would need to know the person and her reason for refusing in order to know how properly to care for her. Perhaps she resents being cared for and feels that having to take pills impedes her freedom and, strange as it might sound, she would prefer to have those seizures than follow a pill regimen. Or perhaps she simply hates swallowing these large and bitter pills—and claims to not care what the consequences are of not taking them. Alternatively, she may not want to squander scarce resources on the medication. She would prefer to use the money to help her children eat better.

The best carers, if they remain convinced that the person would be better off taking the seizure medication, would attempt to find ways around the obstacles. They may, for example, allow the person more control over when and how to take the medication, find sources where the medication can be gotten more affordably, find more palatable alternative medications, or devise ways to make it easier to take this medication. These attempts to overcome obstacles require participation on the part of the cared-for, when the cared-for is capable of engaging with the carer. Not paternalism, but respectful care, is what is needed.

---

[38] I thank Susan Brison for discussions on this last point.

8.3.4.2 Case 7: The Depressed Person

Steven Darwall asks us to consider a person who is depressed and feels unworthy of care or lacks all concern for his well-being. Darwall points out that we would be wrong to deny that person our attention just because the person feels unworthy of care. Is Darwall's case a counterexample and his claim a justifiable case of paternalistic care? My answer is that CARE looks to the long haul. If we know the person, we may know that such depression is not a constant state. But even if the person is a stranger, we know that often depression is not unremitting, and generally can be mitigated, if not cured. We try to do what is consistent with the person's values and concerns when the person is *not* depressed. Most importantly, we try to lift the depression.

It might be, however, that the depression comes at the end of a long and well-lived life. A person might fear or be aware that one's care has become too burdensome for everyone else. One may be experiencing an unrelenting discomfort and pain that takes all joy out of life. Those who care about and for the person may reluctantly come to appreciate that she truly wants her life terminated and that nothing can be done to alter the death wish. In that case, the only caring alternative may be to find a way to oblige the person. Yet again, there may be alternatives that are escaping us, and there may be a way to turn the situation around. This is one of the deeply troubling concerns a carer faces. It is another face of the indeterminacy that so vexes the caring individual.

8.3.4.3 Case 8: The Mature, Conscious, Autonomous Subject Who Refuses to Act in Accordance with Her Objective Good

The most challenging case concerns a mature, autonomous, and capable decision-maker, who resists actions done for her sake and that are objectively good for her (that is, actions that would preserve her life, health, or other objective features of well-being). Case 7 is an instance of this. But Michael Slote presents another twist on this in the following case: "If I prevent my adult child from riding helmetless on a motorcycle, he or she may never acknowledge the value of what I have done, but what one does is good for the child. Should that not count as care?"[39] *Respect* would require that we yield to the decision to ride helmetless, if it is a decision made as a well-informed autonomous person. *Care* would require that we prevent her from riding helmetless. Care and respect seem to come apart here.

---

[39] Personal correspondence, April 5th, 2010. For Steven Darwall this is a classic instance of caring for someone for their own sake, although Darwall may argue that here the attitude we should take toward the person is not care but respect.

One answer is that, without enlisting the adult child's willingness to take up our prohibition as care, the care is at best partial.[40] (If the adult child vigorously protests but does wear the helmet nonetheless, he is probably caring for the parent at least as much as the parent is caring for him.) If he is prevented from riding the bike, or wears the helmet resenting the parents all the while he is wearing it, then, while the parents have cared for his physical well-being—and to the extent the body stays protected, the care has been taken up—there is a sense in which we have failed to care for him as a subject.[41] If the adult child, having gotten into an accident in which the helmet prevented worse harm, later agrees that we did right to insist, then he takes up our admonitions as care. A parent may determine that she would rather have the adult child alive, and live with the child's disapprobation, than the reverse. Other cases where an adult autonomous agent is involved may require a different sort of answer, as we will see in the following section.

8.4 Care, Paternalistic or Respectful

Care is often regarded as fully compatible with paternalism. After all, we often are providing care for those who are not fully autonomous. As it appears justified to treat those who are not autonomous paternalistically, it seems unobjectionable that care is frequently paternalistic. The conception of care (CARE) I am developing, however, is antithetical to paternalism, even when caring for those who are not fully autonomous. Instead it is compatible with respect. CARE, as I shall argue, even *requires* that we respect the person for whom we care.

8.4.1 Care as a Natural Disposition

Justifying paternalism in the name of care appears reasonable only if we consider care itself to be a nonmoral notion, a "natural disposition."[42] CARING however is not, or not simply, a "natural disposition" but a process of morally motivated attention, discernment, and response. And because what counts as CARING is

---

[40] I assume here that I prevent my child from riding a motorcycle without a helmet out of my concern for his well-being and not from a need to control his actions. Then, surely, the action is done from a *desire* to care for the child for the child's own sake.

[41] We might still be right to prevent him from riding helmetless, but this may be for the consequences his possible injuries might have on others.

[42] I am not taking a position on the question of whether paternalism is ever justified, only that it is not justifiable in the name of care, because when we think of care as a fully normative notion, we must take the perspective of the person in need of care, and that is opposed to paternalism whereby another claims to know what *our* good is.

gounded in the person's genuine needs and legitimate wants, this sort of care must take the perspective of the one cared for, and cannot be justified paternalistically. There is no other way to determine right action within an ETHICS OF CARE without also trying to see the situation and the good as the cared-for sees it.

If caring isn't merely a natural disposition but a form of moral deliberation[43] guided by an empathetic concern for the other, then, as in any particularistic ethic, the deliberative process depends on a discernment of what is morally relevant in any particular case.[44] For a care ethics this requires thought and self-examination about one's own capacity to care in this situation for this person, in addition to attention to the other's needs and wants.[45] Self-reflection on the part of the caregiver is needed to ponder whether she, even inadvertently, fails to convey her respect for the cared-for's point of view. Such self-reflection is necessary for the carer to examine whether or not she has used her power qua carer to dominate and impose her own will, whether or not she has the requisite competence to assist in this situation, whether or not she should seek help or advice from another, and so on.

The give-and-take in a caring relationship, along with self-reflection on the part of the carer and the cared-for (when the cared-for is capable of it), can help define what would constitute appropriate action in *this* particular situation with *this* particular cared-for. And if the action chosen succeeds, then the outcome is morally preferable to a coercive paternalism or a neglectful "abandonment" of persons to their putatively autonomous choices, as Onora O'Neill (2002) has put it.

This is not to say that the cared-for's own notion of her good at a particular moment ought *always* to dictate the carer's response. The cared-for may have impaired judgment at the moment they are most vulnerable and need to have another judge as to what is (or will eventually be) conducive to the cared-for's flourishing. The carer may have moral objections to doing what the cared-for

---

[43] See chapter 7 for a discussion of moral deliberation within an ETHICS OF CARE.

[44] One might ask if such moral deliberation depends on the natural disposition of empathy. If it does, does this mean that people incapable of empathy have no moral responsibility within an ETHICS OF CARE? This is too large a question to take on here. For a good discussion of cognitive disabilities, empathetic deficiencies, and moral responsibility, see Shoemaker (2010). See Hoffman (2000) for a discussion of various forms of empathy.

[45] Note that when I say a deliberative process, I include responding in an intuitive and affective manner, where that response is honed by the cultivation of caring responses, and where we determine that the intuitive response is the correct one. Such deliberations can be, and at their best, may be swift and nearly instantaneous. We have learned through cognitive science that quick intuitive responses are themselves the end-product of a sort of cultivation. For a really good, empirically informed philosophical essay that pertains to this point, see Holroyd (2012).

wants.[46] There may be larger forces that constrain the carer's ability to respond as the cared-for desires. But we can intervene in the lives of another *only* because we believe that we are addressing the other's genuine needs and legitimate wants as she does (or would) understand them, even if she herself does not *yet* acknowledge these. As a carer, I must also be prepared to find that I am mistaken in thinking that what I consider to be the cared-for's good is a good as she sees it. Otherwise, I am not caring for *her* in all her particularity.

The tools for the caregiver's moral deliberation are not neatly packaged moral principles—neither the categorical imperative nor injunctions to maximize utility serve us well here. At most, AN ETHIC OF CARE has regulative ideals. As in any particularist ethics in which deliberation does not take us from general principles to particular instances, care involves attention and discernment to understand what right action is in *this* case (Little 2000). It also requires the ability to anticipate needs and a mindfulness, that is, a presence of mind and awareness of one's surroundings, to avoid allowing harm to come to a dependent that the dependent may not be alert to. In sum, the rightness of the action we choose depends on accurate discernment, careful attention to the other, mindfulness, the requisite competencies, and sufficient agility in one's responsiveness—not on a general principle or standard that will apply to all cases which we as carers can paternalistically impose on the cared-for.

8.4.2 Care and Respect

If this way of thinking about care sounds a lot like respect, it is because CARE includes respect. CARE and respect, on this account, share the feature that each has to take up the perspective of the other to understand how to respond, and each aims to give that perspective its due. Clearly, respect and CARE are not identical. Respect involves us in a "thinner" relationship than CARE, one that can tolerate a greater "arm's distance." Although CARE requires respect, respect does not usually commit us to an attitude or labor of care. CARE commits us to respond to the other when appropriate; respect commits us to avoid interfering with another. Both are moral responses.[47] Although both CARE and respect require us to take the perspective of the other, neither *always* requires a total suspension of

---

[46] As I mentioned earlier, the carer has a moral responsibility to be alert to wants and desires that lack legitimacy. Recall that these are legitimate because they do not involve clearly immoral demands, demands that in order to be fulfilled means causing others intentional or foreseeable harms, and needs or wants that require unjust demands on the carer. If the cared-for's perspective requires us to participate, even indirectly, in behavior we know to be immoral, the carer has the moral obligation to refuse. See Sandra Bartky's "Feeding Egos and Tending Wounds" in *Feminity and Domination* (1990).

[47] See Dillon (1992) and Miller (2012).

one's own views nor deference to the other's values when the other's views and values are harmful or morally repugnant.

Although care and respect are not always regarded as compatible, we can see the plausibility of the view I am propounding when we consider that a person cannot take up the actions of a caregiver as CARE if she is left feeling disrespected. Said differently, I cannot feel better off than I was before if I feel humiliated or frustrated by what you do, supposedly on my behalf. Care not administered in a way that preserves and respects the person's dignity is not a care most of us would desire. Indeed, it is a form of care we fear. And on my normative understanding of care, it is not CARE at all.

Interestingly, when we reserve the idea of respect for those who have autonomous decision-making ability, we fail to respect those whose dignity is most at stake, those who need respect the most. John Vorhaus, a philosopher who has spent time working with and educating people regarded as severely and profoundly cognitively disabled, writes the following:

> From the fact that a person does not make use of or understand such terms as "dignity" and "respect," it does not follow that she is not sensitive to behavior that is more or less respectful, since this does not depend upon the ability to recognize oneself under these descriptions. Doubtless there are profoundly disabled people who do not conceive themselves as having dignity and as being owed respect. Yet by their behavior and expressive repertoire they may provide evidence of growing or failing self worth in response to how they are treated. This might be suggested, on the one hand, by a developing preparedness to experiment in a learning environment, and to engage with and learn from their peers; and, on the other hand, a tendency to withdraw from human contact and attempt less and less in the way of novel or even familiar learning activities. (2015, 125)

An important qualification needs to be discussed with respect to individuals who are at very advanced stages of a terminal degenerative condition such as Alzheimer's disease when the subject appears absent most of the time. I remarked in case 1 that sometimes it appears that the best we can do is care for the body, that we have no epistemic access to the subject, and there is no future that can affirm for us that we have properly cared for the individual as a subject. In the literature on Alzheimer's disease, there is much discussion regarding whether the person that the individual once was is the one whom we should be respecting, or whether we need rather to deal with the person as they are now. The situation in which subjectivity is not only altered but increasingly absent is, I believe, a quandary that cannot be resolved. But that it is a quandary means that at the very least we need to be as respectful to the individual before us as it is possible to be.[48] The lack of epistemic access here means that we are also lacking moral access, that is, access to the moral possibilities of interaction with this person.[49]

This qualification, however, does not absolve us from recognizing the agency and subjectivity of a person with severe to profound cognitive disability. An important thing that caring for my daughter has taught me is that wherever there is a subject, there is agency which ought to receive respect and attention: there is a will, a way one wants to feel oneself in the world, an intuitive sense of what is good for oneself. One does not need to demonstrate autonomy to command respect.

That my daughter seems not to be autonomous does not mean that I need not respect her wants and wishes and the demonstrations of her agency. If she turns away from food I consider delicious and nutritious, I have no business forcing that food on her, but I do have a responsibility to find a substitute food that she will eat willingly.[50] This is not respect for some autonomous decision-making capacity, but for her as a subject with her own likes and dislikes and as someone who wants a measure of control in what she consumes. However inarticulate the expression of this agency, "attention must be paid."[51] The carer must pay attention to discern that good, to respond to it, and not to impose an alien one. Another's good can be as ill-fitting as another's garment, as Mill pointed out (1860 [1978]). Mill—had he come into contact with individuals like my daughter—would likely have seen that this pertains to her no less than to himself.[52]

I took away this lesson from a daughter with a cognitive disability, but all parents must grapple with the either/or of a paternalistic imposition on their children of their own views and with a caring that strives to be more fine-tuned to the individual child. Given the scarcity of time, imagination, and patience,

---

[48] I thank Susan Brison for engaging me on this point.

[49] See Kittay (2017) where I introduce the idea of "moral access."

[50] But even presenting one with food might not be respectful in the case of someone who is terminally ill and whose body is shutting down. This is often a mistake people caring for terminally ill people at the very end of life make. Again, my discussions with Susan Brison have been helpful here.

[51] This is said by Willy Loman's wife Linda in Arthur Miller's *Death of a Salesman*, speaking to her sons about her totally despondent husband: "But he's a human being, and a terrible thing is happening to him. So attention must be paid. . . . Attention, attention must be finally paid to such a person." In a passage pertinent to the discussion here, she speaks of her knowledge of her husband's toying with suicide by poisoning himself with gas and her struggle with whether or not to discard the rubber tube by which he might end his life. "Every day I go down and take away that little rubber pipe. But when he comes home, I put it back where it was. How can I insult him that way?" (Miller 1996, 56).

[52] In this respect, one might say, ETHICS OF CARE is a liberal ethics, although the stress on relationality is less a liberal view.

paternalism is the route many parents take. Furthermore, many would argue that it stretches the meaning of respect to say that in caring for the infant we must *respect* him. In the case of an infant, what we no doubt should respect is the infant's right to life, to be adequately fed, and to the sorts of thing that are on any objective list of things we think infants universally need to survive and thrive. These do not involve us in discerning the particularity of *this* infant's wants and needs.

In response, we can note that a very young infant does not (or may not) yet have *individualized* CARES—CARES that are particular to *that* individual. Once such more particular CARES do start to manifest themselves, I don't see why we don't have an obligation to respect them, as long as they are not self-defeating, putting at risk goods we can anticipate the child having as she or he matures, or ones that are harmful to others.

Our thinking about children and their rights has evolved, and we now think it is wrong for parents to treat their child's will as an extension of their own. Even as we deal with young children, we try to discern where their preferences and talents lie, and caring which helps to foster the child's development tries to nurture their preferences as long as they stay within the constraints I have mentioned. Thus, on the view I have defended, even young children are generally better served when they receive not paternalistic care, but are given the respect worthy of CARE.

8.5 Moral Luck

I have argued that, despite all our most arduous efforts to bring our actions to a successful conclusion, we may fail, and that failed good-faith efforts of care may be evidence of a caring disposition or the will to act in accordance with a duty to care, but—in themselves—are neither morally praiseworthy nor blameworthy as CARE. The efforts of CARE require recognition, because one should not want to demoralize one who is dealing with a difficult situation of care more than the situation itself dispirits such a caregiver. I believe that one comfort, though often only a cold comfort, is the recognition that moral luck plays an especially large role in an ETHICS OF CARE. It plays an important part in our ability to be the praiseworthy moral actors we may aim to be.

As Aristotle already understood and in recent times Bernard Williams so elegantly and persuasively argues, moral luck is inevitable in moral life. Williams argues that in many instances we cannot know, as we embark on a course of action, if we really have a moral warrant for choosing to do as we have done. This is because the outcome will turn on matters that are simply beyond our control: given one outcome, it appears as if the choice was morally warranted, but given another it appears to have been a poor moral choice.

We see how pervasive and inescapable moral luck is when we consider moral choices from the consideration of the completion of care. Understanding care from the perspective of the completion of care presents the hard reality that whether or not our action will hit its mark ultimately depends not on us, but on the cared-for and on conditions not in our power to effect. This means that we need to choose carefully whom and what we care about—for to intend to care for and indeed care for someone who does not want our care is to act futilely.[53] It also means that we need the skills, talents, and resources to be effective—not all of which are within our power to attain. And we need the cared-for to interpret our actions as care—if not immediately, then in time. If those for whom we care are not able to respond and for whom the condition that warrants care is terminal, then in the absence of any confirmation on the part of cared-for we need to invoke the counterfactual and hope that the person would interpret our actions as CARE were they able.[54]

Although the caregiver may not be morally blameworthy, and many of her actions and attitudes may display morally praiseworthy virtues, questions will remain for her: Did she have the requisite skills to accomplish this task? If not, was it morally responsible to take on the responsibility—or to take it on without cultivating the necessary skills? Was she sufficiently committed to the caregiving? Did she observe that a given tack was failing and was she suitably motivated to change course as needed? If there is an accident involving a dependent, the caregiver must question if she was sufficiently mindful of dangers lurking in the environment. Many such queries arise at the end of an unsuccessful effort at CARE. Often enough, the answers are indeterminate or underdetermined, and we cannot find a good resolution to the question of praise or blame. Thus when it comes to an ETHICS OF CARE, in which intention cannot be all and a clear conscience is difficult to ensure, nagging guilt may be just one of the occupational hazards of caregiving. In this sense, caregiving is morally hazardous.

Perhaps nothing that I have thus far argued is as difficult to accept as the role that moral luck has within an ethics of care. It is, I think, difficult to accept that someone who prima facie does what we expect of a carer can be deprived of her laurels because the individual for whom she cares fails to take up her acting as caring. That is to say, it may well be just a caregiver's bad luck to have chosen, been assigned, or found themselves by default in a position to care for someone who cannot take up as care what she has done, and for this reason all her efforts at care remain efforts only and not CARE. As disturbing as this is, I shall insist

---

[53] Though possibly not in a morally blameworthy way.

[54] As I noted earlier, care in the face of a terminal illness means allowing the person to die with as much peace, comfort, and dignity as the condition allows.

upon it. Moral luck is as inevitable to an ETHICS OF CARE as care is indispensable to human life.[55]

The fact of moral luck is compounded by the fact that CARE, except in short simple cases, has very complex, as well as ill-defined, results.[56] There are many effects, not all of which we intend even when we intend to benefit the cared-for. A fine example of these complexities is found in the famous 1927 movie *The Jazz Singer*. The son of a long line of cantors happens to have a beautiful voice. For the father, caring for the child means cultivating that voice with an eye to developing the next cantor in a long ancestral line of illustrious cantors. The son, however, wants to use his talents and skills only to be a jazz singer, and with his superb voice training, he is en route to a successful career. It is the bad moral luck of the father to raise a son in the secular cultural context of his day. Beyond this, the father fails to appreciate the depth of his son's desire to sing the secular music the son loves. The father thinks he is offering the best sort of care. But he is wrong. On the other hand, his care in training his son's voice *is* taken up by the son. And, in the very last minutes of the father's life, the son acknowledges his debt to his father and his father comes to understand that the upshot of his care is the gift of song. Not all similar instances have such a Hollywood happy ending.

In a different set of cases, the failure to have our care taken up occurs because certain background conditions required for successful care are not present: the parent lacks the resources to adequately feed her child because of poverty, and there is no third party to take up the responsibilities inherent in the dependency relationship; the caregiver of a disabled person gets no relief and so fails to be able to carry on successfully; the caregiver of a disabled person cannot obtain the needed equipment or other support to adequately care; the mother is the caregiver for a disabled man who is at times violent and aggressive, and she is left alone to try to care for someone who endangers himself and her, but whom she loves; the nurse is stuck in a bureaucracy that places obstacles between her responsibility to her patient and the successful execution of that responsibility— all these cases display what care ethicists have so often emphasized: namely, that rather than being a simply dyadic relationship, the relationship between a carer and a cared-for sits in a set of nested dependencies.

It may appear to be just our bad moral luck when we find ourselves in the dysfunctional, and even sabotaged, situations I just listed, but it is not only moral luck at work. It is often injustice and callous disregard for marginalized people as

---

[55] Michael Slote, in a personal communication, April 10, 2010, noted that this "last point doesn't really make things much better." Agreed, but that it doesn't make things better doesn't make it less true.

[56] Another set of important elements are the background justice conditions that affect the possibility of the success of the care. These will be discussed in *Who is Truly Human?*

well. It is precisely because these situations can help us identify injustices that it is important to insist that, as sad as it may be to say, CARE was not given.

8.6 A Moral Obligation to Receive Care?

Now I want to force a moral question that arises from this analysis: Do we have a moral responsibility to graciously accept care when it is offered in good faith and with the suitable competence to answer a real need? Do we have a moral obligation to consider such efforts at care in assessing our own needs? I speak here of people who can be held morally accountable, which, of course, is not always the case with people in need of care. There are a number of different situations we need to consider.

8.6.1 When an Intended Cared-For Is Absolved of the Responsibility to Accept Care

There are some clear instances where an intended cared-for is not morally obliged to accept proffered care. I discuss three such instances. First, the carer believes there are needs to respond to but is mistaken, and so the efforts to provide care are justifiably refused by the cared-for. Second, the carer may be incompetent, and so even if the care is offered in good faith, the person being cared for is justified in refusing efforts that not only will fail to help her, but also could cause her harm. And third, the cared-for may recognize that the care offered is not offered in good faith, that is, the carer may have motives other than the good of the cared-for that therefore fail to benefit the cared-for in the right way (that is, with caring motives or intentions).

8.6.1.1 Answering to Non-Needs

If another wants to meet needs that I don't want met, I can reply that the point of care is to answer *my* needs and not another's. If I choose to struggle along, that is entirely my affair, and it is paternalism at its worst to insist otherwise. A caregiver may be free to offer care, but the intended recipient is equally free to refuse it. That was essentially the argument I made in the example of the parent who prevents his adult child from riding a motorcyle without a helmet. There I insisted that respect is needed for care. In the case of disabled people, they are expected to be grateful at the offer of help even when these attempts can only frustrate their true needs and desires. This point is a critically important feature of the fully normative sense of care, especially when we consider care in the context of disability. I propose that the problems that scholars of disability and activists have with care is a problem with paternalism, not with CARE in the fully normative sense.

8.6.1.2   *Care Offered in Good Faith But Without the Requisite Competence*

A very common—and potentially dangerous—form of intended care is the one taken on by people who lack the needed skills and competence and, worse still, who do not realize that they lack them. Because care is mistakenly thought to be a "merely natural" capability (especially for women)—one that needs no training, no acquisition of skills or competence—people presume to know what someone else needs and how to meet those needs, when in fact they know neither and know not that they don't know.

It may be as minor as fixing a pillow under the head of a person so frail that most arrangements are discomforting, or knowing how to position a cup of liquid so that a person without the use of his arms and hands might drink without gagging or spilling. Or as major as attempting to treat an open wound or feeding someone using a feeding tube. The degree of discomfort, humiliation, and outright mortal danger of efforts at care that are inattentive, clumsy, or incompetent varies. But the person on the receiving end has no moral obligation to receive care in the hands of an incompetent carer.

8.6.1.3   *The Insincere Carer*

A person has no obligation to accept care from someone who is not actually acting to benefit the cared-for, especially when the cared-for have good reason to believe they are being used or exploited for nefarious purposes. An extreme example is found in *Slum Dog Millionaire*, where a gangster abducts homeless children whom he feeds, clothes, and houses, and he even provides occasional treats to the recently hungry children. But he does it all to win their trust and compliance so that he can then either blind or maim them, turning them into suitably pitiful beggars, or exploit the girls as prostitutes as soon as they mature. These children cannot be accused of being ungrateful when, upon learning about their fate, they run away from the gang.

8.6.2   When the Intended Cared-For Have an Obligation to Receive Care Graciously

Finally, I want to turn to the role of the cared-for.

8.6.2.1 The Refusers

Because care is more complex than the coordinated action of two actors, the care refuser, when the care refuser refuses care that can benefit him, harms not only himself but does an injury to the caregiver and to the relationship between them. When we refuse care offered in good faith and with the requisite competence, we refuse relationship. In the case of people to whom we are close, this can be a painful rejection of our expression of love and concern. In the case of people who are giving care professionally, this is a frustration of their duty and obligation.

8.6.2.2 The Overdemanders

We can also fail to receive care graciously when we demand more than is reasonable. The overdemander subordinates the other's interests to his own. To borrow a phrase from Marilyn Frye (1983, 65–66), he grafts the substance of the other onto his own. When an elderly husband is unsatisfied with any hired help and demands to be cared for only by his wife—also elderly and with needs of her own—he fails to acknowledge the wife as having interests that are equally valid. The lack of graciousness can often show itself in a dismissive attitude toward the needs of the carer. Instead, the cared-for believes himself entitled to impose his will on his caregiver, with little regard for her as a person in her own right. The caregiver's actions are thought of as not issuing from her willingness to care; instead, the cared-for sees the carer's actions as a mere extension of his own will. This is what Rivas (2002) referred to as appropriating the authorship of the caregiver's agency.[57]

The failure to take up care *graciously* is a moral lapse on the part of a cared-for who is capable of making moral choices. But it is one that is facilitated by certain structural social features. Consider the caregiving relationship between a husband and wife in a very traditional marriage. When the wife gives care to a husband who becomes dependent, the subordination of her will to his can be such a normal expectation that any additional efforts of the wife may be invisible to her spouse. The same situation is evident in the case of a paid female caregiver. The image of the cantankerous old man who is an overly demanding, never satisfied patient is a caricature, but the real-life instantiations hang on a scaffold of patriarchal relationships. The situation of the paid personal attendant to a disabled person who wants to be seen as independent, in the sense of self-sufficient, is

---

[57] See discussion in chapter 6 concerning the attitude toward attendants by some of the clients who employ them.

similar. The scaffolding here is a society that refuses to acknowledge the unavoidable dependencies.

In brief, the refuser and the overdemander each short-circuit and so doom to failure the ethical imperative of caring for the needs of those who cannot care for themselves. Caring for those who are meaningful in our lives is one of the most important ethical projects we undertake, and its failure is a great wound, a genuine harm. If the carer's success in caring hinges on the uptake of the cared-for, those cared for have an obligation to receive care (to the extent to which they are in a condition to do so) when it is offered in good faith and with the requisite competence. As Noddings puts it: "How good I can be is dependent, is partly a function of how you—the other—receive and respond to me" (1984, 154).

9

Forever Small

The Strange Case of Ashley X

9.1 The Case and the Parents' Justification

In 2002, the parents of a six-year-old girl with a condition that will require physical care throughout her life, and who had begun to exhibit signs of precocious puberty, requested and were granted permission to have high doses of estrogen administered to induce the premature closing of the long-bone epiphyses, thus maintaining the girl's height at 4′5″.[1] The intention was to facilitate her care by keeping her small. To reduce the uterine bleeding that accompanies the procedure, as well as the risk of uterine cancer, she underwent a hysterectomy prior to the estrogen treatment. To reduce the risk of breast cancer (which was in her family history) and to prevent the growth of large breasts (also a familial trait) her breast buds were removed. Surgeons also performed an appendectomy as a prophylactic, which was unrelated to the other procedures. Knowing only these facts, the reader may find herself outraged—how could a parent do such a thing, and how could doctors agree to carry out such procedures?

But now we add: The girl has severe cognitive disabilities from an unknown cause, which is described as static encephalopathy with marked global developmental deficits, rendering her profoundly intellectually limited as well as incapable of mobility, holding up her head, or doing anything at all for herself. Her physicians made this case public in a medical journal, referring to the procedures in the title of their article as a "New Solution to an Old Dilemma" (Gunther and Diekema 2006).

---

[1] An earlier version of this chapter was published as (Kittay 2011a). I thank Debra Bergoffen and Gail Weiss for their helpful editorial assistance, and Serene Khader and William Pearce for comments on an earlier draft. The catalyst for this article was Benjamin Wilfond and Sara Goering's kind invitation to the Seattle Growth Attenuation and Ethics Working Group and to participate in the publication of the results of the study (Wilfond et al. 2010).

Does the fact of her disability alter the response of outrage? Should it?

This is the notorious case of Ashley X. Following the scientific publication announcing the procedures, the case made the media rounds,[2] and her parents set up a website to tell their story and to promote what they dubbed "the Ashley treatment" (AT) for other children like Ashley.[3] By all accounts, and as they appear in the website, her parents, middle-class and educated professionals, are loving and caring. They want to keep her small because this will permit them to care for her in their home for the longest possible time and allow her to participate in family events and in activities she enjoys, such as going to the beach. They justify the hysterectomy by arguing that their daughter will never be a mother. Without a uterus, she will never become pregnant should she become a victim of sexual abuse—and, as a woman with disabilities, especially cognitive disabilities, her risk is higher than that of other women. They justify the removal of the breast buds by claiming that large breasts will make the straps that keep her in place in a wheelchair uncomfortable, and their absence will also reduce the likelihood that caretakers will sexualize her. In addition, surgery will guard against the slightly increased possibility of cancer in these sexual organs caused by the high-dose estrogen treatments. Despite all the criticisms, the parents actively have defended and continue to promote AT as a way to care for other "pillow angels," as they call Ashley.

Is the rationale sufficient? Should such a procedure be permissible? If not, why not? Many arguments critical of AT have been proffered.[4] I will not avail myself of many of these. Although the removal of breast buds and hysterectomy suggest a strong gender dimension to the case, I will not stress this, since growth attenuation (GA) is an option for boys as well; and in boys, it has also been accompanied with breast bud removal as the estrogen stimulates the growth of breasts. The issue of her hysterectomy, however, is one that bears on the particular sort of harm that has been inflicted on women with cognitive disabilities.

Nor will I argue that this is a procedure done selfishly for the parent's mere convenience.[5] First because, in a relational account, the parent's well-being has a

---

[2] See Burkholder (2007); Caplan (2007); King (2007); Ritter (2007); Saletan (2007a; 2007b); Tada (2007); Tanner (2007); and Verhovek (2007). See also Fitzmaurice (2008) for a bibliography of news commentary on the Ashley treatment.

[3] See Ashley's parents' blog. The original blog is no longer posted. The new blog is http://www.pillowangel.org.

[4] For an exhaustive list of criticisms see Gunther and Diekema (2006). The number of articles and websites are too numerous to cite.

[5] See Lindemann and Lindemann Nelson (2008). Also Dresser (2009). Both reject the idea that this is a valid criticism, because they argue that the well-being of the parents is not irrelevant to deciding the issue. An excellent and balanced discussion is provided by Liao, Savulescu, and Sheehan (2007).

bearing on the child's well-being and the reverse is true as well. Secondly, because I take her parents at their word when they say that they did this *for Ashley's sake.*

I will also not decry the "unnaturalness" of the procedure, for the term "unnatural" has too often been used to impede human progress. Similarly, I refrain from arguing that Ashley's parents did not accept her as she was. There is every reason to think their love was unconditional.[6] My argument instead is that its expression in attempting to keep her small was misguided. Furthermore, while I do agree with opponents or skeptics that the parents, doctors, or hospital should have sought court approval and that court approval should have been mandated for a hysterectomy, I am much more ambivalent than many others in the disability community about the intervention of courts in medical treatment or care of children with parents who are devoted to their well-being.[7] The courts are too adversarial a setting to resolve most such issues; and when there is a genuinely loving family, much harm comes when those not directly affected by a decision intervene in a child's care.

Finally, I do not rely on an argument that the procedure violated Ashley's dignity: not because, as some have argued, Ashley has no dignity to violate (I believe she does and in *Who is Truly Human?* I will make the case that dignity needs to be understood in a way that includes the Ashleys and Seshas of the world). The term 'dignity' has recently been tarred by critics from the left as a tool of the conservative right.[8] I disagree, but if we can argue against AT without engaging that argument, all the better. Instead, I begin with the self-evident truth that AT is an instance of intended care and will look to an ETHICS OF CARE to help determine its justifiability. The care ethics that I will be referencing is one that is informed by the ETHICS OF CARE that I developed in the preceeding chapters. The Ashley case reveals views of human embodiment that have important ethical consequences, ones that are lived in the disabled body of a girl who now will remain forever small. The procedure has since been administered to other children. At stake are two questions: 1) Did Ashley's parents, doctors, and the hospital act ethically? 2) Should AT be made available to all parents of children whose prognosis is severe cognitive disability and nonambulation (SCDN) at an age early enough to make AT effective, that is, when they are two to six years of age?[9] The second question is of special importance, since there are estimates

---

[6] See Asch and Stubblefield (2010). Also ADAPT (2007).

[7] See Savage (2007).

[8] See Kittay and Kittay (2007) for my response. For two prominent critics of the use of the concept of dignity in bioethics, see Macklin (2003) and Pinker (2008).

[9] Note that GA, growth attenuation, also called GAT, growth attenuation therapy, differs from the Ashley Treatment (AT) in that AT includes procedures such as the removal of the breast buds, hysterectomies, and sometimes other organs such as the appendix in addition to the

that as many as sixty-five children have received growth attenuation therapy (GA).[10]

Whether or not all or many of the children also had the other features of the Ashley treatment—a hysterectomy, breast bud removal, and appendectomy—is not included in the information of the report. There are at least three other children (one of whom is a boy) who are publicly known to have received AT: one in New Zealand, one in London, and one in New York. It appears that there is growing acceptance of the procedure in medical circles, even though we know little about its long-term effects and there are no protocols regarding its acceptability or unacceptability. It is not subject to any of the standard procedures of introducing new medical interventions—no studies, no testing. The apparent moral certainty of the parents interviewed is stunning in the face of everything that is objectively unknown about the interventions. Furthermore, some (particularly Ashley's parents) are actively proselytizing for the use of the procedure.

For an issue as morally complex as this, no one argument is likely to be decisive. In making my case, I will rely on the conjunction of four related arguments tied to four questionable assumptions. Although all parties acted in good faith to provide Ashley the best available care, as I argued in chapter 8, good intentions do not suffice. Recall the person who thought she was caring for a wilted plant by pouring in a clear liquid, vinegar, which she took to be water. Ashley's parents surely intended to pour restorative water, but I contend, they may have poured vinegar instead. Moreover, had the available social supports been ready to hand, the option they conceived of might never have been considered.

9.2 A Tale of Two Girls and One Mother's Journey

In the face of the extensive criticism directed at Ashley's parents, proponents responded that those who had not walked in their shoes ought not to judge them

---

growth attenuation. GA (or GAT) refers only to the hormonal treatment to surpress height. Some proponents of GA agree that the hysterectomy undergone by Ashley most likely should have been subject to court approval. See Allen et al. (2008).

[10] In a letter published by *Archives of Disease in Childhood* (Pollock, Fost, and Allen 2015), endocrinologists, at least some of whom are known to be very supportive of growth attenuation therapy (GAT), surveyed a relatively small sample of pediatric endrocrinologists and found more than the number of publicly reported cases of GAT for "non-ambulatory children with severe physical and cognitive disabilities (SPCD)." They write, "In conclusion, paediatric endocrinologists are receiving inquiries regarding GAT from families of children with SPCD more commonly than previously realised and at least 65 children with SPCD have received GAT. Most of the responding paediatric endocrinologists view GAT as an appropriate therapeutic modality in certain circumstances."

(Wilfond et al. 2010). Although I cannot presume to have walked in the shoes of Ashley's parents, I have long traveled in a similar pair.[11]

My daughter, no longer a child but a woman in her forties, is not quite a "pillow angel" in the sense defined by Ashley's parents in their blog.[12] She possesses some motor skills. She learned to hold up her head by the age of two years (instead of the typical age, two months). She did learn to walk—at age five after extensive physical therapy—but retained the wide gait of a toddler. For many years, however, as locomotion on her own became too hazardous because of her seizure disorder and scoliosis of the spine, she has used a wheelchair. Like Ashley, she is very comfortable in bed, but we don't keep her there except to rest. Unlike Ashley, who requires a feeding tube, my daughter Sesha has eaten regular food (which she delights in), but she can at best finger feed.

Like Ashley, she does not toilet herself, speak, or turn herself in bed; she can do no daily tasks of living for herself, and she has no measurable IQ. Like Ashley, she is sweet, loving, and easy to love. A person with Sesha's disposition would easily be called "an angel," *regardless* of disabilities. Sometimes I wonder if Sesha is a special being sent to us from elsewhere, for there is an impossible-to-articulate

---

[11] It should be noted that I am not the only parent of a child similar to Ashley who has objected. One piece appeared in a blog published by *Psychology Today* by "a Dad" (2012).

[12] The blog says:

"'Permanently Unabled' children, who we affectionately call 'Pillow Angels':

- Form a new category of disability, survival was made possible through recent medical advancements
- Constitute less than 1% of children with disability, they are the most vulnerable of society
- Are profoundly dependent on their caregivers & profoundly precious to their families
- Their quality of life is much richer under their family's loving care, versus getting "warehoused in institutions"
- The overwhelming majority of their families & caregivers believe that increased weight & size is their worst enemy
- An extreme condition that calls for individualized options in the hands of parents to help their children."

See http://pillowangel.org/AT-Summary.pdf. This definition is deeply problematic. To mention but a few points: "permanently unabled" indicates a purely medical model view of this disability. Furthermore, although the survival of many people with disability and without disability is possible only through recent medical advances, children like Ashley are not unique in this regard. Consider the person who receives a heart or liver transplant. The second bullet may well be contested by parents who have children with other very significant disabilities or life threatening illnesses. The third bullet suggests that what is precious about these children is that they are profoundly precious to their families, rather than that they are precious in their own right. The fourth bullet implies that there may be some children who are better "warehoused in institutions"—no one is better off "warehoused in institutions." The fifth bullet is what is contested in this chapter. As a parent of such a child who meets other parents of such children, I have yet to meet one who thinks weight and size are their worst enemy. The last bullet is also contestable, and again, that is the point of the current chapter.

sweetness, graciousness, and emotional openness about her—qualities we rarely find in others. I sense from the writings of Ashley's parents that Ashley too has these qualities. Still we try to refrain from referring to Sesha as "an angel" since that has the unfortunate side effect of edging her out of the human community. To love Sesha as she is, it is of critical importance to us that, unlike an angel, Sesha has a body, and, unlike eternal beings, she does age. Especially because it is hard for many to recognize and acknowledge people whose lives are significantly different, we need to reiterate the unqualified humanity of people with serious cognitive disabilities.[13]

On first consideration there appears to be a great difference between parents' expectations and hopes for children with cognitive disabilities (on the one hand) and (on the other) those for their other children. As parents, we don't expect significantly cognitively disabled children to make us grandparents or have a thriving career, and we don't hold them accountable for their actions. But on further consideration, we want the same things for all our children: that they live and stay as healthy as possible, that they have a chance for happiness and joy, that malevolent forces do not disturb their lives, and that they contribute in some way to the lives of others.[14] As I tried to argue in part I, these are features that we generally take to be constitutive of a good life. Despite the special qualities we parents find in our disabled children, and in spite of our curbed expectations, we share with most parents a deep love for our children, a commitment to their flourishing, and a desire to always have them in our lives.

AT was Ashley's parents' innovation, and clearly it was never presented to us as an option for Sesha since no one considered it prior to Ashley's parents. From my position as the mother of a grown woman, I recoil at the thought of doing this to my daughter. (Note the turn of phrase: "to my daughter" not "for" her, even though parents such as the mother of "Charlie"—a New Zealand child who was subject to AT—explicitly say that they did not do this "to" her but "for" her.) Might I have felt differently when Sesha was Ashley's age and showed signs of precocious puberty? At six, Sesha was making progress physically and had started to walk. We could not envision a regression, and so we would have rejected any such suggestion. Could I say the same knowing, as I do today, that as an adult Sesha would not walk independently? Could I say the same if confronted, as were Ashley's parents, with a six-year-old who was developing breasts and sprouting pubic hair? I can certainly imagine being alarmed and fearing what the future held. Still, had I contemplated this option, I can say today that I would have been happy to have had someone talk me out of it.

---

[13] See for example Singer (2008).

[14] These correlate with Sara Ruddick's discussion of a child's demands: preservative love, development of capacities, and social acceptance (1989).

I have already spoken of how difficult it was for us to imagine a grown Sesha—it was incongruous and, quite frankly, very disturbing. People then and now speak more easily and hopefully of children with developmental "delays" or intellectual disability. Still we rarely hear of adults so labelled except as victims of terrible abuse or when some poor fellow with "the IQ of a child" has committed a crime. Things have changed insofar as there is some visible presence of adults with Down syndrome in the media, but the positive images of adults with developmental delays and intellectual disability are scarce. When Sesha was young, I was limited, as I believe are the parents who speak of the children they have subjected to AT, by a "horizon of ability" (Siebers 2008). It is from this horizon that our children appear to be, as Ashley's parents have labeled their pillow angel, "permanently unable."

From the vantage point of the mother of a grown woman, I look back at the pain of those early years. The dominant horizon of ability has given way to a rich acceptance and full appreciation of who she is, of the lovely woman she has become. As much as I loved Sesha from the moment of birth, perhaps I love her still more today. She has acquired her own personality, her own mature beauty. And no doubt, Ashley will as well. And her parents too will have to rethink what they mean by "permanently unable"—unable in what ways? What is permanent and what alters with time and with Ashley's exposure to the world about her?

But what is of particular importance and relevance is that I have grown increasingly humble in what I think I know about my daughter (just as, I may note, I have had to learn how little I know of and understand my nondisabled child). Sesha's otherness is both more and less palpable today. The quality of containment, of mystery that we each present to each other, regardless of ability, is increasingly clear to me. We always see each other through a glass darkly, but when viewing a child with cognitive disabilities, the glass is darker still.

At the same time, I find more and more ways in which her disability is not as much of a difference as I had presumed. Her development will not show up on an IQ test, but she has become increasingly mature emotionally. As in the case of my adult son, the decades have altered her tastes, her understanding, and her responses to the world. All this, I hope to show, is pressingly relevant in considering the ethical dimensions of AT.

9.3 A Care Ethics Framework

Although many arguments against AT have been offered, some more effective than others, we will appeal to an ETHICS OF CARE, as articulated in chapters 7 and 8. Such an ethics is compatible with a complex social model of disability that is attuned to what disability scholar Tobin Siebers called the "complex embodiment" of disability. As such, it is informed by a notion of rights that are of special importance to people with disability, in particular—with reference to AT—the right to bodily integrity.

According to this ETHICS OF CARE, we CARE for another when we are motivated to concern ourselves with the other's flourishing for the other's sake and when we act in such a way that we contribute to the other's flourishing through our intended actions. Because it recognizes that our ethical life includes unequal and dependent parties, an ETHICS OF CARE seems the appropriate moral framework to consider the ethics of AT. For the procedure, beginning with a child diagnosed with SCDN who is incapable of consenting or entering the conversation, involves parties that are asymmetrical in power and dependency. The asymmetry is not only between the power and situation of the child and the parent. The parents who have the standing to provide a "substituted (or surrogate) judgment" are themselves not fully equal and autonomous agents in medical situations. They are dependent on medical personnel for expertise in making the best choice for the child.

An ETHICS OF CARE would demand that the medical personnel recognize their own asymmetrical power. In their role as carers, they have to listen to parents' views and concerns. But the new parent, if not herself disabled or already the parent of a disabled child, is likely to bring her own ableist biases to the situation, her "horizon of ability." Ideally the people upon whom the parent depends can encourage the parent to recognize her prejudice and limited perspective. Unfortunately, physicians tend to view disability as only a medical condition: it is a professional hazard to ignore the many social factors that go into one's understanding of disabled lives. The physician and the parent, in order to be fully capable of caring, need to understand themselves as requiring information from those better situated to provide a perspective from a life lived with disability.

Such information is especially necessary since an ETHICS OF CARE asks that we make ourselves "transparent" to the needs of the other, promoting the interests of the other as that individual experiences those needs—as best as we can ascertain this. As carers, our moral labor demands that we imagine the world from the perspective of the one cared for; that we respond to the cared-for in accordance with her own needs, desires, and interests; and that we attend to ways that our own needs, desires, and interests may color, obscure, or deflect those of the individual cared for. This is already hard when one is dealing with a still-unformed person such as a young child, but it is especially challenging when the person being cared for cannot be explicit in communicating needs and interests. In the case of a child like Ashley, the difficulties seem insurmountable—we can at best get asymptotically close—but it is precisely for someone as vulnerable as Ashley that we need such stringent requirements.

Within the constraints of a CARE ETHICS, all the carers, parents, physicians, and hospital review boards must be informed by the *lived experience* of disability. No doubt this is complex since those who can offer a view are by that fact alone not the target audience for AT. Nonetheless, from within the constraints of a CARE ETHICS, the fact that the judgment of AT from the disability community is decidedly negative carries moral weight, not only because this third party might have an interest in the outcome of this case, but also—and of special importance—because people with disabilities help able parents become more transparent to the needs of their disabled child. One thing that strikes a reader of interviews by parents who have opted for GAT or AT is their surety about what is best for their child. As parents we all want to think that we know what is best for our child. And, in fact, I do believe that parents are exceptionally well situated to know what is best for their child when the parent is a loving one who is concerned deeply (probably more deeply than anyone else) with the child's welfare and sufficiently familiar with this particular child to ascertain what that welfare is for that child.

But, all parents are sometimes wrong—and sometimes very wrong. Sometimes the very strength of their love can itself lead them astray. And when the child is an "apple that falls far from the tree" (to adopt the metaphor Andrew Solomon uses for children who are very significantly different from their parents), the epistemic access of the parent is far more limited than many parents wish to acknowledge. Able parents of disabled children, especially at the beginning of their child's life, are subject to the same ableist assumptions that disabled people have attempted to dislodge. Therefore, the additional judgment of others whose lives are closer to the child's likely adulthood may be the better judge of what that child needs to flourish.

In no way do I doubt that the well-being of a child, assuming a loving family, is critical to the well-being of parents and siblings, just as their well-being is crucial to that of the child. This interdependency is at the heart of Ashley's parents' argument that AT is for Ashley's own sake and makes their argument persuasive to those who might otherwise oppose AT. Yet the porosity of the relational self which is well appreciated in an ETHICS OF CARE condones neither the full merging of selves nor the absorption of the interests of one self by those of another. That selves are relational does not vitiate the need for a self to maintain a certain integrity. On the contrary, for there to be a relationship there must be selves that can maintain their integrity. Otherwise the relationship collapses— there is left only one self that has swallowed another. In chapter 7, we saw how notions of merging were a "temptation" of an ethics of care.

To act CARINGLY toward another is a mean between thinking of the other's interests as identical to our own and thinking of them as entirely distinct. Achieving the mean requires that family members act within certain generally agreed-upon constraints. Consider, for example, a parent who insists that she knows her child better than anyone else and knows that the only way to handle the child's misbehavior is to beat sense into her. But severely beating children contravenes strong moral prohibitions against violating another's bodily integrity, and we insist that a parent's power does not reach that far. The question in the case of AT is whether Ashley's parents' action fell within such constraints or whether they exceeded the legitimacy of their parental power.

Still another consideration that an ETHICS OF CARE alerts us to is the embodied and contextual nature of ethical interactions. From an ETHICS OF CARE perspective, we cannot attend to the body without attending to the person, and we cannot care for a person without attention to their bodily integrity and well-being. Thus respecting the right to the bodily integrity of another is critical to an ETHICS OF CARE. In addition, we cannot care in a fully normative sense without taking into account particular actors, as well as the time, place, and circumstances relevant to ethical deliberation. In the case of Ashley X, although the context of this particular child and this particular family matter, the context of her care has important implications for the care of others, not least because Ashley's parents have made a point of promoting AT. No evaluation of AT within an ETHICS OF CARE can ignore broader contextual features of the case, especially as the population in question historically, and still today, is highly stigmatized, and (as people with such disabilities have been, and continue to be) mistreated and abused.

However, the aspect of an ETHICS OF CARE that I will lean on most heavily is the role of the completion of care, as discussed in chapter 8. Most pertinent is the position that ministrations directed at the other are not CARE until they are taken up by the cared-for as care. As we have yet to see how Ashley and other (unpublicized) cases of AT and GA turn out, the final verdict remains uncertain. But, as we shall see, an ETHICS OF CARE gives us many reasons to be doubtful that AT is CARE, that is, care in the fully normative sense. The contention of this chapter is that despite good intentions, neither Ashley nor other qualified disabled children are well served by AT. Though it was done in the name of care, it appears not to foster flourishing in critical ways and thus falls short.

9.4 The Ashley Treatment's Questionable Presumptions

The arguments that condone AT and encourage its proliferation are joined to what I will show are a questionable set of presumptions. Some are related to questions of embodiment more generally, others to the disabled body and the disabled mind in particular. The first presumption is that we can respect a *person* even as we regard the body as only of *instrumental* importance to that individual. The second is that we can determine a *static* age of the mind of a cognitively impaired individual. A Cartesian mind/body duality, which is (not so) hidden in the first presumption, allows proponents of AT to argue that the procedure simply brings the size of the body into alignment with the age of the mind.[15] The third presumption is that we can avoid the danger that AT or GAT will be used indiscriminately or in some way abused by limiting its use to severely cognitively disabled children who are nonambulatory. The last is that AT solves the difficult problem of caring for Ashley in a way that keeps her close to the bosom of her family. How do these presumptions hold up against a more complete understanding of cognitive disability and an ETHICS OF CARE?

9.4.1 The Body "Instrumentalized"

9.4.1.1 The Right to Bodily Integrity

In an article meant to lay to rest the many criticisms launched at AT, Douglas Diekema and Norman Fost concede a right to bodily integrity, but claim it is a right that a physician may override in certain instances under certain conditions. They may do so, they claim, when they have the permission of the person or a surrogate decision-maker. Even without such permission, they point out, physicians may do so if they determine the presence of "tumors, tonsils, and appendices" that are medically required to be removed.[16] Furthermore, in the case of children with disabilities, physicians "alter physical appearance," insert "gastrostomy tubes and tracheotomy tubes," and perform osteotomies (Diekema and Fost 2010, 34). AT, they contend, is no different. Is AT ethically equivalent? I believe not.

First, even an autonomous patient's permission is not always dispositive. Our body is our own, but we are not thought to have an absolute right to violate it, or to permit others to do so. Ashley did not, because she could not, give her permission. In such cases the surrogate, usually the parent, decides[17]—for

---

[15] Liao et al. (2007, 166), point out the absurdity of this proposition when applied to anyone who becomes cognitively disabled later in life.

[16] I assume that means without the consent of the nonautonomous person, but with the consent of the surrogate, or, in emergencies, without anyone's consent.

[17] Surrogacy may be based on "substituted judgment" or "best interest." Substituted judgment supposes that the surrogate can know what the patient would have wanted, had the patient been able to choose. As Ashley could never make an autonomous decision, the "best interests" standard is likely to apply. See the AMA Code of Medical Ethics (n.d., Opinion 8.081: Surrogate Decision Making).

who is better equipped to determine and to care about the child's best interests than a caring parent? (As a parent, I also do not want others to intervene.) But to determine what is in the child's best interest, one's beliefs—even a parent's—need to rest on a solid foundation. New parents of a disabled child have little sense of the trajectory of that child's life, so their decision rests on shifting sands. Furthermore, their decision is based on a physician's assessment that their child will always "have the mind of a baby." This, I will argue, is misleading.

Are the medical procedures that do not require permission appropriate comparisons? Tumors are removed because they are life-threatening or may interfere with important bodily functions. Tonsils are removed because they heighten susceptibility to infections. Appendices are removed when infected, or likely to become infected, and pose a risk to life. Where there is an imminent danger, physicians can proceed without permission if getting consent involves a risky delay. None of these conditions apply in Ashley's case. And in Ashley's case, three entirely healthy organs were surgically removed: her appendix, her uterus, and her breast buds.

Note that all the procedures enumerated by Diekema and Fost preserve life or ameliorate a health condition. They address specific ailments that need treatment whether or not the child is disabled. That procedures that do not preserve life or affect function are carried out on disabled children raises serious moral questions that require careful consideration. The procedures involved in AT preserve neither life, health, nor function. Diekema and Fost point out that some procedures are perhaps still more problematic than AT and yet physicians do them.[18] But that we do permit some questionable practices is a poor justification for permitting still others.

A proponent of AT may want to retort that intrusions on bodily integrity are ultimately justified in Ashley's case because, like all those mentioned, they are procedures intended to promote the patient's flourishing. AT promotes parental care, and because such care is more important than height for her flourishing, the treatment is justified. Were Ashley's care impossible without these modifications of her body, then . . . Yes.

Ashley's parents have insisted that there are no substitutes for the sort of care that they can give her in her diminutive state. Nurse and philosopher Robert Newsome III who defends AT (albeit hesitantly) nonetheless grants that some of Ashley's parents' claims are overstated, e.g., that the treatment was needed to assure that she would not have to be sent to an institution, that she would not need transfers with cumbersome lifts, that this way she could be kept free of

---

[18] See arguments in Parens (2006).

bedsores, and that she will remain a size where she would be given the hugs that are so meaningful to her. He notes in a blog:

> We do in fact lift, transfer and reposition even bariatric patients on a daily basis. For over a year one of my patients was a lady who weighed over 500 lbs, and she was up, dressed, eating lunch in the dining room and playing bingo every day, thanks to specialized equipment. She was also completely free of pressure ulcers thanks to a special bed. We hugged each other each time I came on duty. Ashley could, obviously, go to school, participate in family and community life, never get a pressure ulcer, receive hugs, and so forth, without growth attenuation. (Newsome 2012)

Yet he continues:

> But, matters do not end there. Caring feels most genuine and rewarding when it is unmediated by the mechanical and the non-human. . . . Human touch is a critical component of human caring. It is comforting in ways that the mechanical is not. . . . It is for this reason that I will confess that I don't like hoyer lifts. I do not like putting patients in a sling and lifting them, like a horse you are transferring from a ship to a barge, with the aide of a machine. What is more, most patients don't really like them either, and will tell you so if you ask. Those who are cognitively intact will tell you so in words; those who are not will let you know in other ways. One also needs to wonder if lifts need to be as awkward as they are. So much equipment has seen improvements as disabled people have demanded better treatment. To use the old barb, "If we can send a man up to the moon . . ."

My experience with Sesha until recently was not helpful in assessing the use of lifts—Sesha had been able to stand and pivot (while being held) and we needed to use a lift only rarely. Since an unfortunate set of hospitalizations for seizure control and complications from epilepsy has left her too weak to stand, we have had to rely on lifts. I confess, their use is less than ideal. However, how much patients object to them is less clear to me. Sesha actually enjoys the ride— which is what we call it. She smiles when she is put in and graps the straps and sort of swings with it. (I think I have more trouble with the lift than she does.) Clearly, as Newsome points out, we can hug a person without the hug being part of being lifted. And what a person being lifted is most concerned with is her own safety—that she not be dropped! I know a young man who lives with Sesha who was dropped when he was lifted by caretakers, many years ago—and he is neither heavy nor tall. According to his mother, he far prefers the mechanical lift for it makes him feel more secure. Sesha is actually hugged when we stand her and pivot her—it is the best way to make sure she doesn't fall. When she is in the mood, she will take it as a hug and not mind it. At other times, she looks uncomfortable in the embrace. A hug is a hug when it is a hug—and is not necessarily experienced as one when it is primarily a means to another end.

Being handled, whether by hands or a mechanical device, is not always welcome, and hands or devices can be used caringly and with care, or not. It may well be that if we have to hire help or rely on equipment to do what parents' hands and arms can do, then there is a loss; but although the ability to care for Ashley without such assistance may be lost, the ability to care for Ashley well, and even to provide that care at home, is not. Learning what services and resources are available, advocating for more services and better equipment (as Newsome himself urges), adjusting to new people and equipment, all take time and energy. And surely raising a child with severe disabilities is demanding enough: I know, I have been there. AT, in particular GAT (growth attenuation), is a shortcut through these difficulties. But, as I will argue, if we believe that no reason justifies restricting the future height of a person to that of a six-year-old when that person does not have severe cognitive disabilities,[19] then, as the procedure neither cures nor mitigates the disability, we should not do it in the case of this disability either.

As one mother, Sue Swenson, put it: "Parents [of disabled children], too, need to operate within the bounds of society." As for the opportunities that open along with the difficulties, she writes:

> It is difficult to care for a son who is legally blind, quadriplegic, non-verbal, autistic, profoundly intellectually disabled, six feet tall and 190 pounds. Heck, if you put it that way, it sounds impossible. . . . We have not been his sole caregivers since he was eleven. . . . Family support helped us learn to let go, and to recognize the man that emerged from behind the face of our baby boy. We needed information and training about raising a severely disabled child: how to position him so he could participate; how to transfer him without lifting; how to support his mobility and find useful equipment; how to figure out what he wanted; how to think about his rights. . . .We love our profoundly disabled son as we love our other sons. Like them, he is a strong, gentle, complex, and interesting person. He is his own man.[20]

---

[19] This, of course, then exempts dwarfs from consideration. An objection to growth attentuation should not be understood as disparaging Dwarfism, which is a human variation.

[20] Personal communication. May 19th, 2010. See also Wilfond et al. (2010).

9.4.1.2 The Inherent Good of Growth and Sexual Development

Diekema and Fost defend GAT by comparing it to another manipulation of a child's growth, namely growth *promotion* therapy. Its acceptance, they contend, is uncontroversial because people mistakenly think its point is to bring a child within a given norm, while people object to growth attenuation because GAT takes the child further from this norm. Instead, they argue, both procedures have nothing to do with norm heights but are manipulations of the body that make it more conducive for certain ends: In the case of growth promotion it is to make the child competitive in the job market and in social interactions. In the case of GAT, it is to make the child small enough to be cared for in the home (Diekema and Fost 2010, 34).

The difference between growth attenuation and growth promotion, however, is that growth is what happens when a child is kept healthy and properly nourished—this is true even of those whose genetic makeup results in short stature. *Children* with achondroplasia who are kept healthy and well nourished grow to the height of an *adult* with achondroplasia. Although some parents do opt for growth promotion to bring their child the social advantages of height within a socially accepted norm, growth attenuation too has been used to bring tall girls into line with a socially accepted norm. In the 1950s and 1960s, a tall girl was at a distinct social disadvantage. The innovative "solution" to this socially constructed "problem" was GAT using high dosages of estrogen. As we move toward gender parity, GAT for tall girls has been cast into the waste-bin of oppressive gender practices. In time, we might look at growth promotion for social acceptance, when there is not a medical reason for a child's inability to grow, in the same way. Attempting to manipulate the height of a child, whether for social acceptance to a rigid norm or for another instrumental purpose, is a questionable behavior that takes the body as a mere instrument, and not as the embodiment of the self.

To signal this instrumentalism of the body, critics have asked (rhetorically) that if the aim of GAT is to produce a size small enough to keep children like Ashley within the family orbit, then why not just remove her legs? Diekema and Fost dignify this rhetorical question with a response, giving as one "nontrivial" reason against limb removal that it reduces the number of sites for intravenous access![21] Even if true, the response is grotesque. Removing healthy limbs is

---

[21] They add that additional reasons include morbidity, which is a risk of limb removal, and appearance, that is, the visual impression created by a person missing limbs. Neither is compelling as the reason to favor GAT by high-dose estrogen. High-dose estrogen for very young children has not previously been tried, and hysterectomy and breast-bud removal carry the risks of surgery. Either procedure will produce an anomalous appearance. But good cosmetic prosthetics are available for those missing limbs.

abhorrent because we value bodily integrity as a crucial intrinsic good. When deciding whether to remove a limb (or attenuate growth), we weigh not only risks and benefits, but also our values. Imagine parents requesting GAT for their talented prepubescent son who passionately wants to be a champion gymnast (or jockey or coxswain, where small size is necessary), and is willing to trade height for the realization of a dream. Surely the request would be denied. To accede to it, some may argue, would be to close the boy's future options; but to refuse him, we foreclose an option for which he has demonstrated passion and talent. Instead, I venture, our moral intuition is that when we regard his body as merely instrumental to a specified ambition or goal, we also treat him as a mere instrument: our bodies are ourselves—what is done to our bodies is done to us.

Diekema and Fost take an equally instrumental stance toward sexual organs. Surmising that the removal of the breast buds might reduce sexually pleasurable sensations, they promptly dismiss the worry since Ashley would never "experience sexual pleasure without being exploited or sexually abused" (Diekema and Fost 2010, 34).[22] Asking "what it is about becoming a woman that would be of interest to Ashley?", they answer: "Most of the usual features that distinguish a woman from a girl—the opportunity to marry, procreate, work, lead an autonomous life—would not have been available to Ashley with or without a uterus, fully developed breasts, or normal stature" (Diekema and Fost 2010, 34).

As the childishness in her face fades, Sesha's body has taken the form of a woman. I don't know if Sesha can rejoice in her breasts, if she notices them at all, if she would miss them, or if she compares herself to other girls. What I do know is only that I don't know. Nothing about Sesha—with all her profound incapacities—tells me that Sesha is incapable of these feelings. I can say that I, as her mother, delight in her womanliness. It is very much a part of Sesha, as she is now.

It's true that Sesha, like Sue Swenson's son, has become harder to handle as she grew to be 5'4" and 120 pounds, and we have had to make accommodations. At forty, she now lives away from us during the week and is at home with us during the weekend not because she is too tall or too womanly, but because at this stage of her life, she has a more varied and fuller existence in the community where she is than she would if confined to our home. At a certain point, we stopped taking her with us everywhere not only because she got bigger, but also because we felt that we needed time with our son, and he needed time to do things with us that Sesha could not share. Had Sesha been petite and skinny, some things would have been easier. What started to make it difficult to bring Sesha with us was the cumbersome wheelchair she needed to keep her well positioned.

---

[22] They do not consider the possibility of a spontaneous orgasm.

Today there are umbrella strollers and beach buggies for strolls and water fun. Do I regret at all that the "keep-her-small solution" was not available to us? No, emphatically not. We stand Sesha up and love that she is just a tad taller than me. "Sesha! You're bigger than Mommy!" Why? Why does anyone enjoy noting how tall one's child has become? We take pleasure and pride in our bodies as they grow and mature just because we do. Full stop. It needs no further justification. It is constitutive of a thriving life. That is not to say that one cannot thrive without breasts and without a uterus, or that short stature can mean only that we have not thrived. But height and the bodily changes of womanhood are among the ways in which human beings thrive, and signal this thriving to others.

9.4.2 "A Better Fit" Between the Disabled Body and the Disabled Mind

Ashley's parents approvingly quote George Dvorsky (2006): " 'The estrogen treatment is not what is grotesque here. Rather, it is the prospect of having a full-grown and fertile woman endowed with the mind of a baby.' " They continue: "Ashley can continue to delight in being held in our arms and will be moved and taken on trips more frequently." They say that professionals tell them: "She will always have the mind of a three-month-old infant." They report: "Unlike what most people thought, the decision to pursue AT was not a difficult one." They go on to say that once they understood the options, the "right course was clear to us."[23] What I believe happened is that once they understood that a child who was an eternal baby would grow into a woman, the course was clear to them.

The diagnosis and prognosis they received is stasis. But it is just this idea that misleads us. To have "the mind of a baby" and the capacities of a baby are not the same thing, for the disabled person may well have an understanding and a set of emotional responses that far exceed her capacity to act. The brain may be impaired,[24] but it is not frozen. Synapses continue to be formed as they do in all brains. The "static" in "static encephalopathy" refers to the fact that hers is not a progressive condition in which the brain deteriorates, not to the impossibility of the brain developing. "Global deficits" similarly do not mean that there can be no development. As the Board of the American Association for Intellectual and Developmental Disabilities writes: "The abundant evidence [is] that *all* [my

---

[23] All quotes from Ashley's parents' blog.

[24] It is important to note that the brain may not be impaired in such a fashion that actually does affect the ability to cognize. See Anne McDonald (2007). See the discussion below.

emphasis] children are able to learn and that the cognitive capabilities of children with severe motor impairments can be grossly underestimated" (AAIDD 2007).

A young woman with Rett syndrome with whom I am acquainted has no more capacities than a very young child, perhaps a baby of three months. But this young woman, when told that her father was dying, would be found by the caregivers sitting quietly shedding tears for weeks. This is not within the understanding of a baby. A dear caregiver joked in front of my daughter that the secret of her youthful appearance was that she had no worries, like paying taxes and bills. I countered by saying that Sesha has a lot to worry about, like not being able to scratch an itch, move out of an uncomfortable position, tell us what she wants, and so on. My daughter turned to face me, gave me an intense look, smiled broadly and reached out to hug me. I was startled, as were all who witnessed this response. Maybe she only grasped the tone, but it is no less possible, indeed plausible, that she understood the words. She had, after all, been listening to human speech for over forty years.

What we know of are the capabilities that allow the brain to direct the rest of the body in certain ways. We do not yet know enough about what is actually going on in the (bodily) brain and the subjective world of people with severe cognitive disabilities. A rather stunning example of this is Anne McDonald. McDonald writes:

> Like Ashley, I, too, have a static encephalopathy. Mine was caused by brain damage at the time of my breech birth. Like Ashley, I can't walk, talk, feed or care for myself. My motor skills are those of a 3-month-old. When I was 3, a doctor assessed me as severely retarded (that is, as having an IQ of less than 35) and I was admitted to a state institution called St. Nicholas Hospital in Melbourne, Australia. As the hospital didn't provide me with a wheelchair, I lay in bed or on the floor for most of the next 14 years. At the age of 12, I was relabeled as profoundly retarded (IQ less than 20) because I still hadn't learned to walk or talk. (2007)

At eighteen McDonald weighed nearly thirty-five pounds, had not developed breasts or menstruated. It was not through medical intervention but through medical neglect that her growth was attenuated. When she was sixteen, she was given access to means of communication, and her life changed. She eventually reached her full height of 5 feet, and matured as a woman. About the AT she writes: ""Been there. Done that. Didn't like it. Preferred to grow."

There are two points to be made here. The first is that we cannot know for certain the capabilities of someone whose motor skills are so impacted that they cannot speak or walk. This is not to say that like Anne Macdonald, Ashley's cerebral palsy has no intellectual involvement. The second is that, even if there is intellectual impairment, even to a very significant degree, we still do not know what she will be able to comprehend and experience.

As Ashley will have hormones produced by intact ovaries, she may well experience the sensations of bodily maturation. What will it mean to her not to have breasts? Do we know? What will it mean to her to be a woman? Do we know? How will she experience bodily growth? Can we say? No, no, and no. It is the misleading image of a fertile, full-grown woman with the mind of a baby that makes us think we know something about which we have, at the current time, not a clue.

Diekema and Fost concede that "some rights claims raise troubling questions" among which are "that Ashley had been robbed of the right to sexual pleasure." They grant that the removal of the breast buds might reduce sexually pleasurable sensations she might otherwise experience, but promptly dismiss the worry. Why? Because it is too worrisome to think of children like Ashley growing into sexual beings.

I deeply appreciate the worry and the fear that such a young woman might be exploited or abused, but removing breast buds and preventing breasts will not guarantee or even reduce these possibilities. If one is perverse enough to sexually abuse such a girl, might he or she even be attracted by the strange history of a child whose parents removed her breast buds? Who can say? Only careful screening, supervision, and respect for these girls and women can offer the needed protection.

Desiring AT for one's child may make sense if "she will always be a child mentally," as an adult body makes meeting her needs (the needs of a child) more cumbersome. Keeping Ashley forever small will, alas, not keep her forever a child. Though difficult to grasp while the child is still young, one learns that, in the case of disability, things don't just fit together in standard ways. Some cognitive skills are minimal, others may go through a relatively "normal development." Because one is incapable of holding up one's head, speaking, or walking does not mean that they cannot understand a slight. Because someone has had no apparent expressive speech does not mean that he or she cannot understand the thoughts of others as they are conveyed through language. The relationships among such capabilities are more complex and less predictable than in those who are species-typical.

From a position of an ETHICS OF CARE, the caregiver needs to be able to understand the world, as far as possible, from the perspective of the cared-for. But this sort of understanding on the part of an able parent of a disabled child requires more than empathy and more than love. It requires understanding and education. It requires time to grow with the disability as the child does. To short-circuit the project is ultimately not conducive to good care. Even if Ashley herself will never understand the growth attenuation as a slight, as a curtailment of her right to grow and develop, is Ashley, or Sesha, or another individual best cared for by always being kept close to Mom and Dad? Having moved through over forty years of the life cycle, I have come to seriously question that proposition. A three-month-old may need only Mom or Dad or Grandma. But a severely cognitively disabled adult needs more, much more: the companionship of peers, of other caregivers, different settings, and experiences that Mom and Dad cannot supply.

9.4.3 Cognitive Disability as the (Sole) Indicator for AT

Proponents recognize that there is always a risk of a misdiagnosis. Furthermore, I have offered reasons to question if the SCDN truly are incapable of all such understanding, even when the diagnosis is correct. Proponents respond that all medical procedures involve some uncertainty; there is always the risk that we are wrong. As in all medicine, we weigh doing the procedure against doing nothing. In the case of breast bud removal, Diekema and Fost ask if we had done nothing and "Ashley suffered frequent yeast infections under her breasts, recurrent biopsies, and fatal breast cancer due to a delayed diagnosis" (Diekema and Fost 2010, 36), would that be preferable to having done nothing? But this retort is not compelling.

Yeast infections are a problem for large-breasted women, yet can be treated with over-the-counter antifungal cream and often are preventable with good care. As unpleasant as recurrent biopsies are, it is hard to imagine anyone choosing breast removal to avoid them. When there is a congenital risk of breast cancer, some women do favor preemptive mastectomy. But so far at least, we have not suggested removing breast buds in all young girls where there is a family history of breast cancer. It is no more urgent in women with very severe cognitive disabilities.

Newsome adds another argument to that of Diekema and Fost. Addressing my objections and those of Asch and Stubblefield (2010), he remarks that while it is surely true that "any medical diagnosis and/or prognosis might be erroneous," he does not think that this gets us very far in the case of prognosis and certainly not in the case of diagnosis. He cites the case of Wilms tumor, which is a rare malignant tumor of the kidney. This develops in childhood and manifests in various indicators and symptoms. But the diagnosis is uncertain—even the presence of a mass on the kidney could be a benign tumor (a metanephric adenofibroma). With respect to the uncertainty of diagnosis, he writes:

If it is, surgery is not a "medical necessity." Still, metanephric adenofibroma is an even more rare condition than Wilm's [sic] tumor, and the consequences of NOT surgically removing a Wilm's [sic] tumor are certain death. In other words, a diagnosis might be wrong, but it would nevertheless be a mistake NOT to accept it as true when deliberating upon what to do. The parent who decides to just HOPE that this is simply a case of metanephric adenofibroma would seem, at least to me, to be more than a little daft. (Newsome 2012)

With respect to prognosis he writes:

Continuing on with the Wilm's [sic] tumor example, even if the tumor is excised while it is "stage 1," the patient is "cured" in over 90%, but less than 100%, of such cases. So, we might not want to say that we "know" the child in question is cured (at least when certain epistemologists and sophomores are in earshot). We might want to say, instead, that we hope this child is cured, and that the hope is not a vain and fanciful one, but rather is based on evidence, and pretty good evidence at that. We would not think, given our collective experience, that a parent who hopes their child is cured is, under these circumstances, simply blinded by parental love and engaged in wishful thinking. (Newsome 2012)

It unclear to me how Newsome's arguments about the uncertainty of a malignant tumor that causes death if untreated is equivalent to the AT. Unlike the case of Wilms tumor, Ashley's condition is not fatal and her parents acknowledge that she is likely to live a long life (indeed, that is part of their justification for the treatment), even if nothing is done. The question about AT is not uncertainty or diagnosis or prognosis per se, but rather what constitutes a reasonable weighing of risks and benefits, of the value of "treating" or not given that nothing in her condition is life-threatening, that not treating does not need to involve a deterioration of her health, and that there are alternative means by which to give her not only care, but good care.

An explicit presumption in the arguments of Fost and Diekema—if not in Newsome's—is that the risks are justification enough *for the nonambulatory severely cognitively disabled child,* as they lack the awareness (and always will) to understand the losses or engage in social interactions where the losses would be felt. Against the complaint that this looks like discrimination, proponents answer that all medical procedures target limited populations. One prescribes antibiotics only to people with bacterial infections; anticonvulsives are limited to epileptics, and so on. Each medical intervention is targeted at particular ills that are dangerous to life, cause pain or ill health, or reduce function. Children with disabilities are subject to many invasive procedures that are limited mostly to people with disabilities. Diekema and Fost cite "tracheotomies to improve airway patency and enable suctioning, tonsillectomy to reduce airway obstruction, fundoplication to reduce gastroesophageal reflux, gastrostomy tubes to aid feeding, spinal fusions to prevent advancement of scoliosis, and tendon releases to reduce the effects of spasticity" (Diekema and Fost 2010, 36).

But all these are also carried out on children not otherwise disabled or they are directed to a *specific medical disorder*, not a *class of persons* per se. Tracheotomies are used for whosoever needs this assistance for breathing; tonsillectomy and spinal fusions are carried out regardless of a person's cognitive or physical capabilities; gastrostomy tubes may be more frequently administered to old and young whose cognitive function is impaired, but only because such impairment is coupled with conditions that impact swallowing and food intake. Severe cognitive disability (coupled with nonambulation) is not an indicator for any of these or any other procedure save AT, for which it is the sole and necessary indicator.

AT is intended for ease in handling the person and preemptively treating sources of pain or discomfort. The disanalogy with all the other cases is that AT alone is not considered as a treatment for any *other* people whose size, or potential size, can pose equivalent difficulties in care or exclusion from family life—for example, for an autistic boy who is likely to turn into a bulky six-footer and to have violent tantrums that will require restraints, but is capable to the extent that he can ambulate.

The main reason for limiting the eligible population in this way is the supposition that these people alone will never know the difference—even if we cannot be sure this is true. But the treatment is not directed at their cognitive disability. It is directed at the difficulty of caring for them—a condition shared by many other populations. Why not subject other difficult-to-care-for individuals to AT? Because they may know the difference.

Then what else might we be able to do to this population on the supposition that they will never know the difference? Aside from the real epistemic quandary (that is, that this prognosis may be wrong), consider that the long, cruel, and gruesome history of people with cognitive disabilities, especially when the disabilities are severe, is strewn with procedures justified on the supposition that these people don't know the difference or can't feel the indignity—that they won't know the difference if a part of their brain is lobotomized, if they are deprived of clothing and left sitting naked in their own excrement, or if they are showered communally by being hosed down. The horrid shame of it all is made that much worse when some who are included are *totally* cognizant of their mistreatment. Yet we also have learned that once we stop supposing that "they don't know the difference anyway," we find out that they were quite capable of knowing, understanding, or at the least experiencing the treatment as mistreatment even if there is cognitive impairment. People with severe cognitive disabilities are often not told when a close family member dies because "they just wouldn't understand." Yet the young women with Rett understood all too well when told. So did another young man, diagnosed as severely cognitively disabled, whom I know. I myself witnessed his howling pain when told of his father's death. I was also told that at a moment when the issue of loss was discussed with the entire group of residents at my daughter's house, my daughter took the noise-making object she favors and placed it onto the tray of her grieving friend. That was her one means of expressing her desire to make him feel better, and she took it.

The uncertainty of us not knowing what these individuals know is a great risk indeed. And the risk of further stigmatizing this group and discriminating against them—doing something to them that would not be done to anyone else—is also far too grave a risk to permit AT or even just GAT to be routinely offered to parents of these children. We reopen a Pandora's box of well-intended salves that turn into nightmares when we allow severe cognitive disability to be the lone and sole indicator for a certain treatment. In medical care as well as parental care, we do balance risks and benefits. Caring is often a matter of making these difficult choices, but if we fail in our care when we do more damage than good, most moral theories,[25] and especially an ETHICS OF CARE, would suggest that some risks are not worth taking, no matter the apparent benefits.[26]

The psychological pain expressed in some other cases where parents have intervened in their child's development while their child was very young and where there was not a medical necessity indicates that AT is not a risk worth taking, especially since the difficulty is ultimately less with the child's body and more with the social response, or rather lack of social response, to the needs of families of a SCDN child.

Moreover, if it is wrong to a person who does know the difference, that is, if it is justified in this case only because these people do not know the difference anyway, then, as Asch and Stubblefield (2010) argue, it is a wrong—whether or not a person is aware of what has been done to them. They point to the ruling in the case of *People v. Minkowski*, in which a gynecologist was convicted of raping his patients after he had engaged in intercourse with them during vaginal exams without their consent, although they were not aware at the time that that was what he was doing. A woman who is unconscious when penetrated without her consent is no less raped than were she awake. And to be raped is to be wronged, whether or not we are aware of it. If we should not do GAT, hysterectomies, or

[25] Utilitarianism may be an exception to this general claim.
[26] See, for example, Dreger (1998); Chase (1999); Feder (2002).

breast bud removals to cognitively able children, then we should not do them to cognitively disabled children.

9.4.4 Doing "Justice to the Scope of the Problem"

Jeffrey Brosco, a pediatrician and medical historian, in one of the best commentaries on the subject, writes sympathetically of the predicament faced by many parents of severely cognitively and physically disabled children. As a practical matter, Brosco (2006, 1077–8) points out that we do not know if AT will work. That is, "will the administration of high-dose estrogen to children with profound disabilities enable them to remain at home under the care of their parents for a longer period? And will this improve the quality of their lives?" His question is particularly relevant for an ETHICS OF CARE because of its strong consequentialist element. Perhaps we would have to wait too long for the Ashley case to provide evidence in either direction. But we have no evidence that smaller individuals are kept at home longer, nor that this is a factor in decisions to place children in out-of-home residences. We also lack evidence correlating smaller size with a better quality of life.

Most importantly, Brosco asks whether the proposed treatment does "justice to the scope of the problem." His assessment is that the most morally troubling feature of the Ashley case is that it "fails to situate the plight of these parents struggling to care for their children, in the larger context of a societal failure to provide adequate social support in this most admirable of undertakings." Instead it offers "simple technical fixes for seemingly intractable problems, which often combine biological and social aspects of human existence" (Brosco 2006, 1077–8).

Many hoped that the case would fuel demands for increased assistance. Equipment (often not user-friendly, reliable, or gainly) and caregivers (often untrained and inexperienced) are expensive and are only occasionally covered by health insurance. In communities where help can be obtained, parents have to scratch and claw their way into the appropriate programs. Although some strides have been made in making equipment easier to use, more reliable, sleeker, and less—well, let's say it—ugly, most equipment is still made for institutional, not home, use. Yet as we pointed out earlier, as imperfect as it is, serviceable equipment exists, and good nonfamilial caregiving is possible. The gains that have been made for people with severe cognitive disabilities have been hard-won—and mostly by families who refused to settle for an inferior life for their child.

Keeping Ashley forever small is quixotic as a "new solution to an old dilemma." While Ashley won't grow in height, her familial caregivers will age, and carrying around a child much bigger than a one- or two-year old becomes increasing difficult. More broadly, the problems of care will continue to exist for those whose growth cannot be attenuated: those already past puberty; those who become disabled through disease, accident, or war; those who are frail, elderly, or no longer able to care for themselves. We cannot pare down their bodies to the leftover functional parts—not, that is, without creating a monstrous society. The Ashley treatment simply fails "to do justice to the scale of the problem."

9.5 The Social Model and Care's Completion

Brosco's appeal to the larger social problems that are the larger context for the Ashley case has an implicit appeal to the social model of disability. Disability activists who have largely decried AT abjure solutions that "fix the person" rather than alter the environment. Diekema and Fost (2010), along with other proponents, acknowledge the social problem, but ask why a family needs to sit around to wait for needed societal changes. If a family can make life better by altering the impaired body, why should an ideological construct such as the social model stand in the way?

If we dismiss the social model as mere ideology, we fail to see that because of it, disabled people have been able to reject the view of themselves as damaged goods, to claim "the right to live in the world" (tenBroek 1966, 843) and to do so as they are. In order to see the world from the child's viewpoint, a parent attempts to cultivate a "transparent self." But as nondisabled parents who try to cultivate a transparent self of an ETHICS OF CARE, we must acknowledge our limited grasp of life lived with disability. As much as we love our children, we are unlikely to see the world from their perspective, and we are likely to continue to harbor biases we retain from an "horizon of ability." The caring physician too needs to acknowledge that it is an occupational hazard to favor a medical model of disability. In the early years of our disabled children's lives, we parents desperately want to believe that with an operation here, a treatment there, the right exercises, the right therapies, the problem will dissolve—our children will live "normal" lives. Clearly Ashley's parent's do not expect Ashley to live a "normal life." But they do want to normalize, to some extent, their interactions with her (for example, not relying on lifts and strangers for her care). In itself, there is nothing wrong with that desire. Nonetheless, parents have to tread a delicate line between refusing resignation on the one hand and—on the other—accepting the child as she is *and as she will become.* When there is no way to "normalcy" or increased function, a change in perspective is more than just "settling": it is positively transformative.[27]

[27] See for example, AAIDD (2007) and ADAPT (2007). For comments from an individual disability activist, see Peace (2007).

When Sesha was six, I shared Ashley's parents' urge to freeze time, to keep her as the child she was then. But no medical intervention can suffice. We age, and what was small when we were young is now not small enough. Siblings, too, mature and will want to do things without any siblings—disabled or not. Even if Ashley herself is cherished within the family, her future caregivers may well feel differently about the parents' choice, disparaging the parents, the child, or both. As they grow older, will Ashley's siblings see what had been done to her as the loving act of parents with a full acceptance of Ashley for who she is? Or will they wonder what conditions attach to their parents' acceptance of them as they are?[28]

The transformation that the social model offers is to be open to possibilities. If we shut off discussion with certainties of what is to be when we face disability, we will make the same mistakes that created Willowbrook, that led to devastating practices like lobotomies, damaging overmedications and such. It is worth pointing out that lobotomies were procedures that parents, seeking help with the care of their disabled children, sought out, that doctors consented to, and that today we look upon with dismay. At the time, it looked like a reasonable solution to Rosemary Kennedy's new acquired bouts of irritability and aggression. Rosemary, daughter of the powerful Joseph Kennedy and sister to the celebrated Kennedy brothers, was "slow." This child, raised lovingly at home, was lobotomized when her behavior threatened to disrupt family life. Frontal lobotomies were new procedures that carried much promise: just remove one small troublesome part of the brain—the rest was left intact—and all would be well again. Especially worrisome in Rosemary Kennedy's case, there was a fear that this beautiful young woman might get lured into sexual contact and get pregnant.[29]

Rosemary, who was believed to have mild mental retardation, was after the procedure very severely cognitively impaired. She was institutionalized; the previously loving family never visited her. They put her as fully out of their lives as they were able, until her sister, Eunice Shriver, brought the family secret out of the closet and began the campaigns that have vastly improved the lives of intellectually disabled people. Defenders of AT do not use frontal lobotomies as a relevant comparison class and insist that AT is far removed from such a barbarity. Most likely that is true, but I suggest that the similarities and differences should be carefully studied, since only hindsight reveals the true contours of many choices.

---

[28] Recall some of the questions my own son raised in chapter 4.

[29] The story of Rosemary is recounted in Larson (2015). How interesting that the fear of a pregnancy is a component in many of the interventions in the bodies of disabled girls and women.

Proponents may reply that this is the old bug-a-boo about the slippery slope. We can put constraints into our ethics guidelines and institute laws that will protect this group. And yet in the arguments presented in this chapter, they themselves rely on that easy glide down the slope of permissible interventions. They argue: "We can do x, y, and z, so why can't we do AT?" It's the oldest trick in the book for further stigmatizing a stigmatized group, and there is precious little that indicates that it will all stop at AT.

The prototypes of the environmental fix that the social model of disability urges are alterations in the physical environment, e.g., ramps, braille on elevator panels. As important as these are, still more important is the environment of inclusion: of welcoming many sorts of bodies and minds, seeing the world as enriched by this diversity, and embracing the possibilities as well as the challenges presented by those who diverge from the norm.[30] If our actions with respect to our children ignore the need to make the environmental transformations— creating a world for them to flourish even when we parents are no longer there for them—there is a generalized way in which we have not done well by them, have not cared as well for them as we might have, had we directed some of our energies to help build a more accommodating world.

The Ashley case should have heralded a movement to secure better services, better equipment, and more attention to the needs of severely disabled individuals and the families who care for them. Instead we now have at least sixty-five Ashleys, male and female. Tragically, our society still fails to sufficiently reduce the unjust burden of their care and so impels the Ashley treatment copycats to shrink their children instead.

9.6 Peter Singer Weighs In

Peter Singer (2007; 2012), defender of animal rights par excellence, has twice had editorials in major media outlets (the *New York Times* and *The Guardian*) about Ashley, and twice I have written responses (Kittay and Kittay 2007), which were not published in those venues. Peter Singer is a fine philosopher and has made extremely important contributions in the areas of animal rights and poverty. His work on people with disability is less distinguished and is consistently disputed by people who live with the conditions of which he speaks.

What astonishes me is that people who know as little about disability as Singer are repeatedly invited to pontificate on the subject. I am also perplexed when I hear the debate about Ashley X framed as one between cognitively able

[30] See Garland-Thomson (2012) for a notion of "eugenic logic," which may be operative here.

disability rights activists and the parents of children with cognitive disability. I understand that many parents have contacted the parents of Ashley, but outside of my participation in the Seattle Children Hospital workshop discussing growth attenuation, I have yet to meet a single parent of very severely and profoundly affected individuals who has any sympathy for the procedure.

While I will address Singer's views on cognitively disabled people more fully in a forthcoming volume, *Who's Truly Human? Justice, Personhood and Mental Disability*, there is one argument he makes defending the AT that I want to address here as a postscript to the main arguments. It centers on the question of dignity, again a subject that I will address in the forthcoming book. Rather than inveighing against dignity per se,[31] Singer maintains that Ashley has no dignity to violate. Singer thinks that neither a very young child nor an older human with comparable intellectual capacities can have dignity. A baby is cute. But dignified? And, argues Singer, we don't attribute dignity to dogs and cats, "though they clearly operate at a more advanced mental level than human infants" (Singer 2007), so why should we attribute dignity to infants or those who have an infant's intellectual capability? A philosophically naïve reader might wonder: what does intellectual ability have to do with dignity? Isn't dignity something that we should give to *all* human beings regardless of how smart they may be? But such a reader would not be familiar with a long tradition of philosophical thought that takes humans' intellectual ability to be the source of human dignity.

I do believe, as do Ashley's parents, that Ashley has dignity. They maintain that while Ashley has no concept of dignity, "We however care a great deal about our daughter's human dignity and feel that the treatment makes Ashley more dignified by providing her with a better quality of life."[32] In this instance, the concept of dignity can give us no purchase whichever side we argue for. But AT does call for a clearer understanding of what dignity means, and particularly what dignity means with respect to individuals such as Sesha and Ashley, who may not have a concept of dignity, but could nonetheless have dignity.

---

[31] As do Ruth Macklin (2003) and Steven Pinker (2008), who respectively have argued that dignity is a "useless" or "stupid" term.

[32] In an interview with Ashley X's father (Pilkington 2012), he maintains: "Her life is as good as we can possibly make it."

Afterword: My Daughter's Body—A Meditation on Soul

Sesha pushes my head to her neck. I find those sweet tender places at the crease of her neck, soft and warm. And she gurgles with pleasure. My daughter's body. Its problems, its mystery, its soul. How very difficult it is to convey all that I experience when I am in her presence, the presence of that lovely, somewhat twisted, wheelchair-user body. It is through my daughter's body that I come to know her.

That I come to know another through her body is an epistemic claim. It is in one sense true for all subjects of human knowledge, and in another, it is particular to people such as my daughter, that is, to people who are restricted in their movements and who have no (or little) expressive language. When we seek and come to know another, we learn who another is by what they say or do, not merely their physical material aspect. Our epistemic access to another is linguistic and behaviorial, not material. Although it goes without saying that both these are grounded in, or the consequence of, our bodies, we discount the bodily as a contigent and not a necessary aspect of who a person (or mind or soul—choose your metaphysics) is. And unless we are lovers, bodies matter little as the source of knowledge of the other. But of course the materiality of the body matters—what is voice but the manifestation of our bodies, what is language but the materialization of mind? We always know each other only through body, but we pretend otherwise. It has been the wisdom of feminism to reveal the displaced body that lurks within the mental, the repressed emotion that lurks within the "rational," the hidden dependence in in-dependence. Yet even many feminists have missed the full extent of how we know the other through their body.

Disability involves us in an immensely complex relationship to our bodies, whether we adhere to a strict version of the social model of disability or accept a more complicated model that does not restrict the term to socially induced disadvantage. While disability can offer an identity, no disabled person wants to be defined exclusively by their impairment. No one wants to be the object of the metonymic mistake of identifying their whole being by means of a singular bodily part, aspect, or function.

Many fail to give the body its epistemic due because, in the absence of illness or impairments, the body responds to our will seamlessly. It becomes transparent to us—we are scarcely aware of it. Only when the body breaks down through accident or illness, when the physical or social environment becomes an obstacle, or when we are physically attacked, does the body become opaque: We cannot relate to our world without being aware of our corporeality.[1] It is at this juncture, when we recognize our inevitable materiality, that we also most acutely feel the need to deny that we are merely our bodies. It is this paradoxical relationship to the body that I also experience in the presence of my daughter's body.

It is through my daughter's bodily limitations and her mental incapacities, not despite them, that I experience my daughter as a person—and, in more mystified terms, as a soul. In fact, what I see in her by means of her body is a beautiful soul. When I say of my daughter that she is a lovely person, a beautiful soul, those who know her do not for a moment hesitate to assent—they do not have to stop to figure out what I mean by this. Sesha's soul is experienced more directly, not through what she does but by how she is.

Yet how can this be the case? We are used to identifying the characteristics of a beautiful soul in terms that require an efficacious body, one that acts and speaks, that reveals the animating self. When I praise another as having a "beautiful soul," I mean to respond to her moral character, or what I can glean of it in the time that I have had to get to know her: the person has an open smile, appears to listen to others, speaks in a kindly manner, and evinces generosity in her actions. We feel pleasure being in that person's company. We predict from these interactions that this is not a person who would do us ill, and they will be sympathetic, perhaps helpful when we face adversity. If we find our expectations are not borne out, we will say, "I thought so-and-so was a lovely person, but I found out differently."

Sesha cannot speak and so cannot say kind words or engage in charming conversation. It is hard to attribute to her acts of kindness and other moral virtues, for her ability to act is very limited. So if I say that she has a "beautiful soul," am I using the term metaphorically? Let's think again about what we are implying when we praise others in this form. There are a host of bodily interactions from which we glean a personality, a soul: an unaffected smile, a gentleness of manner, an openness to (physical) affection, a sparkle in one's eyes. These are bodily comportments that we identify (sometimes incorrectly) with moral attributes

---

[1] This is also true for disabled people who acquire a new disability. Tom Shakespeare, who has achondroplasia, writes of the late onset of back problems, that for the first time in his life, "my impairment caused me serious pain and restrictions" (2006, 5).

and that delight us when we are in that person's presence. Being in the presence of Sesha is frequently a delight. We can enjoy her calm demeanor, her lovely look, the gentleness in her face—which is not to say that she cannot get excited or that she can't yank hard at someone's hair, even when she merely means to pull them over for a kiss. In the case of most people, we use these comportments as indications of something else. In Sesha's case they are something in and of themselves. That "calm" is in her body. That "gentleness" is in her very skin: its softness, its lovely scent, the tenderness of her touch. Sesha shows us how completely we can be what our bodies show us to be.

Fiction writers will not infrequently use the conceit that someone's physicality is a direct manifestation of their character. Dickens's minute descriptions of some facial feature, teeth that are too prominently displayed in a smile for example, tells us all we need to know of the perfidy of Mr. James Carker, the manager in *Dombey and Son*. In *The Picture of Dorian Gray*, Oscar Wilde uses this literary device and turns it on its head. He first creates characters who firmly believe that a person's character is written on his face. The novelist delights in describing every facial aspect to convey the character's inner self. His protagonist, Dorian Gray, however, who engages in corrupt behavior and murderous criminality, nonetheless stays looking young, as lovely as one who could only do good. But the conceit that physical beauty is a direct manifestion of inner goodness is nonetheless sustained by revealing an oil portrait of him painted when he was morally innocent which has been hidden in his house, and which over time records each misdeed by becoming more and more hideous. Although the portrait in the attic is a fiction and a physical impossibility, it captures a belief we live by: that our character and our lives are inscribed in our flesh. Dorian's portrait is not an entire refutation of the idea—for his portrait holds the record of his crimes; but it is also a tale that cautions that we can be grievously deceived by how the body itself appears. Likewise, we are as gullible as Dorian's admirers if we read the nontypical body, with impairments that defy conventional notions of beauty, as manifesting a "damaged" person and unappealing soul.

The portrait of Dorian Gray stands in stark contrast to a portrait of Sesha. Sesha's beauty shines through her nontypical body (as it does in so many who defy conventional beauty). Her body is her. When I am with Sesha, she is fully there, though I can read but a small part of her. As her agency is diminished by her disabilities, to read her I take in every look, whether it is the downcast eyes, a distracted expression, or an intense gaze. She looks into my eyes as if light waves could substitute for sound waves. I take in her sweet smell, the clapping hands, the glistening mouth, and shining hair. The warm womanly body, which she loves to have in an embrace. To read her also means watching her eyes as they glean a tasty morsel on a fork, as they spy the box of chocolates, the cup of morning coffee—all of which she devours with her eyes before they touch her lips. When we see her turn her head slightly to the left as her eyes gaze far off, we know now that she is enthralled by the music that is playing in the background, which I fail to notice until I see her engaged.

But her body can cause distress and anxiety. Her tongue is sometimes prominent in an open mouth, indicating an absence of a socially engaged self, bespeaking to the rest of the world her cognitive deficit. Her bodily needs involve cleaning her free of feces, changing a drenched brief, wiping away drool. Most crucially, we can use only her body—small indicators and extensive seizures—to inform us of what are sometimes mortal dangers. Her inability to control portions of her body and her failure to grasp dangers requires a constant and total vigilance on the part of a carer. I tremble for this vulnerable body, unprotected by the usual means of repelling a menacing world.

No words, no outright actions—just looks, aspects of a face, or bodily comportment—are the means by which we surmise thoughts, desires, pleasures, unhappiness, discomfort. She is all surface and yet mostly mystery. I know her well—better than most, since so few others pay such close attention. At the same time, I know her so little. I don't know what she understands, whether she knows what I say, what I tell her. She gazes deeply into my eyes, waiting for me to understand—but understand what? Sometimes there is a desire I can deduce from the circumstance—a desire for music when there is silence, a desire for a kiss, a desire to tell me she understands. But mostly, what I understand is that there is a soul: an intending, desiring, feeling, comprehending, and unique person. Sesha's body, Sesha's soul. There is no one else I have ever met who makes me utter "soul" as much as this person whose self so fully appears to be her body.

BIBLIOGRAPHY

Acharya, Kruti. 2011. "Prenatal Testing for Intellectual Disability: Misperceptions and Reality with Lessons from Down Syndrome." *Developmental Disabilities Research Reviews* 17 (1): 27–31.

Adams, Rachel, and Benjamin Reuss, eds. 2015. *Keywords in Disability Theory*. New York: New York University Press.

ADAPT. 2007. "ADAPT Youth Appalled at Parents Surgically Keeping Disabled Daughter Childlike." https://groups.google.com/forum/#!topic/news-for-cmcd-folks/WQ58vBZsjWg.

Albrecht, G. I., and G. Devlieger. 1999. "The Disability Paradox: High Quality of Life Against the Odds." *Social Science and Medicine* 48 (8): 977–88.

Alcoff, Linda, and Elizabeth Potter, eds. 1993. *Feminist Epistemologies*. Thinking Gender. New York: Routledge.

Allen, David, Michael Kappy, Douglas Diekema, and Norman Fost. 2008. "Growth-Attenuation Therapy: Principles for Practice." *Pediatrics* 123 (6): 1557–61.

American Association on Intellectual and Developmental Disability. 2007. "Board Position Statement: Growth Attenuation Issue." https://aaidd.org/news-policy/policy/position-statements/growth-attenuation.

American College of Obstetricians and Gynecologists. 2007. "ACOG's Screening Guidelines on Chromosomal Abnormalities." https://www.acog.org/About_ACOG/News_Room/News_Releases/2007/ACOGs_Screening_Guidelines_on_Chromosomal_Abnormalities.

American Medical Association (AMA). nd. "Code of Medical Ethics, Opinion 8.081: Surrogate Decision Making." http://www.ama-assn.org/ama/pub/physician-resources/medical-ethics/code-medical-ethics/opinion8081.shtml.

Americans with Disabilities Act of 1990: 42 U.S.C. ch. 126 § 12101 et seq

Andrews, Lori, Jane Fullerton, Neil Holtzman, and Arno Motulsky. 1994. *Assessing Genetic Risk: Implications for Health and Social Policy*. Washington, DC: Institute of Medicine.

Aristotle. 1908. *Nicomachean Ethics*. Translated by W. D. Ross. Oxford: Clarendon Press.

Arneil, Barbara. 2009. "Disability, Self Image and Modern Political Theory." *Political Theory* 37 (2): 218–42.

Asch, Adrienne, and Erik Parens, eds. 2000. *The Ethics of Prenatal Testing and Selective Abortion: A Report from the Hastings Center*. Philadelphia: Temple University Press.

Asch, Adrienne, and Anna Stubblefield. 2010. "Growth Attenuation: Good Intentions, Bad Decision." *American Journal of Bioethics* 10 (1): 46–48.

Asch, Adrienne, and David Wasserman. 2005. "Where is the Sin in Synecdoche? Prenatal Testing and the Parent-Child Relationship." In *Quality of Life and the Human Difference: Genetic Testing, Health Care, and Disability*, edited by David Wasserman, Jerome Bickenbach and Robert Wachbroit, 172–216. New York: Cambridge University Press.

Baier, Annette C. 1995. "The Need for More than Justice." In *Justice and Care*, edited by Virginia Held, 47–58. Boulder, CO: Westview Press.

Baltes, Margret M. 1995. "Dependency in Old Age: Gains and Losses." *Current Directions in Psychological Science* 4(1): 14–19.

Barnes, Colin. 1990. *The Cabbage Syndrome*. London: The Falmer Press.

Barnes, Elizabeth. 2014. "Valuing Disability, Causing Disability." *Ethics* 125 (1): 88–113.

Barnes, Elizabeth. 2016. *The Minority Body: A Theory of Disability*. Studies in Feminist Philosophy. Oxford: Oxford University Press.

Bartky, Sandra Lee. 1990. "Feeding Egos and Tending Wounds: Deference and Disaffection in Women's Emotional Labor." In *Feminity and Domination: Studies in the Phenomenology of Oppression*, 99–119. New York: Routledge.

Barton, Len, ed. 1989. *Disability and Dependency*. London: The Falmer Press.

Beauvoir, Simone de. 1989 [1953]. *The Second Sex*. Translated by H. M. Parshley. New York: Vintage.

Benhabib, Seyla. 1987. "The Generalized and the Concrete Other: The Kohlberg-Gilligan Controversy and Moral Theory." In *Women and Moral Theory*, edited by Eva Feder Kittay and Diana T. Meyers, 154–77. Lanham, MD: Rowman & Littlefield.

Bernstein, Jane. 2010. *Rachel in the World: A Memoir*. Champaign: University of Illinois Press.

Bérubé, Michael. 1998. *Life As We Know It: A Father, A Family, And An Exceptional Child*. New York: Vintage.

Beyleveld, Deryck, and Roger Brownsword. 2001. *Human Dignity in Bioethics and Biolaw*. Oxford: Oxford University Press.

Bookman, Myra, and Mitchell Aboulafia. 2000. "Ethics of Care Revisited: Gilligan and Levinas." *Philosophy Today* 44 (Issue Supplement): 169–74.

Bourdieu, Pierre. 1990. *The Logic of Practice*. Translated by Richard Nice. Redwood City, CA: Stanford University Press.

Bown, Nicola, Daniel Read, and Barbara Summers. 2002. *The Lure of Choice*. London: London School of Economics and Political Science, Department of Operational Research.

Brickman, Philip, Dan Coates, and Ronnie Janoff-Bulman. 1978. "Lottery Winners and Accident Victims: Is Happiness Relative?" *Journal of Personality and Social Psychology* 36 (8): 917–27.

Brison, Susan J. 1993. "Surviving Sexual Violence: A Philosophical Perspective." *Journal of Social Philosophy* 24 (1): 5–22.

Brison, Susan. 1995. "On the Personal as Philosophical." *APA Newsletter on Feminism and Philosophy* 95 (1): 37–40.

Brison, Susan J. 1997. "Outliving Oneself: Trauma, Memory and Personal Identity." In *Feminists Rethink the Self*, edited by Diana T. Meyers, 13–39. Boulder, CO: Westview Press.

Brison, Susan J. 1999. "The Uses of Narrative in the Aftermath of Violence." In *Essays in Feminist Ethics and Politics*, edited by Claudia Card, 200–25. Lawrence: University Press of Kansas.

Brison, Susan J. 2002. *Aftermath: Violence and the Remaking of a Self*. Princeton, NJ: Princeton University Press.

Brison, Susan. 2010. "The Need for First-Person Narratives in Theories of Personal Identity." Eastern Division APA Meeting, Boston, MA, December 30, 2010.

Brison, Susan J. 2017. "Personal Identity and Relational Selves." In *Routledge Companion to Feminist Philosophy*, edited by Serene Khader, Ann Garry, and Alison Stone, 218–30. New York: Routledge.

British Council of Organisations of Disabled People (BCODP). 1987. Comment on the Report of the Audit Commission. London: British Council of Organisations of Disabled People.

Brock, Daniel. 1995. "The Non-Identity Problem And Genetic Harms—The Case Of Wrongful Handicaps." *Bioethics* 9 (3–4): 269–75.

Brock, Daniel. 2004. "A Response to the Disability Movement's Critique of Genetic Testing and Selection." Princeton University, Princeton, NJ, October 20, 2004.

Brock, Daniel. 2005. "Preventing Genetically Transmitted Disabilities While Respecting Persons with Disabilities." In *Quality of Life and Human Difference: Genetic Testing,*

Health Care and Disability, edited by Jerome Bickenbach, David Wasserman, and Robert Wachbroit, 67–100. Cambridge: Cambridge University Press.

Brosco, Jeffrey P. 2006. "Growth Attenuation: A Diminutive Solution to a Daunting Problem." *Archives of Pediatric and Adolescent Medicine* 160 (10): 1077–78.

Brosco, Jeffrey P. 2010. "The Limits of the Medical Model: Historical Epidemiology of Intellectual Disability in the United States." In *Cognitive Disability and Its Challenge to Moral Philosophy*, edited by Eva Feder Kittay and Licia Carlson, 27–54. Oxford: Blackwell.

Buchanan, Allen E. 2000. *From Chance to Choice: Genetics and Justice*. Cambridge: Cambridge University Press.

Buckley, F., and S. J. Buckley. 2008. "Wrongful Deaths and Rightful Lives—Screening for Down Syndrome." *Down Syndrome Research and Practice* 12 (2): 79–86.

Budig, Michelle J., and Paula England. 2001. "The Wage Penalty for Motherhood." *American Sociological Review* 66 (2): 204–25.

Bull, Marilyn J., and the Committee on Genetics. 2011. "Health Supervision for Children with Down Syndrome." *Pediatrics* 128 (2): 393–406.

Burkholder, Amy. 2007. "Ethicist in Ashley Case Answers Questions." CNN, www.cnn.com/2007/HEALTH/01/11/ashley.ethicist/index.html.

Campbell, Fiona Kumari. 2009. *Contours of Ableism: The Production of Disability and Abledness*. New York: Palgrave Macmillan.

Camus, Albert. 1956. *The Rebel: An Essay on Man in Revolt*. New York: Vintage.

Canguilhem, Georges. 1991 [1978]. *The Normal and the Pathological*. Translated by Carolyn Fawcett. New York: Zone Books.

Caplan, Arthur. 2007. "Is Peter Pan Treatment a Moral Choice? Debate Over Stunting a Disabled Child's Growth Pits Comfort Against Ethics." http://www.msnbc.msn.com/id/16472931.

Card, Claudia. 1991. "The Feistiness of Feminism." In *Feminist Ethics: Problems, Projects, Prospects*, edited by Claudia Card, 3–35. Lawrence: University Press of Kansas.

Card, Claudia. 1994. *Adventures in Lesbian Philosophy*. Bloomington: Indiana University Press.

Card, Claudia. 1995. *Lesbian Choices, Between Men—Between Women*. New York: Columbia University Press.

Carlson, Licia. 2009. *The Faces of Intellectual Disability: Philosophical Reflections*. Bloomington: Indiana University Press.

Carlson, Licia. 2010. "Philosophers of Intellectual Disability: A Taxonomy." In *Cognitive Disability and Its Challenge to Moral Philosophy*, edited by Eva Feder Kittay and Licia Carlson, 315–331. Oxford: Blackwell.

"The Case For Not Mutilating Your Child: One Father's Voracious Opinion." 2012. *Psychology Today*, August 31.

Cavell, Stanley. 1994. *A Pitch Of Philosophy: Autobiographical Exercises*. The Jerusalem-Harvard Lectures. Cambridge, MA: Harvard University Press.

Chase, Cheryl. 1999. "Rethinking Treatment for Ambiguous Genitalia." *Pediatric Nursing* 25 (4): 451–55.

Child Welfare Information Gateway. 2013. "Impact of Adoption on Birth Parent." Last Modified August 2013. https://www.childwelfare.gov/pubs/f_impact/index.cfm.

Clarke, Steve, Julian Savulescu, Tony Coady, Alberto Giubilini, and Sagar Sanyal, eds. 2016. *The Ethics of Human Enhancement: Understanding the Debate*. New York: Oxford University Press.

Cohen, Richard. 1982. "It Depends." *Washington Post*, April 20. B1, Metro Section.

Collins, Stephanie. 2015. *The Core of Care Ethics*. New York: Palgrave Macmillan.

Connors, Joanna. 2009. "Kent State professor Trudy Steuernagel's fierce protection of her autistic son, Sky Walker, costs her her life." Sheltering Sky. *The Plain Dealer*, December 6. http://blog.cleveland.com/metro/2009/12/kent_state_professor_trudy_ste.html

Cowan, Ruth Schwartz. 1994. "Women's Roles in the History of Amniocentesis and Chorionic Villi Sampling." In *Women and Prenatal Testing: Facing the Challenges of Genetic Technology*, edited by Karen H. Rothenberg and Elizabeth J. Thomson, 35–48. Columbus: Ohio State University Press.

Crisp, Roger. 2013. "Well-Being." http://plato.stanford.edu/entries/well-being/.

Cureton, Adam. 2016. "Offensive Beneficence." *Journal of the American Philosophical Association* 2 (1): 74–90.

Dalmiya, Vrinda. 2002. "Why Should a Knower Care?" *Hypatia* 17 (1): 34–52.

Darwall, Stephen. 2002. *Welfare and Rational Care.* Princeton, NJ: Princeton University Press.

Davis, Lennard J., ed. 1995. *Enforcing Normalcy: Disability, Deafness, and the Body.* London: Verso Press.

Davis, Lennard J. 2007. "Dependency and Justice: A Review of Martha Nussbaum's *Frontiers of Justice.*" *Journal of Literary Disability* 1 (2): 1–4.

De Jong, G. 1983. "Defining and Implementing the Independent, Living Concept." In *Independent Living for Physically Disabled People,* edited by Nancy Crew and Irving K. Zola, 4–27. San Francisco: Jossey-Bass Publishers.

Dewey, John. 1993 [1919]. "Pragmatism and Democracy." In *The Political Writings,* edited by Debra Morris and Ian Shapiro, 38–47. Indianapolis, IN: Hackett Publishing Company.

Diedrich, W. Wolf, Roger Burggraeve, and Chris Gastmans. 2006. "Towards a Levinasian Care Ethic: A Dialogue between the Thoughts of Joan Tronto and Emmanuel Levinas." *Ethical Perspectives* 13 (1): 33–61

Diekema, Douglas, and Norman Fost. 2010. "Ashley Revisited: A Response to the Critics." *American Journal of Bioethics* 10 (1): 30–44.

Dillon, Robin. 1992. "Respect and Care: Toward Moral Integration." *Canadian Journal of Philosophy* 22 (1): 69–81.

Downes, Lawrence. 2013. "A Young Man With Down Syndrome, a Fatal Encounter and a Cry for Understanding." *New York Times,* March 18. http://www.nytimes.com/2013/03/19/opinion/ethan-saylors-death-and-a-cry-for-down-syndrome-understanding.html.

Dreger, Alice. 1998. "When Medicine Goes Too Far in the Pursuit of Normality." *New York Times,* July 28.

Dresser, Rebecca. 2009. "Substituting Authenticity for Autonomy." *Hastings Center Report* 39 (2): 3.

Driver, Julia. 2005. "Consequentialism and Feminist Ethics." *Hypatia* 20 (4): 183–99.

Dvorsky, George. 2006. "Helping Families Care for the Helpless." Institute for Ethics and Emerging Technologies. http://ieet.org/index.php/IEET/more/809/.

Eligon, John, and Erik Eckholm. 2013. "New Laws Ban Most Abortions in North Dakota." *New York Times,* March 26. http://www.nytimes.com/2013/03/27/us/north-dakota-governor-signs-strict-abortion-limits.html?pagewanted=all&_r=0.

Ertelt, Steve. 2013. "North Dakota Now First State to Ban Abortions Based on Down Syndrome." *LifeNews.com,* March 26. http://www.lifenews.com/2013/03/26/north-dakota-now-first-state-to-an-abortions-based-on-down-syndrome/.

Estreich, George. 2013. "A Child With Down Syndrome Keeps His Place at the Table." *New York Times,* January 25. http://www.nytimes.com/2013/01/26/opinion/a-child-with-down-syndrome-keeps-his-place-at-the-table.html?_r=1.

"Eugenics." *Dictionary.com.* Accessed May 29, 2018.

Fadiman, Anne. 1998. *The Spirit Catches You and You Fall Down.* New York: FSG.

Featherstone, Helen. 1960. *A Difference in the Family.* New York: Penguin.

Feder, Ellen K. 2002. "Doctor's Orders: Parents and Intersexed Children." In *The Subject of Care: Feminist Perspectives on Dependency,* edited by Eva Feder Kittay and Ellen K. Feder, 294–320. Lanham, MD: Rowman & Littlefield.

Feder, Ellen K. 2007. *Family Bonds: Genealogies of Race and Gender.* Studies in Feminist Philosophy. Oxford: Oxford University Press.

Feder, Ellen K. 2008. "'In Their Best Interests': Parents' Experience of Atypical Genitalia." In *Surgically Shaping Children,* edited by Erik Parens, 189–210. Washington, DC: Georgetown University Press.

Feder, Ellen K. 2014. *Making Sense of Intersex: Changing Ethical Perspectives in Biomedicine.* Bloomington: Indiana University Press.

Ferguson, Philip M. 1994. *Abandoned To Their Fate: Social Policy and Practice Toward Severely Retarded People in America, 1820–1920*. Health, Society, and Policy. Philadelphia: Temple University Press.

Fine, Michael, and Caroline Glendinning. 2005. "Dependence, Independence or Inter-Dependence? Revisiting the Concepts of 'Care' and 'Dependency.'" *Ageing and Society* 25 (4): 601–21.

Fineman, Martha Albertson. 1995. *The Neutered Mother, the Sexual Family and Other Twentieth Century Tragedies*. New York: Routledge.

Fischer, Bernice, and Joan Tronto. 1990. "Towards a Feminist Theory of Caring." In *Circles of Care*, edited by Emily K. Abel and Margaret K. Nelson, 35–62. Albany: SUNY Press.

Fitzmaurice, Susan. 2008. "News and Commentary About Ashley's Treatment." March 13. http://www.katrinadisability.info/ashleynews.html.

Flam, Lisa. 2013. "Waiter Hailed as Hero After Standing Up for Boy with Down Syndrome." *Today.com*, January 23. http://www.today.com/parents/waiter-hailed-hero-after-standing-boy-down-syndrome-1B8038223.

Francis 2015. "Laudato Si': On Care For Our Common Home." Encyclical Letter. http://w2.vatican.va/content/francesco/en/encyclicals/documents/papa-francesco_20150524_enciclica-laudato-si.html.

Frankfurt, Harry. 1988. *The Importance of What We Care About: Philosophical Essays*. Cambridge: Cambridge University Press.

Frankfurt, Harry. 2004. *The Reasons of Love*. Princeton, NJ: Princeton University Press.

Fraser, Nancy. 1989. *Unruly Practices: Power, Discourse, and Gender in Contemporary Social Theory*. Minneapolis: University of Minnesota Press.

Fraser, Nancy, and Linda Gordon. 1994. "A Genealogy of Dependency: Tracing a Keyword of the U.S. Welfare State." *Signs* 19 (2): 309–36.

Fricker, Miranda. 2007. *Epistemic Injustice: Power and the Ethics of Knowing*. Oxford: Oxford University Press.

Friedman, Marilyn. 2003. *Autonomy, Gender, Politics*. Studies in Feminist Philosophy. Oxford: Oxford University Press.

Frye, Marilyn. 1983. *The Politics of Reality: Essays in Feminist Theory*. Trumansburg, NY: Crossing Press.

Gallegos, Lori. 2016. "Empathy's Contribution to Moral Knowledge: Cultivating Agency under Conditions of Social Inequality." PhD diss., Department of Philosophy, Stony Brook University, SUNY.

Garland-Thomson, Rosemarie. 2012. "The Case for Conserving Disability." *Journal of Bioethical Inquiry* 9 (3): 339–55.

Gastmans, Chris, Bernadette Dierckx de Casterlé, and Paul Schotsmans. 1998. "Nursing Considered as Moral Practice: A Philosophical-Ethical Interpretation of Nursing." *Kennedy Institute of Ethics Journal* 8 (1): 43–69.

Gilligan, Carol. 1982. *In A Different Voice*. Cambridge, MA: Harvard University Press.

Gilligan, Carol. 1987. "Moral Orientation and Moral Development." In *Women and Moral Theory*, edited by Eva Feder Kittay and Diana T. Meyers, 19–33. New Jersey: Roman and Littlefield.

Glover, Jonathan. 2006a. *Choosing Children: Genes, Disability, and Design*. Uehiro Series in Practical Ethics. Oxford: Oxford University Press.

Glover, Jonathan. 2006b. *Choosing Children: Genes, Disability, and Design*. Kindle edition. Uehiro Series in Practical Ethics. Oxford: Oxford University Press.

Glynn, Sarah Jane. 2014. "Explaining the Gender Wage Gap." *American Progress: Economic Report*. Center for American Progress. May 19. https://www.americanprogress.org/issues/economy/report/2014/05/19/90039/explaining-the-gender- wage-gap.

Goodley, Dan. 2013. "The Psychopathology of Ableism: Or, Why Non-Disabled People Are So Messed Up Around Disability." Keynote Address to the Nordic Network of Disability Researchers, Turku, Finland, May 29.

Grinker, Roy Richard. 2009. *Isabel's World: Autism and the Making of a Modern Epidemic.* London: Icon Books.

Groce, Nora Ellen. 1985. *Everyone Here Spoke Sign Language: Hereditary Deafness on Martha's Vineyard.* Cambridge, MA: Harvard University Press.

Gross, Terry. 2000. "Interview of Richard Pryor." *Fresh Air,* National Public Radio. October 27.

Gunther, Daniel F., and Douglas Diekema. 2006. "Attenuating Growth in Children with Profound Developmental Disability: A New Approach to an Old Dilemma." *Archives of Pediatric & Adolescent Medicine* 160 (10): 1013–17.

Hanigsberg, Julia E., and Sara Ruddick. 1999. *Mother Troubles: Rethinking Contemporary Maternal Dilemmas.* Boston: Beacon Press.

Harding, Sandra, and Merrill B. Hintikka. 1983. *Discovering Reality: Feminist Perspectives on Epistemology, Metaphysics, Methodology, and Philosophy of Science.* Synthese Library. Dordrecht: Kluwer.

Hartley, Christie. 2009. "Justice for the Disabled: A Contractualist Approach." *Journal of Social Philosophy* 40 (1): 17–39.

Hassall, R., J. Rose, and J. McDonald. 2005. "Parenting Stress in Mothers of Children with an Intellectual Disability: The Effects of Parental Cognitions in Relation to Child Characteristics and Family Support." *Journal of Intellectual Disability Research* 49 (6): 405–18.

Hedley, Lisa. 2006. "The Seduction of the Surgical Fix." In *Surgically Shaping Children: Technology, Ethics, and the Pursuit of Normality,* edited by Erik Parens, 43–51. Baltimore: Johns Hopkins University Press.

Hegi, Ursula. 1994. *Stones From the River.* New York: Poseidon Press.

Heidegger, Martin. 1962. *Being and Time.* San Francisco: HarperSanFrancisco.

Held, Virginia. 1987. "Feminism and Moral Theory." In *Women and Moral Theory,* edited by Eva Feder Kittay and Diana T. Meyers, 111–28. Lanham, MD: Rowman and Littlefield.

Held, Virginia. 1993. *Feminist Morality: Transforming Culture, Society, and Politics.* Chicago: University of Chicago Press.

Heumann, Judy. 1977. "Independent Living Movement." http://www.disabilityexchange.org/newsletter/article.php?n=15&a=134.

Hingsburger, Dave J. 1998. *Do? Be? Do?: What To Teach And How To Teach People With Developmental Disabilities.* Barrie, ON: Diverse City Press.

Hoffman, Martin L. 2000. *Empathy and Moral Development: Implications for Caring and Justice.* Cambridge: Cambridge University Press.

Holroyd, Jules. 2012. "Responsibility for Implicit Bias." *Journal of Social Psychology* 43 (3): 274–306.

Houser, Daniel, John A. List, Marco Piovesan, Anya Samek, and Joachim Winter. 2016. "Dishonesty: From Parents to Children." *European Economic Review* 82: 242–54.

Hull, John M. 1997. *On Sight and Insight: A Journey into the World of Blindness.* Oxford: One World Books.

Hull, Richard. 2009. "Projected Disability and Parental Responsibility." In *Disability and Disadvantage,* edited by Kimberley Brownlee and Adam Cureton, 369–84. Oxford: Oxford University Press.

Individuals with Disabilities Education Act (IDEA). 2004. Pub.L. 101–476.

Jacobs, Harriet. 1861. "Incidents in the Life of a Slave Girl: Written by Herself." In *The Classic Slave Narratives,* edited by Henry Louis Gates, 333–513. New York: Penguin.

Jaggar, Alison M. 1983. *Feminist Politics and Human Nature.* Philosophy and Society. Totowa, NJ: Rowman & Allanheld.

Jaggar, Alison M., and Paula S. Rothenberg. 1978. *Feminist Frameworks: Alternative Theoretical Accounts of the Relations Between Women and Men.* New York: McGraw-Hill.

Jakobson, Roman. 1963. "Linguistique et poctique." In *Essais de linauistique generale,* edited by Roman Jakobson, 209–48. Paris: Edition de Minuit.

Jaworska, Agnieszka. 2007. "Caring and Moral Standing." *Ethics* 117 (3): 460–97.

Jaworska, Agnieszka, and Julie Tannenbaum. 2014. "Person-Rearing Relationships as a Key to Higher Moral Status." *Ethics* 124 (2): 242–71.

Kahneman, Daniel, and Amos Tversky, eds. 2000. *Choices, Values, and Frames*. New York: Cambridge University Press.

Kant, Immanuel. 1902 [1766]. "Dreams of a Spirit Seer." In *Kants gesammelte schriften*. Berlin: Prussian Academy Edition.

Kaposy, Chris. 2013. "A Disability Critique of the New Test for Down Syndrome." *Kennedy Institute of Ethics Journal* 23 (4): 299–324.

Kaposy, Chris. 2018. *Choosing Down Syndrome: Ethics and New Prenatal Testing Technologies*. Basic Bioethics. Cambridge, MA: The MIT Press.

Kent, Deborah. 2000. "Somewhere A Mockingbird." In *The Ethics of Prenatal Testing and Selective Abortion: A Report from the Hastings Center*, edited by Adrienne Asch and Erik Parens, 57–63. Philadelphia: Temple University Press.

Khader, Serene J. 2011a. "Beyond Inadvertent Ventriloquism: Caring Virtues for Participatory Development." *Hypatia* 26: 742–61.

Khader, Serene J. 2011b. *Adaptive Preferences and Women's Empowerment*. Studies in Feminist Philosophy. Oxford: Oxford University Press.

King, Larry. 2007. "The Pillow Angel." January 12, 2007. CNN, *Larry King Live*.

Kingsley, Emily Perl. 1987. "Welcome to Holland." http://www.our-kids.org/Archives/Holland.html.

Kitcher, Philip. 1997. *Lives To Come: The Genetic Revolution and Human Possibilities*. New York: Simon and Schuster.

Kittay, Eva Feder. 1999. *Love's Labor: Essays on Women, Equality and Dependency*. New York: Routledge.

Kittay, Eva Feder. 2000. "At Home with My Daughter." In *Americans with Disabilities*, edited by Francis Leslie Pickering and Anita Silvers, 64–80. New York: Routledge.

Kittay, Eva Feder. 2007. "A Feminist Care Ethics, Dependency and Disability." *APA Newsletter on Feminism and Philosophy* 6 (2): 3–6.

Kittay, Eva Feder. 2011a. "Forever Young: The Strange Case of Ashley X." *Hypatia* 26 (3): 610–31.

Kittay, Eva Feder. 2011b. "A Tribute to an Idea: The Completion of Care." In *Dear Nel: Opening the Circles of Care (Letters to Nel Noddings)*, edited by Robert Lake, section 4. New York: Teacher's College Press.

Kittay, Eva Feder. 2014. "The Completion Of Care." In *Care Professions and Globalization: Theoretical and Practical Perspectives*, edited by Ana Marta González and Craig Iffland, 33–42. New York: Palgrave Macmillan.

Kittay, Eva Feder. 2015. "A Theory of Justice as Fair Terms of Social Life Given Our Inevitable Dependency and Our Inextricable Interdependency." In *Care Ethics and Political Theory*, edited by Daniel Engster and Maurice Hamington, 51–71. Oxford: Oxford University Press.

Kittay, Eva Feder. 2016. "Deadly Medicine: The T4 Project, Disability, and Racism." *Res Philosophica* 93 (4, Special Issue on Disability): 715–41.

Kittay, Eva Feder. 2018. "The Normativity and Relationality of Care." In *The Oneness Hypothesis: Beyond the Boundary of Self*, edited by Philip J. Ivanhoe, Owen J. Flanagan, Victoria S. Harrison, Hagop Sarkissian and Eric Schwitzgebel, 120–141. New York: Columbia University Press.

Kittay, Eva Feder, and Licia Carlson, eds. 2010. *Cognitive Disability and Its Challenge to Moral Philosophy*. Oxford: Blackwell.

Kittay, Eva Feder, and Jeffrey Kittay. 2007. "Whose Convenience? Whose Truth?: A Comment on Peter Singer's 'A Convenient Truth.'" Published on: February 28, 2007, *Bioethics Forum*. https://www.thehastingscenter.org/whose-convenience-whose-truth/

Kittay, Eva Feder, and Leo B. Kittay. 2000. "On the Expressivity and Ethics of Selective Abortion for Disability: Conversations with My Son." In *The Ethics of Prenatal Testing and Selective Abortion: A Report from the Hastings Center*, edited by Adrienne Asch and Erik Parens, 196–214. Philadelphia: Temple University Press.

Kopelman, Loretta M., and John C. Moskop, eds. 1984. *Ethics and Mental Retardation*. Philosophy and Medicine. Dordrecht: D. Reidel.

Kuhn, Thomas. 2012. *The Structure of Scientific Revolutions*. Chicago: University of Chicago Press.

Kuusisto, Stephen. 2015. "Don't Tell 'Em You Can't See, Just Go On Out There . . ." *Planet of the Blind*, December 5. https://stephenkuusisto.com/

Larson, Kate Clifford. 2015. *Rosemary: The Hidden Kennedy Daughter*. Boston: Houghton Mifflin Harcourt.

Lavoie, M., T. De Koninck, and D. Blondeau. 2006. "The Nature of Care in Light of Emmanuel Levinas." *Nursing Philosophy* 7 (4): 225–34.

Liao, S. Matthew, Julian Savulescu, and Mark Sheehan. 2007. "AT: Best Interests, Convenience, and Parental Decision-Making." *Hastings Center Report* 37 (2): 16–20.

Lillehammer, Hallvard. 2009. "Reproduction, Partiality, and The Non-Identity Problem." In *Harming Future Persons: Ethics, Genetics, and the Non-Identity Problem*, edited by Melinda A. Roberts and David T. Wasserman, 231–48. New York: Springer.

Lindemann, Hilde. 2001. *Damaged Identities: Narrative Repair*. Ithaca, NY: Cornell University Press.

Lindemann, Hilde, and James Lindemann Nelson. 2008. "The Romance of the Family." *Hastings Center Report* 38 (4): 19–21.

Little, Margaret. 2000. "Moral Generalities Revisited." In *Moral Particularism*, edited by Brad Hooker and Margaret Little, 276–304. Oxford: Clarendon Press.

Liu, H., Z. Wei, A. Dominguez, Y. Li, X. Wang, and L. S. Qi. 2015. "CRISPR-ERA: A Comprehensive Design Tool for CRISPR-Mediated Gene Editing, Repression and Activation." *Bioinformatics* 31 (22): 3676–78.

Lugones, María. 1987. "Playfulness, 'World'-Travelling, and Loving Perception." *Hypatia* 2 (2): 3–19.

Lugones, María, and Elizabeth Spelman. 1983. "Have We Got A Theory For You! Feminist Theory, Cultural Imperialism And The Demand For 'The Woman's Voice.'" *Women's International Forum* 6 (6): 573–81.

MacIntyre, Alasdair C. 1981. *After Virtue: A Study in Moral Theory*. Notre Dame, IN.: University of Notre Dame Press.

MacIntyre, Alasdair. 1999. *Dependent Rational Animals: Why Human Beings Need the Virtues*. Peru, IL: Open Court Press.

Mackenzie, Catriona, and Natalie Stoljar. 2000. *Relational Autonomy: Feminist Perspectives on Automomy, Agency, and the Social Self*. New York: Oxford University Press.

Macklin, R. 2003. "Dignity Is a Useless Concept." *BMJ* 327 (7492): 1419–20.

Mansfield, C., S. Hopfer, and T. M. Marteau. 1999. "Termination Rates After Prenatal Diagnosis of Down Syndrome, Spina Bifida, Anencephaly, and Turner and Klinefelter Syndromes: A Systematic Literature Review. European Concerted Action: DADA (Decision-Making After the Diagnosis of a Fetal Abnormality)." *Prenatal Diagnosis* 19 (9): 808–12.

McBryde-Johnson, Harriet. 2003. "Unspeakable Conversations." *New York Times Magazine*, February 11.

McBryde-Johnson, Harriet. 2005. *Too Late to Die Young: Nearly True Tales from a Life*. New York: Henry Holt.

McDonald, Anne. 2007. "The Other Story from a 'Pillow Angel.' Been There. Done That. Preferred to Grow." Last Modified June 16. http://www.seattlepi.com/local/opinion/article/The-other-story-from-a-Pillow-Angel-1240555.php.

McMahan, Jeff. 1996. "Cognitive Disability, Misfortune, and Justice." *Philosophy & Public Affairs* 25 (1): 3–35.

McMahan, Jeff. 2003. *The Ethics of Killing: Problems at the Margins of Life*. Oxford: Oxford University Press.

McMahan, Jeff. 2005. "Preventing the Existence of People with Disabilities." In *Quality of Life and Human Difference: Genetic Testing, Health Care, and Disability*, edited by Jerome Bickenbach, David Wasserman and Robert Wachbroit, 142–71. New York: Cambridge University Press.

McMahan, Jeff. 2006. "Is Prenatal Genetic Screening Unjustly Discriminatory?" *Virtual Mentor: Ethics Journal of the American Medical Association* 8 (1): 50–52.

McMahan, Jeff. 2008. "Cognitive Disability, Cognitive Enhancement and Moral Status." Cognitive Disability: Its Challenge to Moral Philosophy, Stony Brook Manhattan, New York, September 20.

McMahan, Jeff. 2009. "Cognitive Disability and Cognitive Enhancement." *Metaphilosophy* 40 (3–4): 582–605.

Mercer, Christia, and Eileen O'Neill. 2005. *Early Modern Philosophy: Mind, Matter, and Metaphysics.* Oxford: Oxford University Press.

Meyers, Diana T. 1989. *Self, Society, and Personal Choice.* New York: Columbia University Press.

Meyers, Diana T. 1994. *Subjection & Subjectivity: Psychoanalytic Feminism & Moral Philosophy.* Thinking Gender. New York: Routledge.

Mill, John Stuart. 1860 [1978]. *On Liberty.* Indianapolis: Hackett Publishing.

Mill, John Stuart. 1869. *The Subjection of Women.* New York: D. Appleton and Company.

Mill, John Stuart. 2001. *Utilitarianism.* 2nd ed. Indianapolis: Hackett Publishing.

Miller, Arthur. 1996 [1949]. *Death of a Salesman.* Viking Critical Edition. New York: Penguin.

Miller, Sarah Clark. 2005. "Need, Care and Obligation." *Royal Institute of Philosophy Supplement* 57 (December): 137–60.

Miller, Sarah Clark. 2012. *The Ethics of Need: Agency, Dignity, and Obligation.* New York: Routledge.

Mistry, Rohinton. 1996. *A Fine Balance: A Novel.* New York: Knopf.

Moore, G. E. 2005 [1912]. *Ethics: and "The Nature of Moral Philosophy."* British Moral Philosophers. Edited by William H. Shaw. Oxford: Clarendon Press.

Morris, Jenny. 2004. "Independent Living and Community Care: A Disempowering Framework." *Disability and Society* 19 (5): 427–42.

Morris, Jenny. 2011. "Rethinking Disability Policy." https://www.youtube.com/watch?v=XHm4b2Y5j_U.

Moynihan, Daniel Patrick. 1973. *The Politics of a Guaranteed Income: The Nixon Administration and the Family Assistance Plan.* New York: Random House.

Mundy, Liza. 2002. "A World of Their Own." *Washington Post.* https://www.washingtonpost.com/archive/lifestyle/magazine/2002/03/31/a-world-of-their-own/abba2bbf-af01-4b55-912c-85aa46e98c6b/?utm_term=.179b1d17e003.

Murphy, E. A. 1972. "The Normal, and the Perils of the Sylleptic Argument." *Perspect Biol Med* 15 (4): 566–82.

Murray, Christopher J. 1996. "Rethinking DALYs." In *The Global Burden of Disease,* edited by Christopher J. Murray and Alan D. Lopez, 1–98. Cambridge, MA: Harvard University Press.

Narayan, Uma. 1997. *Dislocating Cultures: Identities, Traditions, and Third-World Feminism.* Thinking Gender. New York: Routledge.

National Human Genome Research Institute (NIH). 2018. "Learning About an Undiagnosed Condition in a Child." National Institute of Health, accessed September 17, 2018. https://www.genome.gov/17515951/learning-about-an-undiagnosed-condition-in-a-child/.

National Institutes of Health (NIH). 2014. "What Conditions or Disorders Are Commonly Associated with Down Syndrome?" Last Modified April 9, 2014. http://www.nichd.nih.gov/health/topics/down/conditioninfo/Pages/associated.aspx#f1.

Natoli, Jaime L., Deborah L. Ackerman, Suzanne McDermott, and Janice G. Edwards. 2012. "Prenatal Diagnosis of Down Syndrome: A Systematic Review of Termination Rates (1995–2011)." *Prenatal Diagnosis* 32 (2): 142–53. doi: DOI: 10.1002/pd.2910.

Ne'eman, Ari. 2013. "Autism and the Disability Community: The Politics of Neurodiversity, Causation and Cure." Disability Studies Institute Speakers Series, Center for Ethics, Emory University. October 29.

Nelson, James. 2000. "The Meaning of the Act: Reflections on the Expressive Force of Reproductive Decision-Making and Policies." In *Prenatal Testing and Disability Rights,* edited by Adrienne Asch and Erik Parens, 196–213. New York: Oxford University Press.

Newsome, Robert, III. 2012. "The Ashley Treatment: The Philosophy and Ethics of Growth Attenuation." *Psychology Today,* June 29. https://www.psychologytoday.com/us/blog/the-love-wisdom/201206/the-ashley-treatment.

New York Times Editorial Board. 2013. "Down Syndrome and a Death." *The New York Times*, March 27. http://www.nytimes.com/2013/03/28/opinion/down-syndrome-and-a-death.html.

Nietzsche, Friedrich Wilhelm. 1997. *Beyond Good and Evil: Prelude to a Philosophy of the Future*. Translated by Helen Zimmern. Mineola, NY: Dover Publications.

Noddings, Nel. 1984. *Caring: A Feminine Approach to Ethics and Moral Education*. Berkeley: University of California Press.

Nolen, Jeannette. 2014. "Learned Helplesness." Last Modified November 11, 2014. http://www.britannica.com/EBchecked/topic/1380861/learned-helplessness.

Nortvedt, P. 2003. "Levinas, Justice and Health Care." *Medicine, Health Care and Philosophy* 6 (1): 25–34.

Nussbaum, Martha Craven. 2000. *Women and Human Development: The Capabilities Approach*. The John Robert Seeley Lectures. Cambridge: Cambridge University Press.

Nussbaum, Martha. 2002. "Capabilities and Disabilities." *Philosophical Topics* 30 (2): 133–65.

Nussbaum, Martha. 2006. *Frontiers of Justice: Disability, Nationality, Species Membership*. The Tanner Lectures on Human Values. Cambridge, MA: The Belnap Press of Harvard University Press.

Nussbaum, Martha. 2008. "Human Dignity and Political Entitlements." The President's Council on Bioethics, Washington, DC. March, 2008.

O'Connor, Flannery. 1996. "Good Country People." In *The Tyranny of the Normal: An Anthology*, edited by Carol Donley and Sheryl Buckley, 307–26. Kent, OH: Kent State University Press.

O'Neill, Onora. 2002. *Autonomy and Trust in Bioethics*. Cambridge: Cambridge University Press.

Oliver, Michael. 1989. "Disability and Dependency: A Creation of Industrial Societies." In *Disability and Dependency*, edited by Len Barton, 6–22. London: The Falmer Press.

Olsson, M. B., and C. P. Hwang. 2001. "Depression in Mothers and Fathers of Children with Intellectual Disability." *Journal of Intellectual Disability Research* 45 (6): 535–43.

Paraprofessional Healthcare Institute (PHI). 2014. Home Care Aides at a Glance. In *Public Health International*. February 2014. https://phinational.org/wp-content/uploads/legacy/phi-facts-5.pdf.

Parens, Erik. 2006. *Surgically Shaping Children: Technology, Ethics, and the Pursuit of Normality*. Baltimore: Johns Hopkins University Press.

Parfit, Derek. 1984. *Reasons and Persons*. Oxford: Clarendon Press.

Paul, Laurie A. 2015. "Transformative Experience." APA Pacific Division Meetings, April 3.

Peace, William. 2007. "Protest from a Bad Cripple: AT and the Making of a Pillow Angel." Last Modified January 18. http://www.counterpunch.org/peace01182007.html.

Pellegrino, Edmund D., and David C. Thomasma. 1987. "The Conflict between Autonomy and Beneficence in Medical Ethics: Proposal for a Resolution." *Journal of Contemporary Health Law & Policy* 3 (1): 23–46.

Pettit, Philip. 1997. *Republicanism: A Theory of Freedom and Government*. Oxford: Oxford University Press.

Piepmeier, Alison. 2013. "Outlawing Abortion Won't Help Children with Down Syndrome." Motherlode Blog. http://parenting.blogs.nytimes.com/2013/04/01/outlawing-abortion-wont-help-children-with-down-syndrome/.

Pilkington, Ed. 2012. "The Ashley treatment: 'Her life is as good as we can possibly make it.'" Interview with Ashley X's father. The Guardian, March 15. https://www.theguardian.com/society/2012/mar/15/ashley-treatment-email-exchange.

Pinker, Steven. 2008. "The Stupidity of Dignity." *The New Republic*. May 28. https://newrepublic.com/article/64674/the-stupidity-dignity.

Pollock, Allison J., Norman Fost, and David B. Allen. 2015. "Growth Attenuation Therapy: Practice and Perspectives of Paediatric Endocrinologists." *Archives of Disease in Childhood*, Last Modified July 22, 2015. http://adc.bmj.com/content/early/2015/07/22/archdischild-2015-309130.

Rachels, James. 1998. *Ethical Theory: Theories About How We Should Live*. Oxford: Oxford University Press.

Rachels, James. 1990. *Created from Animals: The Moral Implications of Darwinism*. Oxford: Oxford University Press.

Rapp, Emily. 2011. "Notes From a Dragon Mom." *New York Times*, October 15. http://www.nytimes.com/2011/10/16/opinion/sunday/notes-from-a-dragon-mom.html.

Rapp, R. 1998. "Refusing Prenatal Diagnosis: The Meanings of Bioscience in a Multicultural World." *Sci Technol Human Values* 23 (1): 45–70.

Rawls, John. 1971. *A Theory of Justice*. Cambridge, MA: The Belknap Press of Harvard University Press.

Reinders, Hans S. 2000. *The Future of the Disabled in Liberal Society: An Ethical Analysis*. Revisions: A Series of Books on Ethics. Notre Dame, IN: University of Notre Dame Press.

Reinders, Hans. 2008. *Receiving the Gift of Friendship: Profound Disability, Theological Anthropology, and Ethics*. Grand Rapids, MI: Wm. B. Eerdmans Publishing.

Ressner, Susan L. 2008. "Genetic Counseling." In *Encyclopedia of Counseling*, edited by Frederick Leong, 229–31. Thousand Oaks, CA: Sage Publications.

Reynolds, Joel Michael. 2016. "Infinite Responsibility in the Bedpan: Response Ethics, Care Ethics, and the Phenomenology of Dependency Work." *Hypatia* 31 (4): 779–94.

Rich, Adrienne. 1995. *Of Woman Born: Motherhood as Experience and Institution*. New York: Norton.

Ritter, J. 2007. "Forever a Girl . . . Destined to Grow Up." *Chicago Sun-Times*, January 12.

Rivas, Lynn May. 2002. "Invisible Labors: Caring for the Independent Person." In *Global Women: Nannies, Maids and Sex Workers in the Global Economy*, edited by Barbara Ehrenreich and Arlie Russell Hochchild, 70–84. New York: Henry Holt.

Robertson, John A. 1994. *Children of Choice: Freedom and the New Reproductive Technologies*. Princeton, NJ: Princeton University Press.

Robinson, Fiona. 1999. *Globalizing Care: Ethics, Feminist Theory, and International Relations*. Feminist Theory and Politics. Boulder, CO: Westview Press.

Rollins, Judith. 1987. *Between Women: Domestics and Their Employers*. Philadelphia: Temple University Press.

Ruddick, Sara. 1989. *Maternal Thinking*. New York: Beacon Press.

Ruddick, Sara. n.d. *Sarah Ruddick, Feminist Philosophers: In Their Own Words*. FemPhil Productions.

Ryle, Gilbert. 1984 [1949]. *The Concept of Mind*. Chicago: University of Chicago Press.

Sainsbury, Clare. 2000. *Martian in the Playground*. Bristol: Lucky Duck.

Saletan, William. 2007a. "Girl, Interrupted: The Power to Shrink Human Beings." http://www.slate.com/id/2157861/.

Saletan, William. 2007b. "Arresting Development." *Washington Post*, January 21.

Saloviita, T., M. Itälinna, and E. Leinonen. 2003. "Explaining the Parental Stress of Fathers and Mothers Caring for a Child with Intellectual Disability: A Double ABCX Model." *Journal of Intellectual Disability Research* 47 (4–5): 300–12.

Sandel, M. J. 2009. *The Case Against Perfection: Ethics in the Age of Genetic Engineering*. Cambridge, MA: Harvard University Press.

Savage, T. A. 2007. "In Opposition of AT." *Pediatric Nursing* 33 (2): 175–78.

Savulescu, Julian. 2001. "Procreative Beneficience: Why We Should Select the Best Children." *Bioethics* 15 (5/6): 413–26.

Savulescu, Julian, and Guy Kahane. 2009. "The Moral Obligation To Create Children With The Best Chance Of The Best Life." Bioethics 23 (5): 274–90.

Scully, Jackie Leach. 2011. "'Choosing Disability,' Symbolic Law, and the Media." *Medical Law International* 11 (3): 197–221.

Sen, Amartya. 1990. "Gender and Cooperative Conflicts." In *Persistent Inequalities: Women and World Development*, edited by I. Tinker, 123–49. Oxford: Oxford University Press.

Sen, Amartya. 2002. *Rationality and Freedom*. Cambridge, MA: The Belknap Press of Harvard University Press.

Shakespeare, Thomas W. 2006. *Disability Rights and Wrongs*. London: Routledge.

Shakespeare, Thomas W. 2011. "Choices, Reasons and Feelings: Prenatal Diagnosis as Disability Dilemma." *ALTER, European Journal of Disability Research* 5 (1): 37–43.

Shakespeare, Thomas W. 2013. "Nasty, Brutish, and Short? On the Predicament of Disability and Embodiment." In *Disability and the Good Human Life*, edited by F. Felder, J. Bickenbach, and B. Schmitz, 93–112. Cambridge: Cambridge University Press.

Shakespeare, Thomas W. 2014. *Disability Rights and Wrongs Revisited*. Second ed. London: Routledge.

Shakespeare, Thomas, and Nicholas Watson. 2001. "The Social Model: An Outdated Ideology?" In *Exploring Theories and Expanding Methodologies: Where We Are and Where We Need to Go*, edited by Sharon N. Barnartt and Barbara M. Altman, 9–29. Amsterdam: JAI Pres.

Shoemaker, David. 2010. "Responsibility, Agency, and Cognitive Disability." In *Cognitive Disability and Its Challenge to Moral Philosophy*, edited by Eva Feder Kittay and Licia Carlson, 201–24. Oxford: Blackwell.

Siebers, Tobin. 2008. *Disability Theory*. Ann Arbor: University of Michigan Press.

Siebers, Tobin. 2010. *Disability Aesthetics*. Corporealities Discourses of Disability. Ann Arbor: University of Michigan Press.

Silberman, Steve. 2010. "Exclusive: First Autistic Presidential Appointee Speaks Out." *Noemi concept*. September 22. https://www.noemiconcept.eu/index.php/departement-informatique/meteo-noemi/crise-japon-mesure-taux-radiation-radioactive/5767-exclusive-first-autistic-presidential-appointee-speaks-out.html?fontstyle=f-larger.

Silvers, Anita. 1994. "'Defective' Agents: Equality, Difference and the Tyranny of the Normal." *Journal of Social Philosophy* 25 (s1): 154–75.

Silvers, Anita, and Leslie Pickering Francis. 2000. "Introduction." In *Americans with Disabilities*, edited by Leslie Pickering Francis and Anita Silvers, xiii–xxviii. New York: Routledge.

Silvers, Anita, and Leslie Francis. 2005. "Justice through Trust: Disability and the 'Outlier Problem' in Social Contract Theory." *Ethics* 116 (1): 40–76.

Silvers, Anita, and Leslie Francis. 2010. "Thinking About the Good: Reconfiguring Liberal Metaphysics (or Not) for People with Cognitive Disabilities." In *Cognitive Disability and Its Challenge to Moral Philosophy*, edited by Eva Feder Kittay and Licia Carlson, 237–60. Oxford: Blackwell.

Simplican, Stacy Clifford. 2015. "Care, Disability, and Violence: Theorizing Complex Dependency in Eva Kittay and Judith Butler." *Hypatia*, 30 (1, Special Issue: New Conversations in Feminist Disability Studies): 217–233.

Singer, Peter. 1979. *Practical Ethics*. Cambridge: Cambridge University Press.

Singer, Peter. 1994. *Rethinking Life and Death: The Collapse of Our Traditional Ethics*. New York: St. Martin's.

Singer, Peter. 2007. "A Convenient Truth." *New York Times*. http://www.nytimes.com/2007/01/26/opinion/26singer.html.

Singer, Peter. 2008. "Q&A Session." Conference panel, Cognitive Disability: Its Challenge to Moral Philosophy. Stony Brook University, NY, Sept 19.

Singer, Peter. 2009. "Speciesism and Moral Status." In *Cognitive Disability and Its Challenge to Moral Philosophy*, edited by Eva Feder Kittay and Licia Carlson, 331–34. New York: Wiley Blackwell.

Singer, Peter. 2012. "The 'Unnatural' Ashley Treatment Can Be Right For Profoundly Disabled Children." *The Guardian*, March 16.

Singer, Peter, and Helga Kuhse. 1985. *Should the Baby Live? The Problem of Handicapped Infants*. Studies in Bioethics. Oxford: Oxford University Press.

Single Dad, "The Case For Not Mutilating Your Child: One Father's Voracious Opinion." 2012. *Psychology Today*, August 31.

Slote, Michael. 2007. *The Ethics of Care and Empathy*. New York: Routledge.

Solinger, Rickie. 2002. "Dependency and Choice: The Two Faces of Eve." In *The Subject of Care: Feminist Perspectives on Dependency*, edited by Eva Feder Kittay and Ellen K. Feder, 61–88. Lanham, MD: Rowman & Littlefield.

Solomon, Andrew. 2012. *Far From The Tree: Parents, Children And The Search For Identity*. New York: Scribner.

Spelman, Elizabeth. 1988. *Inessential Woman: Problems of Exclusion in Feminist Thought*. New York: Beacon Press.

Spinoza, Benedict de. 1996a. "Ethics." In *A Spinoza Reader*. Vol. 1, 408–620. Princeton NJ: Princeton University Press.

Spinoza, Benedict de. 1996b. "Treatise on the Improvement of the Human Understanding." In *A Spinoza Reader*. Vol. 1, 7–45. Princeton, NJ: Princeton University Press.

Stramondo, Joseph, and Stephen Campbell. 2015. "Disability, Well-Being and the Complicated Question of Neutrality." Choosing Disability, University of Pennsylvania Medical School, Philadelphia, November.

Tada, Joni. 2007. "The Pillow Angel." cnn.com/TRANSCRIPTS/0701/12/lkl.01.html.

Tanner, S. 2007. "Outrage Over Girl's Surgery." *Monterey County Herald*, January 12.

Taylor, Sunny. 2004. "The Right Not to Work." *Monthly Review* 55, no. 10. http://monthlyreview.org/2004/03/01/the-right-not-to-work-power-and-disability/.

tenBroek, Jacobus. 1966. "The Right to Live in the World: The Disabled in the Law of Torts." *California Law School Review* 54: 841–919.

Thomson, Donna. 2010. *The Four Walls of My Freedom*. Toronto: McArthur and Co.

Tronto, Joan. 1994. *Moral Boundaries: A Political Argument for an Ethic of Care*. New York: Routledge.

Vanacker, Sabine. 2013. "The Story of Isabel." In *A Good Death? Law and Ethics in Practice*, edited by Lynne Hagger and Simon Woods, 167–76. Aldershot: Ashgate.

Vanier, Jean. 1982. *The Challenge of l'Arche*. London: Darton, Longman, and Todd.

Vargas, Theresa. 2013. "Maryland Man With Down Syndrome Who Died In Police Custody Loved Law Enforcement." *Washington Post*, February 19. https://www.washingtonpost.com/local/md-man-with-down-syndrome-who-died-in-police-custody-loved-law-enforcement/2013/02/19/10e09fe0-7ad5-11e2-82e8-61a46c2cde3d_story.html.

Veatch, Robert M. 1986. *The Foundations of Justice*. New York: Oxford University Press.

Vehmas, Simo. 1999. "Newborn Infants and the Moral Significance of Intellectual Disabilities." *Research and Practice for Persons with Severe Disabilities* 24 (2): 111–21.

Verhovek, S. 2007. "Parents Defend Decision to Keep Disabled Girl Small." *Los Angeles Times*, January 3.

Vorhaus, John. 2015. *Giving Voice to Profound Disability*. London: Routledge.

Wade, Nicholas. 2005. "Explaining Differences in Twins." *New York Times*, July 5. http://www.nytimes.com/2005/07/05/health/05gene.html.

Weicht, Bernhard. 2010. "Embracing Dependency: Rethinking (In)dependence in the Discourse of Care." *Sociological Review* 58 (s2): 205–24.

Whitehead, Alfred North. 1938. *Modes of Thought*. New York: The Free Press.

Wilfond, Benjamin, Paul Steven Miller, Carolyn Korfiatis, Douglas Diekema, Denise M. Dudzinski, Sara Goering, and Seattle Growth and Attenuation Workshop. 2010. "Navigating Growth Attenuation in Children with Profound Disabilities: Children's Interests, Family Decision-Making, and Community Concerns." *Hastings Center Report* 40 (6): 27–40.

Williams, Bernard. 1976. "Persons, Character, and Morality." In *The Identities of Persons*, edited by Amelie Rorty, 197–216. Berkeley: University of California.

Williams, Bernard. 1981. *Moral Luck: Philosophical Papers, 1973–1980*. Cambridge: Cambridge University Press.

Winch, Peter. 1958. *The Idea of a Social Science and its Relation to Philosophy*. London: Routledge & Kegan Paul.

Wittgenstein, Ludwig. 1921. *Tractatus Logico-Philosophicus*. London: Routledge & Kegan Paul.

Wittgenstein, Ludwig. 1973. *Philosophical Investigations*. New York: Macmillan.

Wolf, Susan, ed. 1996. *Feminism and Bioethics: Beyond Reproduction*. New York: Oxford University Press.

Wolfe, Katharine. 2016. "Together in Need: Relational Selfhood, Vulnerability to Harm, and Enriching Attachments." *Southern Journal of Philosophy* 54 (1): 129–48.

Wolfensberger, Wolf. 1972. *The Principle of Normalization in Human Services*. Toronto: National Institute on Mental Retardation.

Wong, Sophia Isako. 2008. "Justice and Cognitive Disabilities: Specifying the Problem." *Essays in Philosophy* 9 (1). https://commons.pacificu.edu/cgi/viewcontent.cgi?article=1307&context=eip

World Health Organization (WHO). 2002. *Towards a Common Language for Functioning, Disability and Health (ICF Beginner's Guide)*. Geneva: World Health Organization.

Young, Iris Marion. 1990. *Justice and the Politics of Difference*. Princeton, NJ: Princeton University Press.

Young, Iris Marion. 2002. "Automy, Welfare Reform, and Meaningful Work." In *The Subject of Care: Feminist Perspectives on Dependency*, edited by Eva Feder Kittay and Ellen K. Feder, 40–60. Lanham, MD: Rowman & Littlefield.

Young, Iris Marion. 2005. *On Female Body Experience: "Throwing like a Girl" and Other Essays*. New York: Oxford University Press.

Zola, Irving Kenneth. 1988. "The Independent Living Movement: Empowering People With Disabilities." *Australian Disability Review* 1 (3): 23–27.

INDEX